# TRANSFORMATION OF HEALTHCARE WITH INFORMATION TECHNOLOGIES

# Studies in Health Technology and Informatics

This book series was started in 1990 to promote research conducted under the auspices of the EC programmes Advanced Informatics in Medicine (AIM) and Biomedical and Health Research (BHR), bioengineering branch. A driving aspect of international health informatics is that telecommunication technology, rehabilitative technology, intelligent home technology and many other components are moving together and form one integrated world of information and communication media.

The complete series has been accepted in Medline. In the future, the SHTI series will be available online.



Volume 105

*Recently published in this series*

Vol. 104. R. Latifi (Ed.), Establishing Telemedicine in Developing Countries: From Inception to Implementation
Vol. 103. L. Bos, S. Laxminarayan and A. Marsh (Eds.), Medical and Care Compunetics 1
Vol. 102. D.M. Pisanelli (Ed.), Ontologies in Medicine
Vol. 101. K. Kaiser, S. Miksch and S.W. Tu (Eds.), Computer-based Support for Clinical Guidelines and Protocols – Proceedings of the Symposium on Computerized Guidelines and Protocols (CGP 2004)
Vol. 100. I. Iakovidis, P. Wilson and J.C. Healy (Eds.), E-Health – Current Situation and Examples of Implemented and Beneficial E-Health Applications
Vol. 99. G. Riva, C. Botella, P. Légeron and G. Optale (Eds.), Cybertherapy – Internet and Virtual Reality as Assessment and Rehabilitation Tools for Clinical Psychology and Neuroscience
Vol. 98. J.D. Westwood, R.S. Haluck, H.M. Hoffman, G.T. Mogel, R. Phillips and R.A. Robb (Eds.), Medicine Meets Virtual Reality 12 – Building a Better You: The Next Tools for Medical Education, Diagnosis, and Care
Vol. 97. M. Nerlich and U. Schaechinger (Eds.), Integration of Health Telematics into Medical Practice
Vol. 96. B. Blobel and P. Pharow (Eds.), Advanced Health Telematics and Telemedicine – The Magdeburg Expert Summit Textbook
Vol. 95. R. Baud, M. Fieschi, P. Le Beux and P. Ruch (Eds.), The New Navigators: from Professionals to Patients – Proceedings of MIE2003
Vol. 94. J.D. Westwood, H.M. Hoffman, G.T. Mogel, R. Phillips, R.A. Robb and D. Stredney (Eds.), Medicine Meets Virtual Reality 11 – NextMed: Health Horizon
Vol. 93. F.H. Roger France, A. Hasman, E. De Clercq and G. De Moor (Eds.), E-Health in Belgium and in the Netherlands
Vol. 92. S. Krishna, E.A. Balas and S.A. Boren (Eds.), Information Technology Business Models for Quality Health Care: An EU/US Dialogue
Vol. 91. Th.B. Grivas (Ed.), Research into Spinal Deformities 4

ISSN 0926-9630

# Transformation of Healthcare with Information Technologies

Edited by

Mariusz Duplaga

*Jagiellonian University Medical College,*
*Krakow, Poland*

Krzysztof Zieliński

*AGH University of Science and Technology,*
*Krakow, Poland*

and

David Ingram

*Centre for Health Informatics and Multiprofessional Education,*
*UCL, London, UK*

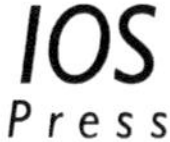

Amsterdam • Berlin • Oxford • Tokyo • Washington, DC

ISBN 1 58603 438 3
Library of Congress Control Number: 2004109131

*Publisher*
IOS Press
Nieuwe Hemweg 6B
1013 BG Amsterdam
The Netherlands
fax: +31 20 620 3419
e-mail: order@iospress.nl

*Distributor in the UK and Ireland*
IOS Press/Lavis Marketing
73 Lime Walk
Headington
Oxford OX3 7AD
England
fax: +44 1865 750079

*Distributor in the USA and Canada*
IOS Press, Inc.
4502 Rachael Manor Drive
Fairfax, VA 22032
USA
fax: +1 703 323 3668
e-mail: iosbooks@iospress.com



PRINTED IN THE NETHERLANDS

# Preface

The final phase of the PRO-ACCESS project coincides with the accession of ten new member states to the European Union. This exciting moment in European history brings great opportunities for the entrant countries, but it also means they will have to face new challenges.

The accession process demands considerable effort on the part of new member states, aimed at developing common policies and strategies. Over the last two years we have tried to encourage the community of medical informatics professionals and researchers from Central and Eastern European countries to undertake these challenges and join European activities in the field of e-health. We are aware of the fact that only common standards and procedures will enable full integration of this region with the main stream of Information Society developments, currently accelerating all over Europe.

The PRO-ACCESS project aims at carrying modern e-health perspectives to new EU member states. We are proud that a considerable number of papers presented in this book have been prepared by authors from these countries. This should prove encouraging for all those who believe in the great potential of this European region. This book also reports on the results of cooperation between researchers and centres representing both new EU entrants and those countries, that have been part of the Community for a long time.

The European Commission has consistently fostered the strategy of e-health development over the past decades. Yet, the economic transformation underway in Central and Eastern European countries does not favour rapid development in this domain. Healthcare systems all over the region are being transformed in search of more effective mechanisms of financing. Even though the e-health environment brings many opportunities related to improved resource management and better quality of care, its potential cannot currently be fully explored, due to the difficult economic situation and the lack of a well-developed information infrastructure.

One of the main motivations for publishing this book was the editors' conviction that only continuous effort to trigger activities, exchange ideas and share experience can speed up e-health services development in Central and Eastern countries. Transfer of knowledge and technology is surely one of the key mechanisms through which these new EU member states can integrate themselves with the Community. Such transfer brings a chance of achieving synergy during the expansion process and bodes well for the increased competitiveness of the enlarged European Union.

We would like to express our thanks to all authors, colleagues and partners from the PRO-ACCESS project, who supported our efforts to prepare this Book.

Mariusz Duplaga Krzysztof Zieliński

# Contents

# 1. E-Health Strategies

*Transformation of Health Care with Information Technologies*
*M. Duplaga et al. (Eds.)*
*IOS Press, 2004*



# Value-Driven Management in e-Healthcare

Małgorzata PAŃKOWSKA
*Information Systems Department University of Economics*
*Bogucicka 3, 40226 Katowice, Poland*

**Abstract.** Web systems present executives with a new variant of an old problem: determining "What am I getting out of this communication technology implementation?" The creation of a set of value criteria is vital. The main aim of the paper is to modify the approach suggested by Kaplan-Norton, emphasizing the value chain processes and other development aspects important for e-healthcare (patient satisfaction, finance, knowledge and technology). The paper contains the definition of the value generated in an e-healthcare system. The paper develops M. Porter's value chain approach and contains a model value chain for an e-healthcare organisation. This approach explains the activities behind the generation of value.

## Introduction

The convergence of the accelerating capabilities of computers, the expanding reach of a ubiquitous standards-based network like the Internet, and the increasing ability to capture and leverage knowledge in a digital form are primarily responsible for driving e-healthcare today. e-healthcare is defined as goods and services provided by healthcare professionals or organizations to patients/customers/end-users via the Internet or other telecommunications pipelines. This definition includes such delivery mechanisms as electronic home monitoring, on-line pharmacies, Web-based distributors of pharmaceuticals and medical devices such as contact lenses or on-line diagnostic services.

Motivated by access to new channels and lower operating costs, many companies are moving from traditional physical sales and service operations towards conducting their business electronically. On the one hand organizations should not think they must provide e-healthcare just because "everyone has a Web site these days"; on the other hand, however, they should not decide that the marketplace has no value just because their competitors haven't moved in this direction.

The Internet and e-healthcare present a new variant of an old problem: determining "What am I getting out of this technology investment?". The creation of a set of value criteria is therefore vital. These criteria form the basis of the business case upon which the e-healthcare process is developed. Evaluation criteria should include the following problems: financial impact, competitive leadership, market, technology and service. The value criteria are developed and compiled into an Internet effectiveness scorecard. This scorecard allows metrics to be developed specifically for each of the criteria. The data capture for the metrics may involve the recording of traditional organizational performance measures such as cycle time or cost per unit. The analysis of the activity against the projected organizational forecast or industry best practice allows for rating the effectiveness of the e-healthcare initiative to be considered.

## 1. Values in e-Healthcare

Since e-healthcare is a product/service package, it is necessary to identify those aspects of the service that are critical to customer perception. Knowing what the customer expects, however, is necessary but not sufficient for satisfying customers who would return for repeat service and provide positive comments to their peers. The principal features important to customers include reliability, responsiveness, assurance, empathy and tangibility. Generally speaking, online service providers have little opportunity to impress customers with their facilities and personnel. The only information most customers of Web sites have available for analysis is what they see on their computer monitor. Therefore, attractive Web site design and presentation of data is of paramount importance for e-healthcare Web site developers. Developers must do all they can to ensure customers form a positive impression of the e-healthcare organization and its personnel.

In e-healthcare the use application and development of information and communications technologies are primarily to enhance and promote health. Promoting health in the population and enhancing effectiveness and efficiency of the healthcare system are the main goals of e-healthcare. e-healthcare development is thus targeted at reducing, rather than exacerbating, inequalities in health. The e-healthcare system must ensure the citizens and healthcare professionals have access to health information which is up-to-date, of high quality, evidence-based and appropriate to their needs.

In 1776 Adam Smith introduced the notion of value in use. He held a view that value was determined by labour costs (or production costs). Looking more closely at the question of user value in healthcare, the following characteristics can be identified:

- cost: the remuneration required from the user (client, patient) in terms of money, time, risk, or self-esteem,
- schedule: the delivery of customer-valued features in the correct quantity, time and place,
- security: price guarantees, personal data protection,
- convenience: reduced preparation times, availability,
- performance: quality features that enhance the customer's health status and self-esteem,
- economy: relative price advantage – initially or over the life cycle of the service,
- ethics.

A patient value criterion may be defined as an attribute (or characteristic) of a service considered by a purchaser to be the primary reason for selecting a specific service because it enhances the value of the patient's output or improves/preserves his/her life status. Value delivery comprises all the activities involved in delivering the service attributes that are considered to be necessary to create customer satisfaction and to maintain an ongoing, long-term relationship with customers and in so doing, build a competitive advantage.

Value is a preferred combination of benefits compared with acquisition costs. From an organization's perspective, the response to customer expectations is a value proposition, which is a statement of what value is to be delivered to the customer. Externally, the value statement is the means by which the organization positions the offer to the target client. Internally, the value statement identifies how the value is to be produced, communicated, delivered and maintained. The internal statement specifies processes, responsibilities, volumes and costs to be achieved if the customer and each of the other stakeholders are to attain satisfaction.

Healthcare value is subjectively assessed by healthcare customers, who base their evaluation of value on their perceptions of the usefulness of the service. The total monetary value is the amount the patient is prepared to pay for the product. Exchange value is realised when the product is sold. It is the amount paid by the buyer to the service producer for the perceived use value. Exchange value, the price paid and the costs of producing the product or service determine the achievable profit.

Within the Information Communication Technology (ICT) sector, value-driven management can be helpful to ensure that commercially necessary and sufficient service levels are provided for users. The failure of e-commerce projects (especially large complex software delivery projects) is an endemic problem in the ICT industry. Even when projects succeed, there are often huge doubts about the realization of promised benefits. The management of e-healthcare is to maximize the value derived from ICT investments. Value management as a concept goes way back to the 1940s and 1950s when Lawrence D. Miles pioneered value analysis techniques. He was primarily concerned with product cost reduction. Since then, value management has enlarged its view to include increases in performance and improving commercial outcomes.

The Institute of Value Management states that one of the root principles of value management is focusing on objectives and targets prior to seeking solutions. The goal of ICT and healthcare alignment is to focus the limited ICT resources on maximizing the delivery of value from ICT products and service delivery by focusing on priority social needs. The Institute of Value Management also states that a basic principle of value management is the continuous awareness of value for the organization, establishing measures or estimates of value, then monitoring and controlling them. The key benefits of success of ICT for e-healthcare organizations are:

- improved ICT investment decisions resulting in demonstrably highest value-adding projects taking precedence and leading to improved profitability,
- improved probability of delivering programs and projects that add optimum value to the customers as early as possible,
- improved probability of delivering ICT services that add optimum value to the customers,
- minimization of performing work that has low (or no) commercial justification; in turn freeing time to focus on work, which demonstrably has and sustains high commercial justification.

Value-driven ICT management would be helpful to ensure that all ICT services are derived from the most effective suppliers, whether internal or external.

## 2. Value Chain in Healthcare

Activities creating value for customers constitute a value creating system. These activities are carried out using sets of human (tangible and intangible) resources. They are linked by flows of material, information, financial resources and influence relationships. Final customers not only receive and consume the value created but can also participate in value-creating activities. Focusing on organisations leads to the classification of activities on the basis of their position in the value chain of individual organizations, rather than on the basis of their economic structure and their contribution towards the creation of value for the final user.

The value chain approach provides an organization with the opportunity to evaluate a number of options that either increase value-in-use (by enhancing the attributes of the consumer surplus) or increase the producer surplus (by optimizing operations costs), or perhaps achieve changes in both. Value in use is the consumer value delivered in response to the identified opportunities. It represents a package of benefits comprising the quantitative attribute, price and qualitative features that often are specific to the customer or customer segment.

Value chain analysis extends across industries and organizations and it is useful to consider both when and where the value strategy is being evaluated. Value chain analysis also identifies sectors of the value chain that are underserviced or which offer opportunities for improving contributions to add value to participants by directing companies towards sectors of the value chain to which their competencies could be applied effectively. Within the model of audit of the value chain, the main areas of inquiry are:

- the concept of the served market,
- revenue, profits, productivity and cash flows,
- processes and activities,
- configuration of core competencies,
- awareness and adaptability to change and flexibility.

Value chain analysis traditionally starts with a view of the assets and core competencies of an organization and then moves towards inputs and other raw materials to the delivery mechanisms and finally to the consumer. Thus it begins with skilled staff, specialist equipment, suppliers and services then it finds a way to make the assets into a product or service that fits a template important to the customer.

Customers maximize value when they select the option for which customer value criteria exceed customer acquisition costs. Both the value criteria and acquisition costs are influenced by external features, such as the significance of expenditures, the strength of the vendor's brand (reputation), the client lifestyle characteristics and their purchasing expectations (the benefits to be delivered). They should perhaps also include opportunity costs, as these are often significant in choice situations.

Any organization, if it is to be successful, should have a set of core competencies or possess the key success factors necessary to compete successfully in its markets. Typically these relate to its competencies (described by capabilities and capacities), its cost structures (economic characteristics) and the technology it has available.

Customer value expectations, together with the key success factors, combine to produce a value proposition that identifies what is to be delivered to the customer and by what means. In other words, the value proposition identifies the benefits and costs for the customer and the internal activities (or processes) necessary to produce the benefits (value). In healthcare, the end-users' criteria are clear. They seek pain relief, mobility, functionality and training on how to better manage their lives. A value benefit that is delivered, of which they may not be initially aware, is the re-establishment of self-esteem and the ability to reassert control of their lives. Their costs are those related to treatment and the psychological impact of changing attitudes towards their conditions.

Competitive advantage depends on what services the hospital will offer, how they will be promoted to its customers and how the services will be delivered. Thus, three types of influence can be derived: knowledge management, relationship management and technology management (Figure 1). Knowledge management is suggested as the organizational capability, which identifies, locates (creates or acquires), transfers and converts knowledge into competitive advantage. Knowledge management in healthcare has a number of facets. Research into causes and treatment of specific conditions is an obvious concern. Other problems include developing an understanding of both efficacy and costs of treatment methods, which are essential for managing current options and for planning future activities (involving facilities, staff and extent of treatment services). Partnerships with pharmaceutical companies that conduct drug trials add financial viability and allow research departments to expand its activities. Healthcare technology management includes treatment procedures as well as equipment. Technology management in healthcare typically focuses on surgical and clinical techniques. Developments in ICT have improved communications among healthcare institutions (e.g. hospitals), customers and other stakeholders (government agencies). Relationship management is concerned with what is required to identify, establish, maintain and reinforce relationships with customers, suppliers, and other partners with complementary capabilities and capacities so that the objectives of the hospital and of its partners can be met.

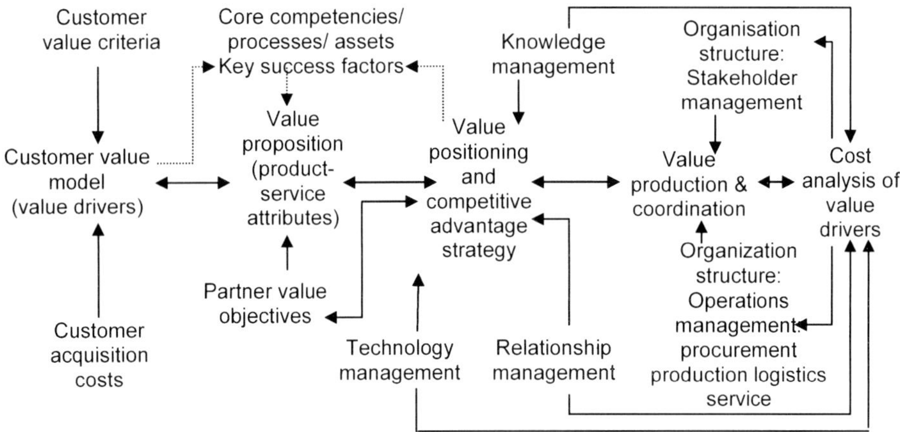


**Fig. 1.** Value determinants in healthcaresource [25]

Value production and coordination are the operational functions which ensure that value positioning and strategic decisions are implemented successfully. There are two considerations: the organisational structure for stakeholder management and the organizational structure for operations management. Stakeholders include: customers (patients), governmental agencies, suppliers (equipment and drug companies), the internal market (nursing staff and administrators), influencers (patient groups), insurance companies, health service agencies, medical and nursing recruitment agencies and investors (government and other funds providers). The second source of influence on value production and coordination is the organization structure, which implements operations management tasks and concerns the management of procurement, production, logistics and services.

In healthcare, the value chain processes are focused on patient care. Process management combines the tasks and inputs comprising value delivery and structure required (regardless of ownership) into an effective value delivery system. Taking into account the generic value chain model proposed by M. Porter, the following processes in healthcare are specified:

- procurement of consumables: both surgical equipment and patient support equipment are subjected to inventory management and procurement routines;
- logistics: this area covers a combination of patient core processes, patient logistics (moving patients through the hospital) and materials logistics (the flow of equipment, drugs and information). It aims to manage patient flow through treatment activities, manage and match equipment availability, manage and match staff availability, as well as manage information flows. Efficient logistics management ensures appropriate matching of facilities with planned patient requirements and enhances system productivity. EDI in logistics supports managing information flows and provides increasingly useful information for patient care process management;
- design and development: they cover research on treatment programs and pain management, cooperative research with pharmaceutical companies, research

programs for enhancing the quality of life and self-social management. Healthcare design and development processes are research-led and are directed towards improving the effectiveness or lowering the costs of treatment programs. Hospitals cooperate with pharmaceutical companies and other suppliers to ensure that treatment not only reflects current knowledge but it is also at the forefront of knowledge development. Research into methods by which patients' quality of life and self-ability for social management are improved forms part of the design and development process;

- production patient care processes: these comprise diagnoses of condition and establishing of patient goals by the treatment team, preadmission clinics and discharge planning. Patient care processes relate to the diagnosis of the patients' conditions, treatment requirements and their implementation by a treatment team;
- marketing: the aim here is to maintain strong care relationships with patients (CRM), to communicate with funding organisations, publish research output to peers, and communicate research and applications to referral organizations. Marketing acts as a conduit between a hospital and its customers' suppliers, peers and competitors to ensure that its research activities are widely recognised;
- services: these cover preadmission clinics, availability of equipment, educational activities, and accommodation.

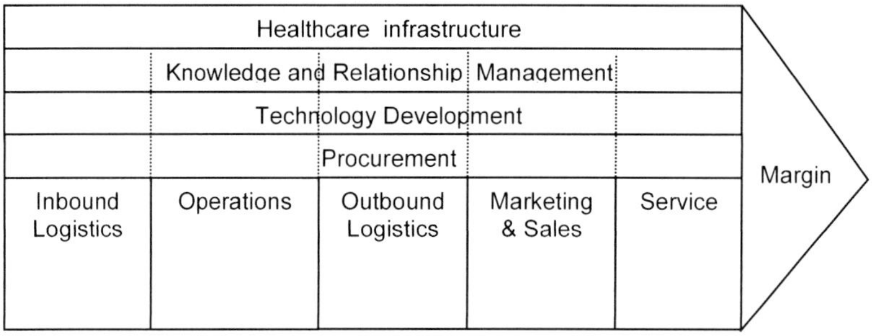

Healthcare infrastructure
Knowledge and Relationship Management
Technology Development
Procurement
Inbound Logistics
Operations
Outbound Logistics
Marketing & Sales
Service
Margin

**Fig. 2.** Modified Generic Porter's Value Chain

The aim of the value chain model delivered by M. Porter [21] is to disaggregate an organization into its strategically-relevant activities in order to understand the costs as well as the existing and potential sources of differentiation. An organization gains competitive advantage by performing these strategically important activities more cheaply than its competitors, and it gains scientific advantage by performing these activities on a more knowledge-intensive basis than its competitors.

Although value activities are the building blocks of competitive and scientific advantage, the value chain is not a collection of independent activities but a system of interdependent activities. These advantages frequently derive from linkage among activities. Linkage may exist not only within an organization's value chain but also between an organisation's value chain and the value chains of suppliers and channels. These links are similar to connections within the value chain itself – the way supplier or channel activities are performed affects the cost of performing the organization's activities.

## 3. Valuation in e-Healthcare

e-healthcare organizations seek independent business valuation for a variety of reasons. The most common reason is to obtain support for decisions regarding the development of a network system or other healthcare information system components. Other reasons are to support the sale or purchase of e-healthcare products or to support financing of a business component. In addition, e-healthcare valuation is being used to evaluate the ongoing strength and growth potential of e-healthcare assets and patient treatment lines. In e-healthcare, an accurate and reliable assessment of the value of business assets will depend on the choice and application of the valuation approaches and methods, the assessment of intangible value, the use of supported and realistic growth rates.

By incorporating both financial and non-financial measures, the Balanced Scorecard (BSC) enables a system of corporate performance measurement that is significantly superior to systems based on purely financial measures of success. Balanced Scorecard was originally developed by R. Kaplan and D. Norton in order to assist companies in turning strategy into action [18]. By supplementing traditional financial measures of performance with three additional perspectives (customers, internal business processes, innovation and learning) the BSC is able to translate strategy into measures that uniquely communicate the vision to the organization. The many advantages of the BSC system of performance measurement include:

- the use of both financial and non-financial measures of success to ensure alignment of strategy with performance drivers,
- the immediacy of the system, which enables companies to modify strategies to reflect real-time learning,
- more effective measurement and management of business performance,
- focus on drivers of future profitability as opposed to simple reflections of past profitability.

Although Kaplan and Norton suggest to consider all four above mentioned perspectives, they do not demand specific measures to be applied; therefore case studies and state-of-art elaborations are full of different exemplary measures or even different perspectives are deployed, as in Aitken's work [1]. Generally there are two categories of measures used in the BSC: the leading indicators or performance drivers and the lagging indicators or outcome measures. Performance drivers enable the organization to achieve short-term operational improvement while outcome measures provide objective evidence of whether strategic objectives are achieved. The two group measures must be used in conjunction with one another to link measurement throughout the organization, thus providing insight into the organization's progress in achieving strategic goals through information resource management and process improvement initiatives.

Kaplan and Norton BSC should be applied to equally balance inputs (the supplier's side) and outputs (the recipient's side). Value is the product of both the supply side view ("Are the e-healthcare system's functions run economically, efficiently and effectively?") and the demand side view ("Do the e-healthcare system's functions deliver quality services that add value to the healthcare organization and result in satisfied customers?"). Therefore the Financial Perspective analysis (Figure 3) aims to answer how cost-efficient the ICT functions are at delivering services. The core financial measures for the BSC include return on investment, economic value added, profitability, revenue growth and cost reduction. The financial focus is to maximize profitability. Profitability, growths in the market or survival are the critical success factors considered within this perspective.

The core measures for the Customer Perspective include market share, customer retention, customer acquisition and customer satisfaction. These core measures are used in conjunction with one another to evaluate and profile the status of the customer base of an e-healthcare organisation. Customer base is the most essential component of the Customer Relationship Management (CRM) system implemented to develop and maintain the best relations among the e-healthcare institution and its customers. Customer relationship development depends on software quality of the e-healthcare system and reliability and security of distributed information (Figure 3).

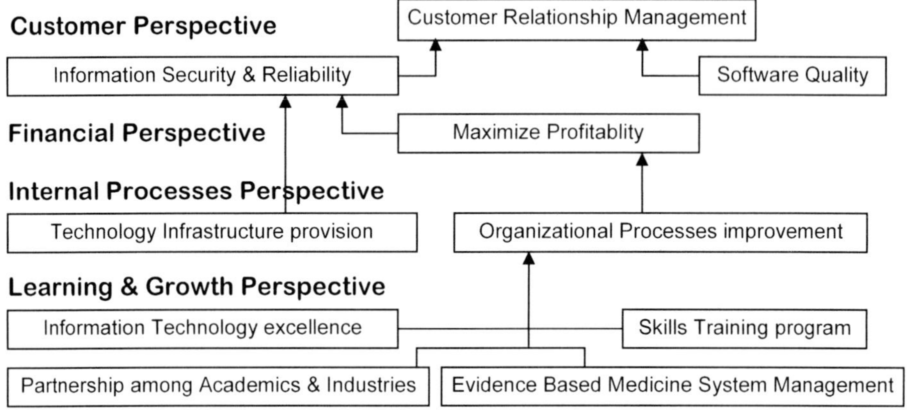


**Fig. 3.** Balanced Scorecard for e-healthcare

The internal business process measures have focused on key factors of process definition and improvement paradigms. Process improvement frameworks have included Total Quality Management or the Software Engineering Institute's Capability Maturity Model (CMM). All of these efforts share a customer focus of measurable business process improvements that result in cost reductions and cycle time improvements. The key resource in deploying effective business processes is knowledge and information technology. Learning and growth perspective supports the creation of the necessary infrastructure to achieve the strategic goals of the organization. The key factors in the perspective are identified as innovativeness, knowledge resources maximization and diversification. The knowledge is suggested for inclusion in Evidence Based Medicine (EBM) systems and highly dependent on training programs, accessibility of ICT infrastructure, as well as interorganizational relationship development.

## 4. Comments

The Internet and network technologies have led to a new perception of value for individuals and organisations. In the network economy the number of possible interactions grows exponentially. Value in the network economy is exhibited as opportunities of relationships among customers, healthcare institutions and their suppliers. In the digital age, e-healthcare value is no longer dependent on tangible assets alone. Whereas in traditional healthcare value is derived mainly from investment in people and in tangible assets (i.e. buildings, medical devices etc.), in the digital economy smart resources such as information, knowledge, brands, relationships and ICT capabilities become indispensable.

## References


[1] Aitken I. (2003) *Value-Driven IT Management*, Butterworth-Heinemann, Oxford.

[2] Anderson J.C., Narus J.A. (1998) Business marketing: understanding what customers value, *Harvard Business Review*, November/December.

[3] Armit R., Zott, C. (2002) Value Drivers of e-Commerce Business Models, [in:] Ch E. Hitt M A., Amit R., Lucier Ch.E., Nixon R.D (2002) *Creating Value Winners in the New Business Environment*, Blackwell Publishing, Oxford.

[4] Boisot M.H. (1998) Knowledge Assets, Securing Competitive Advantage in the Information Economy, Oxford University Press, Oxford.

[5] Bowman C., Ambrosini V. (2000) Value creation versus value capture: towards a coherent definition of value in strategy, *British Journal of Management*, Vol 11. March.

[6] Brandenburger A.M., Stuart H. (1996) Value-based business strategy, *Journal of Economics and Management Strategy*, 5.

[7] Brohman M.K, Parent M., Pearce M.R., Wade M. (2000) The Business Intelligence Value Chain: Data-Driven Decision Support in a Data Warehouse Environment: An Exploratory Study, *Proceedings of the 33rd Hawaii International Conference on System Science.*

[8] Byrd T.A., Turner D.E., (2000), Measuring the flexibility of Information Technology Infrastructure, Exploratory Analysis of a Construct, *Journal of Management Information Systems*, Summer, vol.17, No.1.

[9] Chan Y.E. (2000) IT Value: The Great Divide Between Qualitative and Quantitative and Individual and Organizational Measures, *Journal of Management Information Systems*, Spring, Vol.16, No 4.

[10] Chircu A.M., Kauffman R.J. (2000) Limits to value in electronic commerce-related IT investments, *Journal of Management Information Systems*, Fall, vol.18. No 4.

[11] Cisco S.L., Strong K.V. (2000) The Value Added Information Chain, *IEEE Engineering Management Review*, Third Quarter.

[12] Eickelmann E. (2002) Defining Meaningful Measures of IT Productivity With the Balanced Scorecard Van in: Grembergen W (2002) Information Systems Evaluation Management, Herschey. IRM Press.

[13] Fitzgerald G., (1998) Evaluating information systems projects: a multidimentional approach, *Journal of Information Technology*, 13.

[14] Guide to a Balanced Scorecard Performance Management Methodology, Procurement Executives' Association, 2000, *http://www.statebuy.inter.net/bsc.htm* accessible Jan 2002

[15] Hardey M (2001) E-Health: The Internet and the transformation of patients into consumers and producers of health knowledge, *Information, Communication and Society*, 4:3.

[16] Johnson R.E. (2001) *Shareholder Value – A Business Experience*, Butterworth Heinemann, Oxford.

[17] Johnston D., Pan E., Middleton B. (2002) Finding the Value in Healthcare Information Technologies, Center for Information Technology Leadership, *www.citl.org/news/Interop* accessible Jan 2004.

[18] Kaplan R.S, Norton D.P. (1992) The Balanced Scorecard: Measures That Drive Performance, Harvard Business Review, January-February.

[19] Nixon R.D. (2002) Creating Value Winners in the New Business Environment, Blackwell Publishing, Oxford.

[20] Parolini C. (1999) The Value Net A Tool for Competitive Strategy, Wiley, Chichester.

[21] Porter M. (1985) Competitive Advantage, creating and sustaining superior performance. The Free Press, NY, London.

[22] Raupp M., Schober F. (2000) Why Buyer-Supplier Chains Differ: A Strategic Framework for Electronic Network Organizations, *Proceedings of the 33rd Hawaii International Conference on System Sciences.*

[23] Rayport J.F., Sviokla J.J. (1998) Exploting the virtual value chain, *Harvard Business Review*, 73.

[24] Remenyi D., Money A., Sherwood-Smith M. (2000) *The effective measurement and management of IT costs and benefits*, Butterworth Heinemann, Oxford.

[25] Walters D. (2000) Implementing value strategy through the value chain , *Management Decision* 38/3.

[26] Walters D. (2002) *Operations Strategy*, Palgrave Macmillan, Houndmills, Hampshire.

[27] Wright W.F., Smith R., Jesser R., Stupeck M. (1999) Information Technology, Process Reengineering and Performance Measurement: A Balanced Scorecard Analysis of Compaq Computer Corporation, *Communications of the Association for Information Systems*, Vol 1.

# Technical Aspects of Portal Technology Application for E-health Systems

Joanna KOSIŃSKA, Paweł SŁOWIKOWSKI
*Department of Computer Science*
*AGH University of Science and Technology*
*e-mails: {kosinska, ps}@agh.edu.pl*

**Abstract.** E-health is an emerging field on the intersection of medical information technologies, public health and business, referring to health services and information delivered or enhanced through the Internet and related technologies. Portal technology, allowing services to be accessible over the Internet is a perfect tool for providing e-health services. The use of portal technologies has had deep influence on the architecture of the whole e-health system, both regarding new subsystems and older ones which we want to integrate with the portal. Portals provide new possibilities for creating novel types of e-health applications as well.

In this paper we provide a brief overview of e-health systems and portal technologies, and present many technical aspects of portal technology application for e-health systems such as the architecture of portal-based e-health systems, graphical user interfaces, access to various e-health systems' resources, personalization, security and privacy

## Introduction

Internet technologies are most frequently used to communicate with other people, purchase goods, gather information and explore services. One of the most important areas where these activities occur is related to healthcare [17]. It is not necessary to convince anybody of the benefits of e-health applications. By analogy with other e-applications, they improve access, efficiency, effectiveness, and quality of clinical and business processes utilized by healthcare organizations, practitioners, patients, and consumers in an effort to improve the health status of patients [18]. E-health applications can be combined together to form an e-health system, gathering the features and functionality of all those applications. Apart from harnessing the benefits of particular applications, such a system should avoid the drawbacks of illegibility and being flooded with unnecessary information. The ability to exchange data between applications and to automate reactions to changes in other applications would also be desirable.

This paper addresses e-health systems aiming at the provision of health services and information through a portal. A portal technology, allowing services to be accessible over the Internet, is a perfect tool for providing e-health services. Moreover, portal platforms provide many ready-to-use mechanisms, such as access to databases, personalization, security, support for different types of display devices etc. that are required or at least desirable in e-health systems. Portal technologies allows all these aspects to be integrated in a consistent manner. There are many ways to use portal technologies for e-health systems: developing new portal-based e-health applications, integrating different e-health applications existing within the organization, integrating e-health systems of different organizations, etc.

In this paper we discuss the use of portal technologies for developing e-health systems, focusing on their technical aspect. We omit all the legal issues related to privacy and security in e-health systems. The remainder of the paper is organized as follows: in section 2, we present an overview of different e-health systems; section 3 describes portal technology architecture; then, in section 4, we present different technical issues involved in portal technology application in e-health systems. Finally, section 5 summarizes the paper.

## 1. E-health Systems

There are many definitions of e-health but in general we can assume that e-health is an emerging field at the intersection of medical information technologies, public health and business, referring to health services and information delivered or enhanced through the Internet and related technologies [9]. The growth of e-health systems is related to the evolution of the Internet. As the Internet becomes more widespread, friendly, and faster, the range of its uses is widening.

E-health systems are a front-end for both healthcare consumers and healthcare providers. E-health systems include numerous different types of applications [16]; among others:

- teleradiology – transmitting radiographic images over a distance for use in remote diagnostics and treatment,
- telepsychiatry – the use of live interactive bidirectional audio-video communication in psychiatry,
- telepathology – exchanging of medical information for assisting healthcare professionals at a remote location and/or without proper expertise, with experts knowledge,
- teledermatology – the use of communications technology for dermatology consultations,
- home telecare – health services for patients at home, e.g.: remote monitoring, delivering healthcare from a distance.

Some e-health systems are designed to support an e-health organization e.g. a clinician appointment system or a medical services booking system [15]. A lot of portals provide general health and medical information.

Another important aspect of e-health systems is distributing patient information over different system components. The idea of the Electronic Patient Record (EPR) is becoming very popular and numerous EPR systems already exist [12]. EPR gathers records from different healthcare organizations (hospitals, physicians etc.), so that heterogeneous and distributed information is available centrally. EPR allows providers, patients and payers to interact more efficiently.

## 2. Overview of Portal Technology

The short definition of a portal is "a multi-thematic Internet service". The portal provides to its users a broad spectrum of interesting information – as Yahoo, Altavista or Lycos do. Those are portals in the traditional meaning, based mainly on standalone PHP and JSP pages. On the other hand, there are also portal systems based on Portal Server Technologies where the content of each page is formed by (usually) one servlet, making a decision upon many aspects: who is viewing the page (an anonymous user or a user identified by the system), what information the user wants to see, what information the user is granted to see, etc. Portal Servers provide technologies that simplify locating, connecting, presenting, aggregating, communicating, personalizing, notifying and delivering content [1]. Nowadays, there are lots of Portal Server products available on the market (Oracle 9ias Portal, Sun Java Enterprise Portal System, IBM WebSphere Portal, Microsoft SharePoint), however all of them share the same idea – to make portal creation and management as simple as possible. Below is a description of a Portal Server (abbr. PS) based on the Sun Java Enterprise System (abbr. SJES) solution.

### *2.1 Architecture Overview*

The architecture of the Portal Server is not complex in principle. The product consists only of the following items:

- desktop – the main servlet processing all requests from clients, responsible for overall page layout and contents,
- netmail – a service implementing the mail clients, allowing users to access mail servers,
- rewriter – an engine performing URL transformation in markup languages and Javascript code (expands relative URLs to absolute URLs, prefixes the gateway URL to an existing URL),
- search – engine supporting search and browsing interfaces.

Portal Technology systems consist not only of the Portal Server, but also of additional integratable software components from which the portal leverages functionality and services. The complete architecture of SJES PS is depicted in Figure 1.

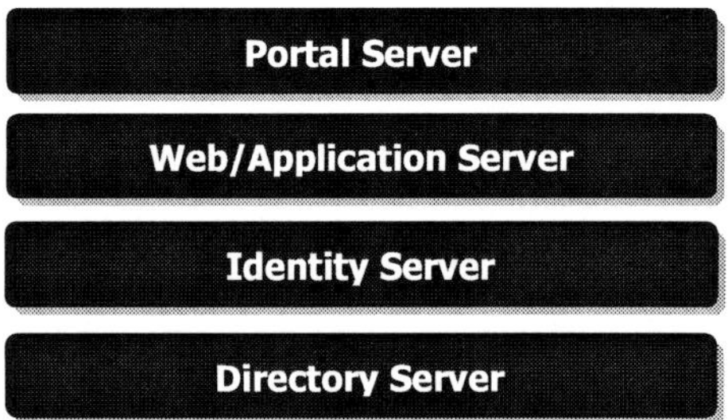


**Fig. 1.** Portal System architecture

As shown in Figure 1, the Portal Server exists on top of other SJES products. The Web or Application Server is a runtime environment of the portal's Web applications. The Desktop Servlet operates in the context of a J2EE-compliant Web container. The next component – Identity Server – provides a comprehensive solution for managing identities and for enforcing authorized access to network services and resources [4]. Identity management allows the definition of user profiles, roles, rights, and other rules to be defined [3]. Those definitions allow us to authenticate and authorize the user through available modules (Certificate, Radius, Unix, HTTP Basic, etc.) The lowermost component – the Directory Server – acts as a data store for information gathered and managed by the Identity Server, hence the other name of the Identity Server is the Directory Server Access and Management Environment.

From the short description provided above one can conclude that the Portal Server acts as a front-end to any kind of application (not necessarily a Web-based application). The developer's aim is simply to implement user interfaces for those applications.

Systems based on Portal Technologies are consistent with the Model-View-Controller (abbr. MVC) design pattern. The model represents enterprise data and the business rules that govern access to and updates of this data. In other words, this layer contains the Directory Server, the Identity Server and other additional databases as well as J2EE beans that communicate with those databases. JSP pages are used to render the view and present it in the user's browser. The controller layer, composed of the Desktop Servlet, is a mediator between the View and the Model layer. It delegates HTTP requests to appropriate handler (portlet – see subsection 3.2) that acts as an adapter between the request and the model.

## 2.2 *Accessing a Portal*

The portal, being a Web application, is accessed through a Web browser. The primary interface for the user to access portal contents is the desktop (generated by the Desktop Servlet). The desktop consists of channels, called end-user portlets, that are in fact pre-built connections between the Portal Server software and third-party applications, services and tools. Usually, a portlet is visualized as a distinct area on the page, surrounded with borders and having a title bar (see Figure 2).

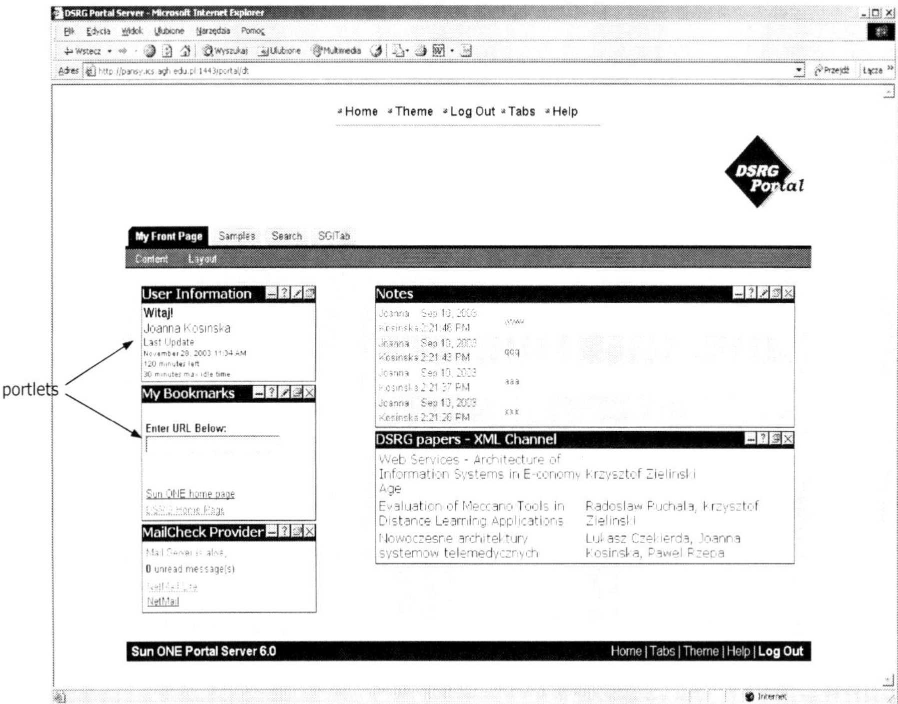


**Fig. 2.** Example of a Desktop

Once a user tries to retrieve the portal's content, he is authenticated via Identity Server modules, then the Desktop Servlet references the display profile which stores information on all available portlets for that particular user and on this basis generates the content of the user's Desktop. The display profile is stored as LDAP attributes in the Directory Server at various levels and contains configuration parameters for portlets.

## 3. Portal Technology in E-health Systems

The use of Portal Technologies in the context of e-health systems is absolutely desirable. Portals can combine live audio, video and monitoring technologies with a variety of medical peripherals, providing the flexibility needed to create patient-specific home telehealth systems [7]. Medical staff can manage more patients more efficiently with confidence, knowing that care is delivered in an efficient manner. Automatic notification mechanisms enable rapid intervention when the patient suffers a sudden, dangerous condition, and facilitate the exchange of information in that eventuality.

### *3.1 Architecture of e-Health Systems*

The three-layered architecture of a portal-based e-health system is depicted in Figure 3. The topmost (presentation) layer assumes a thin client model: the user only needs a Web browser to access all applications provided within the system. Modern e-health systems should be available for any kind of user connecting from any kind of device regardless of its hardware parameters. The Mobile Access extension pack of the SJES Portal Server recognizes and supports hundreds of devices, multiple mark-up languages (HTML, xHTML, WML), protocols and standards, and has the ability to deliver to these devices user-specific applications, content and services [5]. This is a very important feature in the medical environments where medical staff is always on the move from one place (eg. a hospital, where access is provided by a desktop computer), to another (eg. a traffic accident, where access relies on wireless devices such as PDAs, TabletPCs, cellular phones).

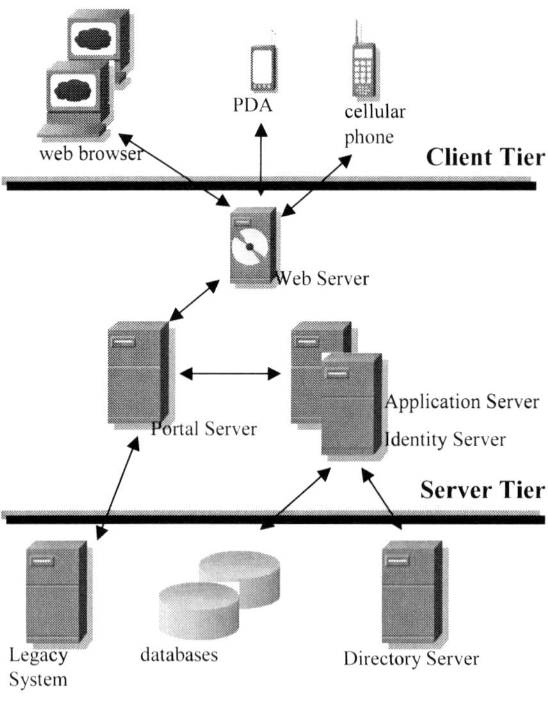


**Fig. 3.** Architecture of a portal-based telecare system

The information (user preferences, profiles) necessary to render the desktop is all stored in the Directory Server and never in the files on the client side. The user is not tied to a concrete machine, as all applications can configure themselves from parameters hosted on the Directory Server.

The second layer encompasses the server layer – both WWW servers preparing documents for the presentation layer and servers realizing authentication, authorization, business logic and those ensuring integration with the data layer. Apart from core Portal Technology components there are additional SJES products that enhance the value of e-health systems. These products include the Calendar Server – enabling users to manage schedules, share resources, and schedule events or appointments collaboratively, and the Instant Messaging Server – enabling secure real-time collaboration including chat, conferences, alerts, polls, and news channels.

The data layer is a repository of all kinds of data gathered by the e-health system and also by legacy e-health applications that already existed and still produce some important data. The databases are included in the third layer as they often collect written information, such as patients examination results, that would slow down the Directory Server performance.

### *3.2 Personalization*

The first function of a portal solution is to create an aggregated pool of information and resources available to multiple users [3]. The purpose is to provide one user interface, available from a Web browser, to any number of services. This reduces the anxiety among people over having to learn numerous applications, usually built according to different schemes.

The portals personalization capabilities enable users to design their own content reducing the problem of overloading users with too much information. A common situation is that users are flooded with a mass of diverse topics and cannot find the relevant information, making system usage a burden. Initial personalization must therefore be performed by the e-health system itself. By recognizing who is logged into the system, the system can provide only the contents that matches the user's profile. Diabetes patients do not require portlets that are referred to patients following a coronary attack. All portlets that are presented to a patient can be rearranged (minimalized, moved or removed) by her/him to suit her/his demands.

Another aspect of portal adjustment to users preferences is internationalization, that is, the process of designing an application so that it can be adapted to various languages and regions without engineering changes. With internationalization capabilities, the e-health system can be valuable for users in different countries and the addition of new languages should not require application recompilation. All that needs to be done is to add locale-specific components and to translate the appropriate text.

In order to deliver personalization functionality, the portal requires to be capable of identifying its users. User identification, authentication and access control to portal resources allow for delivering portal services adequately, securely, and privately.

### *3.3 Security and Privacy Issues*

Information stored by e-health systems is, by its nature, especially sensitive. It often concerns private and confidential health details regarding specific individuals. An example of that type of information is the Electronic Patient Record [12]. Other resources of e-health systems are e-health services. Sometimes they need to fulfill additional requirements, such as being available at all times, e.g. in critical situations, when someone's health may be threatened. A security breach of a e-health system could cause catastrophic loss for a healthcare organization and individuals in the case of unauthorized disclosure or alteration of the individual's health information [11], or denying access to a service.

In order to convince individuals to use e-health systems, it is necessary to instill in them a feeling that their information is well protected and privacy is guaranteed. Privacy means the ability of an individual (or organization) to decide whether, when, and to whom personal (or organizational) information is released [10].

Security policy, i.e. specific security rules for the system, is a foundation of the e-health system's security and privacy. In order to ensure an appropriate security policy, security mechanisms must be involved. Many of these mechanisms are typically provided by portal technology, e.g. authentication, single sign-on, access control, audit, encryption. An important component of portal technology and security infrastructure is the identity server, which helps organizations manage identities and enforce security access to their network services and Web-based resources.

Let's take a closer look at SJES. Security provided by SJES is related to Sun One Identity Server (abbr. IS). To obtain access to a portal e-health system (i.e. information and services) an individual has to pass through an authentication process. Authentication means verifying the identity of an individual. There are many ways to authenticate individuals. Authentication can be, among others, based on: user name/password pairs, PKI digital certificates, physical devices such as smart cards, RF cards or biometrics. IS currently provides the following authentication modules [13]:

- anonymous – allows a user to log on without specifying a user name/password pair,
- certificate – allows a user to log on through a personal digital certificate,
- LDAP – allows for authentication using the LDAP bind, an operation witch associates a user ID password with a particular LDAP entry,
- membership – allows a new user to register themselves for authentication with a login and password as well as other fields such as first name, last name, etc.,
- NT – allows for authentication using a Windows NT server,
- RADIUS – allows for authentication using an external Remote Authentication Dial-In User Service (RADIUS) server,
- SafeWord – allows for authentication using Secure Computing's servers and tokens,
- Unix – allows for authentication using a user's UNIX identification and password.

IS also allows plugging-in custom authentication modules.

To ensure secure transmission of data through the Internet, security protocols are applied. Two of the most popular (and almost always supported by portals) are: Secure Socket Layer (abbr. SSL) and Secure Hypertext Transport Protocol (S-HTTP). These protocols are complete solutions that ensure confidentiality and integrity of data sent over the Web. They also allow mutual authentication of sender and receiver.

Once the individual is authenticated, the system is able to recognize him/her whenever he/she is a source of a request. IS provides a single sing-on (SSO) mechanism which ensures that successive attempts by an individual to access protected resources will not require them to provide authentication credentials for each attempt. SSO mechanism relies on cookies –information packets generated by Web servers and stored by a Web browser on the visitor's computer.

After logging into the portal, the individual can request access to the portal system's resources: services and information. IS allows defining conditional policies for authorization and access control. IS also enables protection for different types of resources, although currently it only supports policies based on URLs. This mechanism works in the following manner: the Web browser request a URL that resides on a Web server. The URL represents a requested service or a piece of information. It is intercepted and the SSO token of the originator is extracted. If the token is not valid, the user is redirected to a login page. Following validation of the token, all policies assigned to the user are checked. Based on the evaluation of policies, the individual is either allowed or denied access to the resource.

IS supports role-based access control [14]. Such control expresses security in terms of the individual's role in the organization's structure. Permissions are directly assigned to roles and not to individuals. If an individual is in a role then he/she gains that role's permissions. Individuals are also not directly assigned to roles - they are grouped into subjects (for flexibility's sake).

One of the IS components is the Logging Service. It allows recording information about user activity, traffic patterns and authorization violations. This information may be used for detecting, reporting, and responding to security incidents. All information is recorded in one centralized location to improve the administration of the system.

Most SJES components are provided with APIs that allow them to be integrated with other subsystems (not necessarily with portal-based ones). All APIs are based on XML and provided as Java and C libraries.

### *3.4 Integration of Different e-Health Applications*

Portal solutions easily integrate with existing infrastructure; there is no need to replace existing applications regardless of vendor. The aim is to create a Web interface for each application. Depending on how the application is implemented, some servlets and JSP pages will have to be written, or to make the application more universal, its functionality may have to be exposed in the form of a Web service [8]. Out-of-the-box portal software typically includes universal portlets to present those interfaces (JSPProvider, WebServiceProvider [2]) in the portal system.

E-health system components created from scratch are easier to integrate with the system compared to legacy ones. First of all, they can share the same organizational structure, access the same information and use their own services. The issue is to adequately use the Portal platform components, beginning with system design from the lowest layer (Figure 1). The Directory Server provides global directory services and information to a wide variety of applications [6]. Instead of using separate databases for each application, the global Directory Information Tree provides a single repository of information about the e-health organization in question, typically including users of the system (patients, medical staff, guests), equipment (ultrasound systems, USG devices, RTG devices), application data (configuration parameters), role and policy configuration, etc. All this data is necessary to authenticate users with e-health systems and to render their desktops.

The available mechanisms facilitate creating new e-health services. First of all, there is no necessity to provide authentication and authorization modules as the ones supplied with the Identity Server can be used and the Portal Server also possesses adequate portlets. The whole identity management process (creation, remove, modification) is done through the Identity Server Web-based *amconsole* tool. The majority of e-health services can make good use of SJES products. The Clinical Appointment System and the Equipment Reservation System can leverage from the Calendar Server - an extensible collaboration platform for managing events, tasks, appointments, resources, even with automatic e-mail notifications, reminders, etc. In fact, there is no need to create the logic of these systems, apart from user interfaces. Other technical aspects of portal technologies for e-health systems include search engines for locating – among others – guides for home telecare, encyclopaedias, bookmark portlets for saving links to other e-health sites and news portlets for publishing information on important events.

## 4. Conclusions

E-health systems are becoming more and more popular. The evolution of the Internet has allowed for new generation of e-health systems, based on portal technologies. Summarizing the paper, portal technologies supply the developer with a platform that facilitates the creation of e-health systems. This platform has already implemented some mechanisms that modern systems should possess. Developers of e-health systems are released from implementing many parts of the system. It is, for example, no longer necessary to manually implement communication, security, localization or transaction mechanisms. Developers may focus on the systems' business logic. The use of portal technologies facilitates both developing new e-Health systems and integrating existing ones.

An interesting aspect that known portal technologies do not currently address is self-adaptability. This issue merits further investigation. An e-health system equipped with this functionality would adjust to the users' behavior, providing them with the context they left during last logon and gathering information related to the users' interests.

## References

[1] Administrator's Guide. Sun ONE Portal Server. Version 6.2, November 2003

[2] Developer's Guide. Sun ONE Portal Server. Version 6.2, December 2003

[3] Sun ONE Portal Server 6. Meeting the challenges of enterprise portals. A white paper by DreamSoft. Sun Microsystems 2003.

[4] Introduction. Sun ONE Identity Server. Version 6.1, 2003

[5] Sun ONE Portal Server, Mobile Access 6.2: *http://www.sun.com/software/products/portal_ma/index.html*

[6] Sun Microsystems: A Technical Overview of the Sun ONE Directory Server 5.2. White Paper. July 2003.

[7] AmericanTeleCare. Practical Solutions. Positive outcomes: *http://www.americantelecare.com/*

[8] L. Bizon, M. Rozenau: *Zastosowanie Web Services w integracji systemów informatycznych*, praca magisterska, Akademia Górniczo-Hutnicza im. Stanisława Staszica w Krakowie, Wydział Elektrotechniki, Automatyki, Informatyki i Elektroniki, Katedra Informatyki, Kraków, czerwiec 2003.

[9] G. Eysenbach: What is e-health? [editorial]. Journal of Medical Internet Research 2001;3(2):e20 *http://www.jmir.org/2001/2/e20/*

[10] J.H. Saltzer, M.D. Schroeder: The protection of information in computer systems, Proceedings of the IEEE 63 (9), 1975

[11] P. Słowikowski, M. Jarząb: Security Aspect of Medical Portals, International Conference on E-health in Common Europe, Kraków, Poland, June 5-6, 2003

[12] D. Gordon, G. Geiger, N. Lowe, J. Jickling, "What Is An Electronic Patient Record?"Proceedings of the AMIA Annual Fall Symposium, 240–244, 1998

[13] Programmer's Guide. Sun ONE Identity Server. Version 6.0, 2002

[14] D. F. Ferraiolo, R. Sandhu, S. Gavrila, D. R. Kuhn, R. Chandramouli: Proposed NIST Standard for Role-Based Access Control, ACM Transactions on Information and System Security. 2001. *http://csrc.nist.gov/rbac/*

[15] K. Zieliński, D. Radziszowski, P. Rzepa: Access to medical databases through Internet tools – International Conference on TELEMEDICINE, Jabłonna, 2002

[16] B. Kwolek, K. Zieliński: Scalable Telemedicine Solutions - Research Directions of KCT, Biomedical Conference Engineering, Kaunas, October 2003. *http://www.ics.agh.edu.pl/papers/ScalableTelemedicineSolutions.pdf*

[17] Meg Broderick, D.H. Smaltz: E-Health defined, May 2003.

[18] Jennifer Marconi: E-Health: Navigating the Internet for Health Information Healthcare, Advocacy White Paper. Healthcare Information and Management Systems Society, May, 2002.

*Transformation of Health Care with Information Technologies*
*M. Duplaga et al. (Eds.)*
*IOS Press, 2004*



# Medical Information Asymmetry in the Cyberworld of Manuel Castells

Piotr KASZTELOWICZ
*Ludwik Rydygier Hospital Torun, Poland*
*e-mail: Piotr.Kasztelowicz@am.torun.pl*

**Abstract.** Before 1997, the Internet was strongly associated with universities and higher education, including medical research. There were only small virtual communities at that time, but all their members had equal access to the entire body of information placed on the net. Each networking participant was able not only to retrieve but also to create and distribute medical information. This state was a symmetry, of sorts, between passive and active Internet usage. Since that time, however, significant commercialization of the Internet (including the medical domain) has been increasing its asymmetry.

We currently observe a division into providers, serving and distributing medical information on the net, and consumers, who receive pre-prepared "products". This brings new challenges for both academic and practicing e-health physicians. First, while all large-scale initiatives to certify medical portals have so far failed, the public must be educated to chose valuable, high quality medical information themselves. Secondly, this imbalance favors abusive commercial behavior, such as spam, spreading viruses and advertising without content-related information. Stimulating a restoration of the previous idea of the Internet for non-profit activities seems to be best way to avoid the continuation of Internet "degeneration". Manuel Castells has defined future industrial and postindustrial progress of humanity as activity in global virtual communities, interchanging ideas, knowledge and information. The role of medical professionals seems to be to educate patients and their families on how to search for quality medical information and to stimulate other medical professionals, researchers as well as patients' supportive groups to be active themselves. Reducing the medical information asymmetry will provide a positive influence on the progress of e-health in the future. Open source software may help reduce costs by creating adequate resources.

## 1. Reality and Vision

The amount of noise in the virtual world can be measured by the amount of spam – unsolicited messages delivered to our mailboxes every day. While searching for interesting information unfortunately we must also read through advertising, including promotion of drugs such as viagra or anabolic hormones. Sophisticated viruses are also spreading, which must be scanned by antiviral software, which of course slows down the operating systems of our servers and workstations, and calls for improvements in the quality of antiviral technology.

```
make[2]: Entering directory `/export/home/pekasz/src/clamav-0.67/libclamav'
source='mbox.c' object='mbox.lo' libtool=yes \
depfile='.deps/mbox.Plo' tmpdepfile='.deps/mbox.TPlo' \
depmode=gcc3 /bin/bash ../depcomp \
/bin/bash ../libtool --mode=compile gcc -DHAVE_CONFIG_H -I. -I. -I.. -I.. -
I./zziplib    -g -O2 -c -o mbox.lo `test -f 'mbox.c' || echo './'`mbox.c
rm -f .libs/mbox.lo
gcc -DHAVE_CONFIG_H -I. -I. -I.. -I.. -I./zziplib -g -O2 -c mbox.c -MT mbox.lo
-MD -MP -MF .deps/mbox.TPlo  -fPIC -DPIC -o .libs/mbox.lo
gcc -DHAVE_CONFIG_H -I. -I. -I.. -I.. -I./zziplib -g -O2 -c mbox.c -MT mbox.lo
-MD -MP -MF .deps/mbox.TPlo -o mbox.o >/dev/null 2>&1
mv -f .libs/mbox.lo mbox.lo
source='message.c' object='message.lo' libtool=yes \
depfile='.deps/message.Plo' tmpdepfile='.deps/message.TPlo' \
depmode=gcc3 /bin/bash ../depcomp \
/bin/bash ../libtool --mode=compile gcc -DHAVE_CONFIG_H -I. -I. -I.. -I.. -
I./zziplib       -g   -O2   -c   -o   message.lo   `test   -f   'message.c'   ||   echo
'./'`message.c
rm -f .libs/message.lo
gcc -DHAVE_CONFIG_H -I. -I. -I.. -I.. -I./zziplib -g -O2 -
```

**Fig. 1.** Fragment of the compilation process of a known free (GPL license) antiviral software clamav-antivirus 0.67 on Unix using the gcc 3.2 compiler

A wholly separate story involves system hacking and violations of computer data secrecy. An important question is how to fix this virtual world and how to restore to e-health its appropriate substantial and ethical character? Latest trends show that the Internet, including e-health, takes on the shape of other mass media – with large content providers (first of all big clinical portals) and clients, i.e. medical professionals searching for helpful information and education. This has resulted in an asymmetry characteristic to traditional media, although the Internet as we know it gives all participant equal privileges to be "consumers" as well as "creators". Manuel Castells in his trilogy on the problems of humans in cyber-world has sait: "the space of flows has introduced a culture of real virtuality which is characterized by timeless time and placeless space. Timeless time ... the dominant temporality in our society, occurs when the characteristics of a given context, namely, the informational paradigm and the network society, induce systemic perturbation in the sequential order of phenomena performed in that context" [1]. Replacing traditional media by new e-media also changes this traditional division. Moreover, when such a division exits, it is exhibited in our brains (consciousness) rather than in the code of new technology. The Vision, resulting from M. Castell's papers advises to increase the power of good, independent and "non-profit" initiatives in telemedicine, created for networking societies of doctors, patients and support groups. Large-scale education is at the core of success. A better educated patient is less susceptible to Internet fraud, advertising or violations.

```
received: from cr80.neoplus.adsl.tpnet.pl (HELO am.torun.pl) (80.54.214.80)
  by dorota.am.torun.pl with SMTP; 28 Feb 2004 10:58:54 -0000
From: your@domain.com
To: "xxxx"@am.torun.pl
Subject: information
Date: Sat, 28 Feb 2004 11:58:47 +0100
MIME-Version: 1.0
Content-Type: multipart/mixed; boundary="33812802"
X-Qmail-Scanner-Message-ID: <107796594252627244@dorota>

--33812802
Content-Type: text/plain; charset=us-ascii
Content-Transfer-Encoding: 7bit

do you?
```

```
--33812802
Content-Type: application/x-zip-compressed; name="msg.zip"
Content-Transfer-Encoding: base64
Content-Disposition: attachment; filename="msg.zip"

UEsDBAoAAAAAAFdXXDBdbrAiAFYAAABWAAAALAAAAbXNnLmRvYy5zY3JNWpAAAwAAAAQAAAD/
/wAAuAAAAAAAAAABAAAAAAAAAAAAAAAAAAAAAAAAAAAAAAAAAAAAAAAAAAAAAACAAAAADh+6
DgC0Cc0huAFMzSFUaGlzIHByb2dyYW0gY2Fubm90IGJlIHJ1biBpbiBET1MgbW9kZS4NDQok
AAAAAAAAAFBFAABMAQMAWfQwQAAAAAAAAAAA4AAPAgsBAjgAUAAAABAAAABAAQDQkAEAAFAB
AACgAQAAAEAAABAAAAACAAAEAAAAAAAAAAQAAAAAAAAAALABAAAQAAAAAAAAAgAAAAAAEAAA
```

**Fig. 2.** Fragment of a computer virus attached to an e-mail with MIME, stopped by the mail-scanner system on the dorota.am.torun.pl mailserver

Safer Internet is one of the principles of the European Union [2], implemented in medicine by the MedCIRCLE project, which is the brainchild of G. Eysenbach [3], developed under European auspices. In Poland, an important discussion on a medical Internet quality certification system took place during the 5th. Polish Medical Internet Conference in Poznan [4] where the author represented a group of enthusiasts propagating such a certification system. About 64% members of the Internet community, gathered on a medical mailing list for patients and their families in two independent studies, have voted "for" certification, but during the 1st E-health conference held in Krakow one year ago the author confronted skeptical opinions regarding the possible success of such a method [5]. Even Eysenbach's [6] initiative is still at the conceptual stage. If a project which creates voluminous rating systems, assessing information about millions of websites, fails to operate, then Internet users cannot be sure how to rank any service as being good or bad. The reason for failures of such ideas seems to be trivial. Every day all the world accumulates more medical information than can ever be evaluated by a team of authorities. This fact has changed my opinion in relation to this topic. I am currently inclined to promote user education rather than forcibly creating certifying institutions, working at tortoise speed. In this era of progress, the commercial Internet seems to emerge as a real as well as potential risk for conflicts of interests between aspiration (to achieve maximal financial benefit) and the need to present quality medical information.

```
Date: Sat, 28 Feb 2004 21:32:19 -0800
From: Overheats S. Nymphomaniacs <astronomer@three-iron.com>
To: Lek <lek-med@achilles.wam.lodz.pl>
Subject: Explore top-rated Super ViagrDa! =] A skeeters rehabilitator
weighshaft.

    [ Part 2.2: "Attached Text" ]

How do you do?
It is not possible for a man to be elegant without a touch of femininity.
CialiWs (Regalims), at cheap prices.
Most zones charge $20, we charge $4.95. Quite a differennce.

Ciali8s is knnown as a Super ViagTra or Weekend Viagwra because its efcfets
start soeonr and last much loegnr.

Shipped worldwide.

Here you will find it: http://www.***
-----
If you do not wish to be hendecoic 8-]
The really great novel tends to be the exact negative of its author's life.
```

**Fig. 3.** Spam advertising Viagra, sent to the mailing list *lek-med@achilles.wam.lodz.pl* (about 500 subscribers) and stopped by list moderator from reaching the list

## 2. Informationalism in Medicine – a New Stage of the Information Paradigm[1]

Network societies, as a driving force [7] of world progress, opening new possibilities for the glocal society have emerged from traditional structures (including the physician/patient relation), formed through the centuries by social evolution. Now it is emphasized that the paternalistic relation model in relations between doctors and patients should be replaced by a partnership to achieve the desired target – health restoration. This cooperative model may change the role of medical professionals in modern urban societies, but in my opinion has not yet defined the place of medical professionals and patients in the information-age society. It can be said that replacing the paternalistic model with one based on partnership is not sufficient to "set free" all the possibilities offered by e-health. To understand this process, we can present four models of relations. The first, ***traditional*** relation, whether *paternalistic* or *based on a partnership*, uses formalized structure care models, such as the insurance model, public or private healthcare systems with first-contact physicians, referencing systems (for hospital care) and regionalism. The patient is inside the model and decisions are made on his behalf by traditional healthcare system institutions supervised by government or local authorities.

The second, ***anarchic*** relation represents a transient form, between traditional and more "mature" models of the information age. Patients can learn about their disorders from the Internet, giving them additional knowledge and benefits, but at the same time the patients possess no ability to evaluate the casual/accidental information, picked up from net. The anarchic model is characterized as being "without a target", including casual, unconfirmed information, a disorganized method of data collection, minimal help of medical professionals and, potentially, many mistakes. It is easy to recognize that this model is unsafe and may provide the patient with false information. The remaining two models are parallel, coexisting mature relations – ***dispersed/altruistic/non-profit*** and ***targeted/business/commercial***. Crucial to furthering the idea of harmonious progress of e-health is, in my opinion, a stable balance between both, which I will confirm in the remaining part of my presentation. The first (dispersed/altruistic/non-profit) relation is based on a hacker (in the positive meaning of this term) culture dispersed on net, consisting of medical professionals with altruistic intentions to help patients, their families and support groups and to present them, first of all, with quality information.. Medical information created by such groups includes Web pages, electronic journals, fora, cooperation on medical mailing lists and usenet groups. There are no government or local authorities supervising this model, but like at universities and within the scientific society, natural forms of control emerge, which (as I will mention in the next chapter) put stress not on certification, but on education (i.e. how to use the medical knowledge from the net). Medical scientific societies may also be involved in this model, substantially improving the value of non-profit initiatives. In Poland, a good example is the Polish Cardiac Society's initiative to create free medical Web pages for physicians as well as for patients, i.e. the KARDIO-L (common with the Polish Society of Arterial Hypertension) mailing list and an "internet cafe", which hosts discussions with renowned professors of cardiology. The second model (targeted/business/commercial) is the result of activity of e-business-oriented people. This model is characterized first of all by the use of advanced technology, targeting selected group of people (consumers) with selected forms of interactions (services). Investors look to achieve financial benefit and the activity of medical portals (the portal is the most frequent form of e-technology) is legitimized usually neither by authorities nor scientific supervision, but by market rules – portal users can become potential advertisers themselves. Some portals combine altruism (high quality medical information) with market

---

[1] Subtitile taken from Bo. Groenlund "The Urba Question and The Rise of the Network Society Manuel Castells confronted" – *http://hjem.get2net.dk/gronlund/Castells.html*

rules, increasing the confidence of consumers (including professionals) in information served by such portals. Good examples are the Canadian Docguide *(http://www.docguide.com)* and MedWeb *(http://www.medweb.com)*.

## 3. Asymmetry

Unfortunately, such examples of the ability to combine medical professionalism and "moneymaking" seem to be rare. This same imbalance between "non profit" and "business" modes does not favor development of e-health based on evidence-based medicine and substantial knowledge.

Because commercial institutions possess resources as well as a precise and stable organizational form – we are observing the process of squeezing out non-profit e-health initiatives by commercial ones. Paradoxically, it should be remembered that the Internet gives all users equal right along with an incentive to enhance resources as well as to create new ones. Yet, the social process described above, which consists of converging the Internet and traditional media, where (traditionally) the division between producers and consumers is essential, continues. I call this process and its effects for medical e-health the **medical information asymmetry in the cyberworld**. It is, generally and from a social viewpoint, clarified in different papers by M. Castells [8], as suggested in the title of this paper. An ideal situation would be to maintain balance between "producing" and "consuming" medical information in the cyberworld. The asymmetry is caused first of all by amplification of the commercial model and squeezing out "non profit"/altruistic activity on the net. The patients' lobby of patients (families, support groups and doctors), including European Union countries, can promote non-profit Internet initiatives in new EU entrants, to change this unfavorable situation (i.e. imbalance). The result of the imbalance is the uncontrolled flow of unsolicited information, including spam, advertising, fraud, viruses, etc. At present, the market itself cannot sufficiently regulate these issues. Perhaps the Internet is still a young (immature) community with extant anarchic trends of progress and the market cannot fully regulate such branches as medicine (others, too).

## 4. Education of Health-oriented e-Communities

Internet has changed the pattern of interpersonal contacts. It is characterized by a very anarchic structure, and the lack of the possibility of regulation. Additionally, as described by Castells, *timeless time* and *space of flow* produce a culture of "real virtuosity". If as suspected, it is not possible to certify medical resources (i.e. all resources present on the Web), another method of empowering consumers (patients, families and support groups) seams to be education. In my opinion, it is not sufficient to create information pages informing how to choose good medical information and reject bad information. There should also be training programs directed at anyone interested in e-health or at selected groups suffering from particular diseases, or interested about any particular problem. From my observation and practice, it is not sufficient to create "passive" documents, which teach the proper use of e-health – we should strive for the actual presence of doctors and other medical professionals on mailings lists and groups, where patients, families and support groups meet.

It seems an urgent necessity to create educational programs for patients, their families and support groups on how to seek quality information on the net. The weight attached to this kind of information on the net is, in my opinion, insufficient. The presence in e-health of oriented communities of doctors and other medical professional not serving any medical business and independent from e-commerce, playing the role of "gurus" and "tour guides", is an important step towards making e-health more useful and safe for all. The European countries as well as the European Union should support such initiatives.

## 5. Reducing Asymmetry

Manuel Castells in "The Internet Galaxy" has characterized the information age culture by describing different groups of people, who play here substantial roles in spreading this innovation. This division has also other aspects than those cited in Roger's "diffusion of innovation", but first of all the aim is to promote non-profit initiatives, particularly those associated with university or medical societies. The European Union and its member states should finance telemedical projects, whose outcomes can be suitable for use in the public health sector. That sector can be, in the future, supported by many e-health activities, improving standards of care. The first step is creating large-scale education programs for patients, families and support groups as well as medical professionals. In the future, it will become necessary to solve many problems associated with medical practice in the information age (including, for instance, the issue discussed on the "SIM" mailing list about purchasing drugs on the net [9]).

## References


[1] Felix Stalder, The Network Paradigm: Social Formations in the Age of Information *http://felix.openflows.org/html/netparadigm.html*

[2] *http://www.europa.eu.int/information_society/programmes/iap/text_en.htm*

[3] Collaboration for Internet Rating, Certification, Labeling and Evaluation of Health Information *http://www.medcircle.org/about.php*

[4] P. Kasztelowicz, Certifikaty moje zdanie "za" (Certify my opinion "yes")

[5] P. Kasztelowicz, Doctors – the role of creating and promoting high quality medical information on the Internet, Presentation on "E-health in Common Europe 2003", Krakow – *http://www.am.torun.pl/~pekasz/Kasztelowicz-ehe.pdf*

[6] Gunther Eysenbach, Gabriel Yihune, Kristian Lampe, Phil Cross, Dan Brickley "Quality Management, Certification and Rating of Health Information on the Net with MedCERTAIN: Using a medPICS/RDF/XML metadata structure for implementing eHealth ethics and creating trust globally" J Med Internet Res 2000;2(suppl 2):e1 *http://jmir.org/2000/3/suppl2/e1/*

[7] M. Castells "The Internet Galaxy" 2001

[8] Bo Groenlund "'The Urban Question' and 'The Rise of the Network Society' – Manuel Castells confronted – *http://hjem.get2net.dk/gronlund/Castells.html*

[9] *http://hilist.au.dk/pipermail/sim/2004-February/thread.html*

*Transformation of Health Care with Information Technologies*
*M. Duplaga et al. (Eds.)*
*IOS Press, 2004*



# Web-Based Health Services and Clinical Decision Support

Darius JEGELEVICIUS, Vaidotas MAROZAS, Arunas LUKOSEVICIUS, Martynas PATASIUS
*Biomedical Engineering Institute, Kaunas University of Technology, Studentu 65, Kaunas, LT-51369, Lithuania*
*e-mail: darius.jegelevicius@ktu.lt*

**Abstract.** The purpose of this study was the development of a Web-based e-health service for comprehensive assistance and clinical decision support. The service structure consists of a Web server, a PHP-based Web interface linked to a clinical SQL database, Java applets for interactive manipulation and visualization of signals and a Matlab server linked with signal and data processing algorithms implemented by Matlab programs. The service ensures diagnostic signal- and image analysis-sbased clinical decision support. By using the discussed methodology, a pilot service for pathology specialists for automatic calculation of the proliferation index has been developed. Physicians use a simple Web interface for uploading the pictures under investigation to the server; subsequently a Java applet interface is used for outlining the region of interest and, after processing on the server, the requested proliferation index value is calculated. There is also an "expert corner", where experts can submit their index estimates and comments on particular images, which is especially important for system developers. These expert evaluations are used for optimization and verification of automatic analysis algorithms. Decision support trials have been conducted for ECG and ophthalmology ultrasonic investigations of intraocular tumor differentiation. Data mining algorithms have been applied and decision support trees constructed. These services are under implementation by a Web-based system too.

The study has shown that the Web-based structure ensures more effective, flexible and accessible services compared with standalone programs and is very convenient for biomedical engineers and physicians, especially in the development phase.

## Introduction

The modern healthcare management paradigm is based on friendly, seamless, secure and cost-effective use of advanced technologies, especially Information and Communication Technologies (ICT). Healthcare facilities presently use ICT to support a wide variety of administrative, laboratory, and pharmacy activities [1]. The purpose of the ICT is to free the physician from administrative, technical and other work not directly related to his medical activities, and also to provide a comprehensive decision support wherever it is needed. Therefore, ICT must ensure effective services (rather than standalone programs), computers and other equipment maintained in the workplace.

The development of the Internet and World Wide Web (WWW) provide a new area and tools for the development of more flexible services for clinical (not only administrative) applications. New possibilities are used for creation of Internet-based medical services for clinical signal (ECG [2]) and image (pathology [3] or ultrasound [4]) analysis, and also for decision support [5]. By permeating medical practices, such services are changing concept of *telemedicine* (as medicine delivered at a distance) to the concept of *e-health* [6].

Despite the existence of many software tools for medical purposes in the market, there are still areas and means for further developments. Web-based tools provide more flexibility for developers and for medical practitioners: compatibility with different computer platforms, better service and response to needs, better access using available Internet connections, etc. Web-based tools can be used in an effective way when combined with signal and data processing tools such as Matlab (*The Mathworks, Inc.*). This synthesis can provide flexible results, especially in the system development phase.

In the present paper, pilot Web-based services and trials for clinical decision support development by the Kaunas University of Technology Biomedical Engineering Institute are presented.

## 1. Decision Support and Web-Based Health Services

A clinical decision support system is understood as an information system that supports and assists healthcare professionals in clinical decisionmaking tasks like diagnosis, therapy planning and monitoring [1]. The structure of such a system can be represented by several functional blocks, as shown in Figure 1. Real implementations can be performed in many ways and on various levels of complexity and versatility.

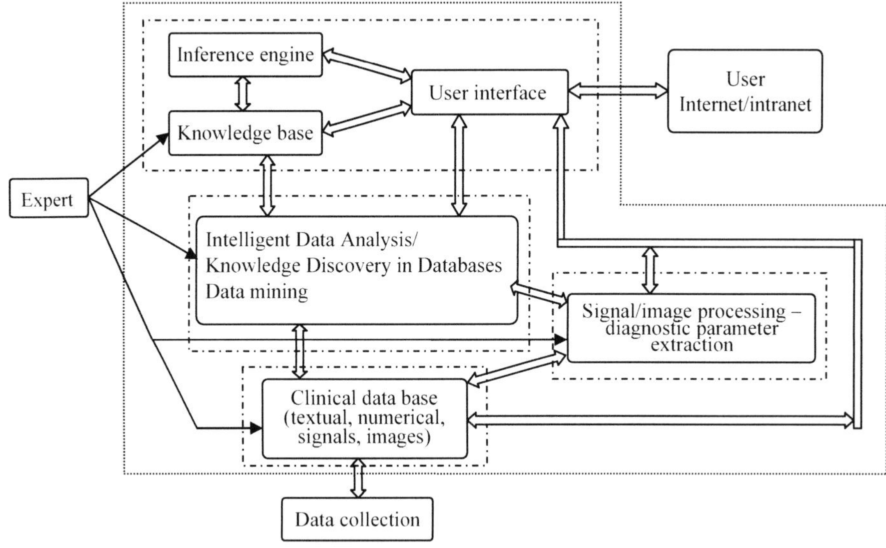


**Fig. 1.** Clinical decision support system

The main components of the decision support system (as outlined in Figure 1) are the clinical database, signal processing, data analysis, a knowledge-based inference engine and a user interface. The raw material submitted to the system constitutes clinical data. Decisions regarding diagnosis and treatment are based on the interpretation and analysis of this data. Data collection can be done integrally within a hospital information system and then linked to the decision support system. Specific clinical data, such as signals and images, is usually interpreted by a physician and only rarely using signal processing systems. Yet, signal processing and the results of this process can yield very valuable information. In some cases such analysis can be directly called "decision support".

The clinical data collected in the database is raw and ready for further processing. Data processing is called "intelligent data analysis", "knowledge discovery in databases" or "data mining". All these names are often used as synonyms [7]. Data processing is the extraction of implicit, previously unknown, and potentially useful information from data. The term "data processing" refers to using a variety of techniques to process large amounts of information in order to discover knowledge which would be useful for decision-making. This covers a number of different approaches, such as clustering, data summarization, learning classification rules, finding dependency networks, analyzing changes, detecting anomalies, and so on. One of the successful applications of data mining techniques for medical diagnostic purposes is illustrated in [8]. The diagnosis of breast tumors by data mining with the effective use of decision trees is described in this work. The See5.0 (C5.0) data mining tool [9] has been used in this instance. The accuracy of the data mining for the breast tumor diagnosis was 96% compared to 86% for physician diagnosis [8]. This impressive result has encouraged us to search for other applications and validate algorithms with actual data from the areas of ophthalmology [13] and cardiology.

Data mining results can be used for diagnostic decision support and for new knowledge discovery. The borderline of such differentiation is subjective and depends on the clinical data preparation and result interpretation. The use of these different approaches is shown in following chapters, applying decision-tree induction for ophthalmologic and cardiologic data. Data mining in ophthalmology was done for diagnostic purposes and data mining in cardiology was done for knowledge discovery to find relations and dependencies between parameters for better understanding of physiological processes.

The kernel of the decision support system is the knowledge base. This base concentrates all knowledge delivered by data analysis and expert advice. This knowledge is used for interpretation of patients' data and for inference of clinical decisions. The role of the expert is very important, especially in medical decision support systems. Experts are involved in almost all decision support system processes on different levels and at various times, depending on the system structure. The knowledge base contains and manages various forms of knowledge [1]: scientific and experiential knowledge. The first type represents the understanding of scientific principles and relationships between pathophysiological conditions as well as disease symptoms. Experiential knowledge helps the physician diagnose diseases based on his experience.

Decision support systems can be implemented in numerous ways. Web-based services offer ease of use, as well as widespread availability. Such implementations allow users to reach services using common Web browsers, centralizing information and management. A Web-based system is easy to maintain as it only provides one application, common for every user, and guarantees user access to the latest, most recent versions. Web-based clinical decision support systems can be represented as interconnection of four elements (see Figure 2, right side): a Web server, a signal/image processing server, a data mining server and a database server. The user connects to the Web server using a Web browser. The Web server acts as a user interface and as a coordination server for data flow between other parts of the system. For interaction and data feed control, the Web server uses PHP, Java applets or other programming techniques. The task of the signal/image processing server is to apply necessary signal processing for received signals and images. Such processing can be performed online or as a background process for data already stored in the database and not requiring an immediate response. The database server is used for data storage and is a source of signal and data processing. The data mining server is a very important part of the system, as it is used for data abstraction, processing, knowledge base formation and inference.

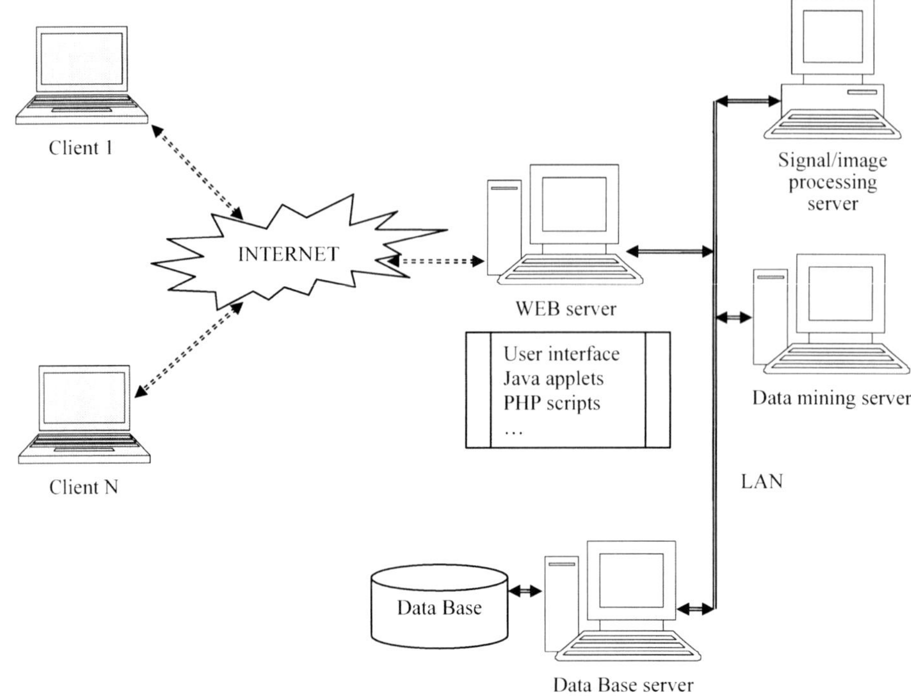


**Fig. 2.** Web-based clinical decision support system structure

The whole system is complex and depends on the decision support task. Building the decision support system can originate from one server containing all or only some system components. In the next chapters, we will describe three case studies from our own practice. Neither of them matches Figure 2 completely, but each contains some elements of a decision support system, in the development phase.

## 2. Case Study: Web Service for Pathology

The main goal was to create a convenient Web-based service for automatic calculation of quantitative parameters of pathology images. This idea arose in a joint Lithuanian-Swedish project Litmed2, dedicated to telemedical cooperation in the area of clinical pathology.

One of the quantities that are determined during immunohistochemical analysis of pathology samples is the proliferation index. This index (also called the "labeling index" (LI)) shows the spread of cancerous cells in the tissue, as well as the degree of tumor malignancy. LI is a number of imunohistochemically labeled cells per 100 cells. Usually it is expressed as a percentage, based on analysis performed on at least 1000 cells [10]. The counting is performed in the region of the tumor with the greatest density of staining [10] or in a randomly-selected area [11]. It is known that manual counting of LI is subjective to considerable intra- and interobserver variability regardless of its high validity [10]; also, it is a time-consuming task. Therefore, LI might be calculated automatically through computerized image analysis. The main task in such an analysis is image segmentation and evaluation of the total number of cells (or the area occupied by cells, proportional to their number).

Components of the Web service for LI calculation are shown in Figure 3. Technologies used in the Web service system include Apache and IIS Web Servers, PHP, MS SQL Server 2000 and MATLAB. The client can use any Web browser to contact the server that runs both Apache and IIS Web Servers. Two servers are used for security reasons. The Apache Web Server is used to run PHP programs that receive user input and it communicates with MS SQL Server 2000 to read and change data in the databases. The IIS Web Server is used to run MATLAB. It is done by executing the matweb.exe file, which in turn uses the "matlabserver" service to locate and run the MATLAB engine, then creates an HTML form containing results [12].

The kernel of the server part is one of the components of MATLAB - the MATLAB Web Server (see Figure 3). It works according to the CGI standard - it processes data taken from the HTML form and returns an HTML page with results (created according to a template) to the client [12]. The MATLAB Web Server cannot read files directly from the local filesystem of the client, so the file in question has to be transferred to the server using the PHP scripting language. This makes it possible to save the system from potentially harmful files (the filename has to correspond to a predefined set of rules). MATLAB executes image processing functions and returns the LI result. The physician can then choose to save those results to the database, created using the MS SQL Server 2000 database management system.

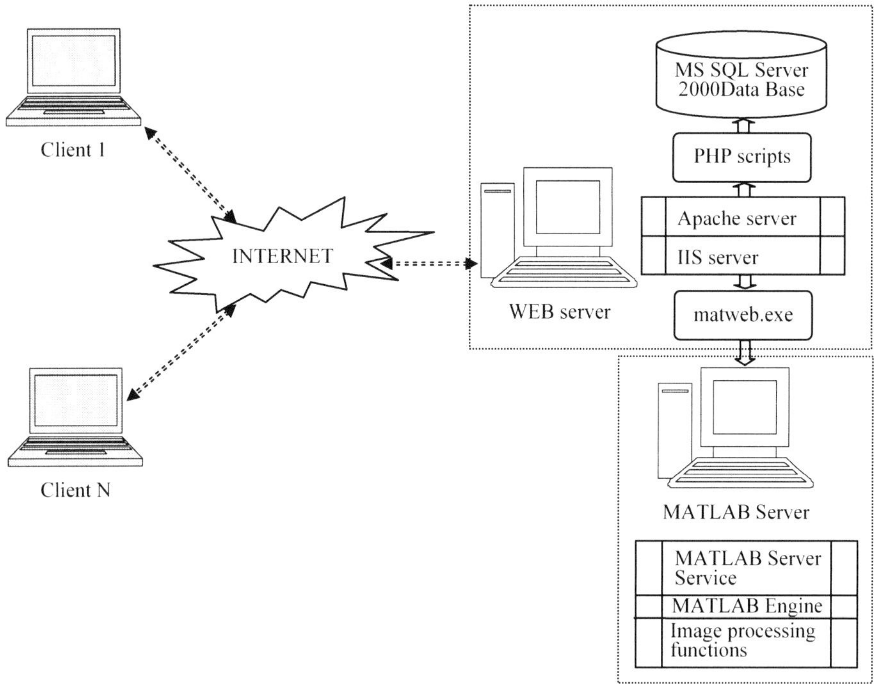


**Fig. 3.** Components of a Web-based service for pathology

Figure 4 represents use case diagrams for the Web-based service for pathology.

User identification is done by entering to the "user" or "administration" pages and providing a login and a password. The pathologist can then browse the system for images on the local computer and upload these images to the server. Subsequently, a Java applet is used to display images. The applet allows outlining regions of interest (ROI), as well as zooming in or out. After the ROI is outlined and sent to the server, calculation of LI can be started by pressing the corresponding button. Following some delay, the server returns the calculated LI and a separate image with marked cells. The user can then add the image to the database and, optionally, to recommend this image for inclusion in the reference database. The reference database is used for image processing algorithm development. Additionally, the user can enter his own subjective estimation of LI.

By logging in as administrator, the user can look at the logs of uploaded and processed files, manage reference files, manage user accounts, and view results of image evaluations by experts.

The images evaluated subjectively by pathologists are used as a kind of "gold standard" for estimation of LI calculation algorithms. These results are stored in a database and are used as a reference for automatic algorithm improvement. The administrator can read estimations of LI for reference images as well as their statistical characteristics (mean and standard deviation), and compare them with the automatic LI evaluation results for each image. New versions of the automatic algorithm can be immediately verified against the reference database with subjective estimates.

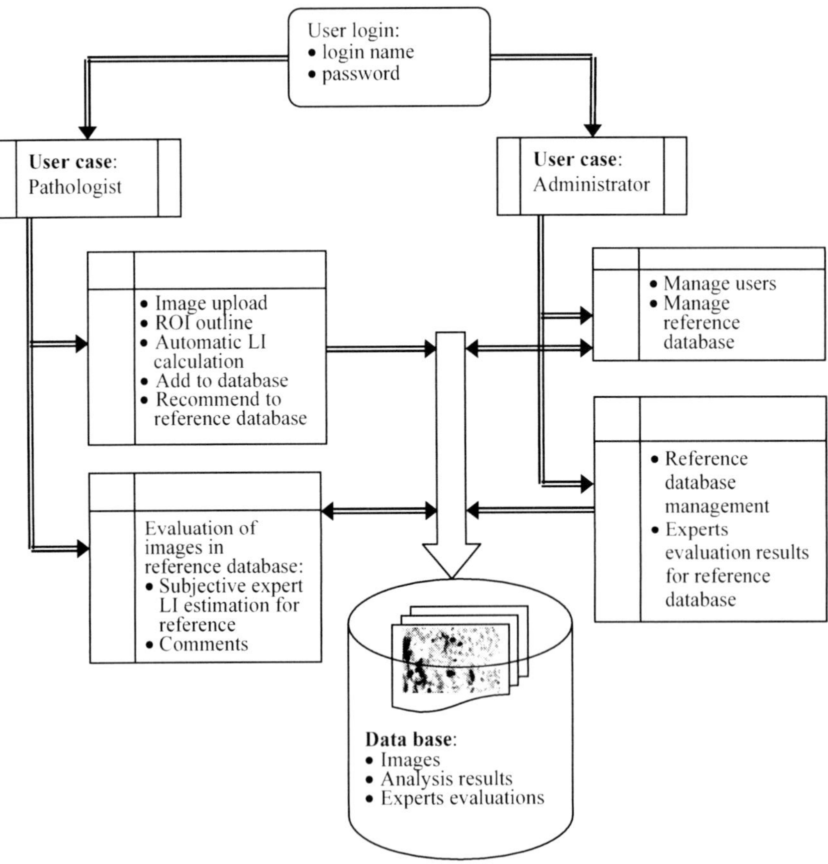


**Fig. 4.** Use cases in the Web-based service for pathology

The Web service being described is installed at the Kaunas University of Technology Biomedical Engineering Institute server, under the following address: *http://www.bmii.ktu.lt/~webservices/pathology*. Figure 5 shows a view of the Web service.

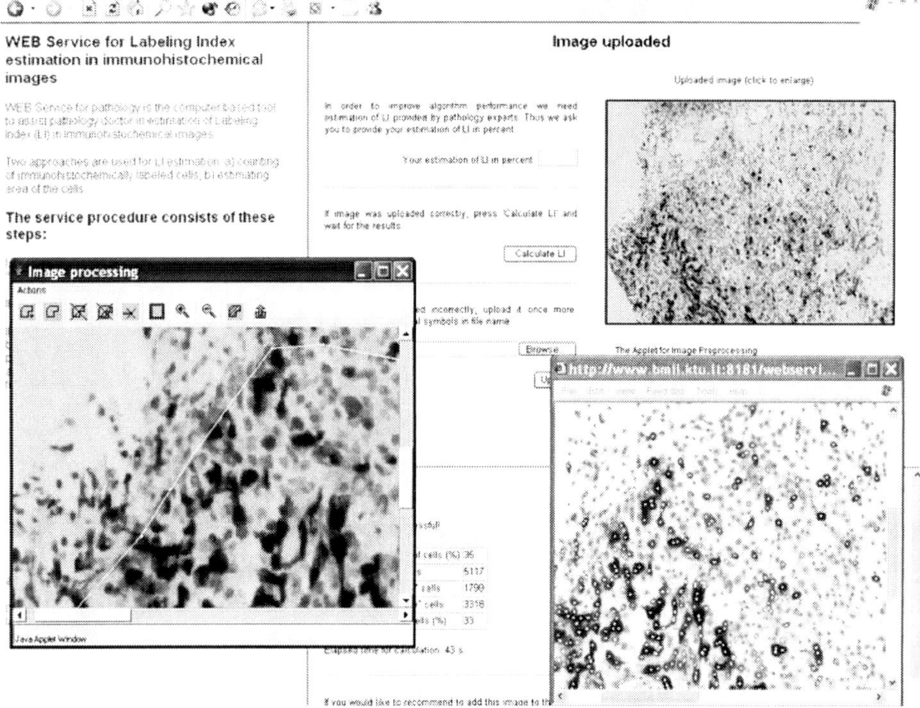


**Fig. 5.** Screenshot of the Web-based LI estimation tool

## 3. Case Study: Ophthalmology

In cooperation with the Ophthalmology Department of the Biomedical Research Institute of the Kaunas University of Medicine, a trial study for application of data mining methods for decision support in ophthalmology has been conducted [13].

Eye tumors were the object of the investigation. Localization, dimensions, shape and morphological type of the tumor are the main parameters in diagnosis, prognosis and choice of treatment for the patient. Evaluation of the morphological type of the tumor is possible only after removal of the eye containing the tumor or after diagnostic biopsy; however A/B ultrasound techniques enable us to diagnose the cell morphology of malignant intraocular tumors in a prospective manner [14]. The A/B ultrasound method allows the physician to localize, measure the prominence and the basis of the tumor, and to evaluate its shape, choroidal excavation, complications (retinal detachments, hemorrhages) and internal reflectivity. Malignant uveal melanoma and metastasis are fairly rare among cancers (only 0,2 percents of all human cancers) but they are the most frequent malignant eye tumors and represent one of the most lethal diseases seen in the ophthalmologic practice [15]. Early diagnosis and differentiation of the eye tumor is important for effective treatment of the patient.

We have used the See5.0 system [9] for the analysis of data related to eye uveal melanoma. The aim of the study was to test decision support algorithms for differential diagnosis of intraocular tumors using parameters from eye ultrasound B-scan images obtained by ultrasound examination. Diagnostic parameters of the tumors were calculated from B-scan ultrasound images.

89 patients with intraocular pathology have been investigated. 9 diagnostic parameters were calculated and prepared for data mining with See5.0. The diagnoses of intraocular findings were known a priori, with three types of diagnoses identified: tumor, metastatic tumor and no tumor (echoscopically resembling a tumor). The See5.0 system had recognized 6 diagnostic parameters for decision tree synthesis. There were 6 diagnostic errors (6.7 %) in the test set using the decision tree model presented in Figure 6. The threshold and sequence of parameters for optimal classification of intraocular tumors into three groups are presented in the decision tree. The prognosis and probability of accurate diagnosis is provided by See5.0 as an answer for the physician. For example, the diagnostic case of a detected tumor with a height of 6,88 mm, a base width of 11,76 mm, a mushroom shape and a 1,22 regularity coefficient is evaluated as an intraocular tumor with the probability of 0,92.

```
Decision tree:
              HBratio <= 0.258:
              :...base <= 12.02: NotTumor
              :   base > 12.02: Metastasis
              HBratio > 0.258:
              :...shape = Polygonal: Tumor
                  shape = Lobular: NotTumor
                  shape = Mushroom:
                  :...reguliarity <= 2.74: Tumor
                  :   reguliarity > 2.74: NotTumor
                  shape = Dome:
                  :...choroidalexcavation = Yes: Tumor
                      choroidalexcavation = Unclear:
                      :...base <= 9.7: NotTumor
                      :   base > 9.7: Tumor
                      choroidalexcavation = No:
                      :...reguliarity > 1.53: NotTumor
                          reguliarity <= 1.53:
                          :...height > 3.14: Tumor
                              height <= 3.14:
                              :...HBratio <= 0.2738: Tumor
                                  HBratio > 0.2738:
                                  :...HBratio <= 0.5306: NotTumor
                                      HBratio > 0.5306: Tumor
```

**Fig. 6.** Decision tree for intraocular tumor diagnosis using ultrasound examination results

Despite a fully automatic decision tree synthesis, it is easily readable. This is another positive feature of our approach, when compared with neural networks, logistic regression and other methods. The reliability of decision support would increase with the addition of new reference cases.

## 4. Case Study: Cardiology

In cooperation with the Institute of Cardiology at the Kaunas University of Medicine, a decision tree induction trial study has been performed using stress electrocardiography (ECG) data. The aim of the study was to evaluate the changes, which appear in the human organism after lasting physical training, and to try to evaluate the functional physical state of the subjects as well as their physiological processes. Three healthy age groups have been investigated, with both genders equally represented: 20-30 years, 30-40 years and 40-50 years; 316 persons overall. The examination parameters measured during bicycle ergometry tests involved arterial blood pressure, heart rate and other parameters, derived from ECG analysis. Measurements were performed at beginning and after 15-16 months of training in fitness groups. The overall number of parameters measured and calculated for each person was 130.

The data mining experiment was performed using See 5.0 decision tree induction software [9]. The purpose of data mining was to find relations between parameters and the functional state of the person. The functional state was evaluated by a so-called "summary value". This value is based on a human organism model, reflecting the behavior of action, regulatory and supply systems during load conditions [16]. All persons under investigation were grouped into three groups ("poor", "normal" and "good") depending on their summary values. Decision trees were built for these groups, using measured and calculated parameters. These decision trees were then used for test data set evaluation and they were interpreted by physicians. An example of a decision tree is shown in Figure 7. The resulting decision trees (separate for men and women) provide an accuracy of 22% and 25% (respectively) for correct physical state prediction using 6-7 parameters. However, the main purpose of this study was to discover and extract new knowledge as well as understanding about the behavior of the human physiological system. The tree-like structure and dependencies of parameters represented in this structure provide new insight for physicians. In this study we have noticed very clear differences between decision tree structures for men and women.

```
Decision tree:
               n.k.(HR) <= 0.44: poor
               n.k.(HR) >= 0.45:
               :...2 -Stc <= 0.74:
                   :...3 -ST <= -0.07: good
                   :   3 -ST >= -0.05: poor
                   2 -Stc >= 0.75 (0.745):
                   :...100W HR >= 156: poor
                       100W HR <= 143:
                       :...n.k.(HR) >= 0.59: good
                           n.k.(HR) <= 0.58:
                           :...Nmax/m >= 3.01: good
                               Nmax/m <= 2.86:
                               :...weight <= 92:
                                   :...1 JTRR <= 322: good
                                   :   1 JTRR >= 342: normal
                                   weight >= 96:
                                   :...Nmax/m <= 2.08: normal
                                       Nmax/m >= 2.5: good
```

**Fig. 7.** Decision tree for physical state evaluation

## 5. Conclusions

A complete framework for implementation and further development of Web-based e-health services for clinical decision support has been outlined. The advantages of Web-based e-health service solution are: ease of use and access for the user, ease of testing and improvement for the developers, centralized information storage and management. Web-based systems are easy to maintain as they only present one common application for every user and guarantee user access to the latest, most recent versions. Constructing a decision support system can originate from one server containing all or only some components of the system. By "decision support" we understand a wide variety of services which can help physicians make their decisions.

A trial service has been implemented as a Web-based tool for pathology. The service is used for automatic calculation of the labeling index in pathology images providing physicians with a numerical estimation for each clinical case. In this implementation, we have integrated the MATLAB computing environment with a Web service to provide effective image processing.

Decision support trials have also been conducted in ophthalmologic ultrasonic investigations of intraocular tumor differentiation and stress-test ECG. Data mining algorithms have been applied and decision support trees constructed. These services are under implementation by a Web-based service too.

We believe that the proposed framework of development, implementation and testing of e-health services could be used in other medical specialties, such as dermatology, neurology, ultrasound echoscopy and others.

**Acknowledgements.** We would like to acknowledge the help and fruitful collaboration with medical personnel: Prof. Henryk Domansky (Lund University Hospital, Sweden); Kaunas Medical University Hospital (Lithuania) Darius Pranys, M.D. and Inga Gudinavičienė, M.D. (Pathological Anatomy department), Prof. Alvydas Paunksnis (Eye department) and Prof. Alfonsas Vainoras (Institute of Cardiology). We also owe thanks to the Litmed2 project (Sweden – Lithuania, Project Manager: Mr. Lars-Olof Almquist , TietoEnator Trigon AB) for financial support.

## References

[1] Bronzino Joseph D. (editor) The Biomedical Engineering HandBook. Second Edition. Boca Raton, CRC Press LLC, 2000, 2912 p.

[2] García J., Martínez I., Sörnmo L., Olmos S., Mur A., Laguna P. Remote processing server for ECG-based clinical diagnosis support. *IEEE Transactions on Information Technology in Biomedicine*, 2002, Vol. 6, pp. 277-284.

[3] M. de Boer, Manner R., Mattes J., Komitowski D. Tele Image Analysis System (TIAS), an Environment for Image Analysis Using the WWW. In: *Proc. of the 12'th IEEE Symposium on Computer-Based Medical Systems*, 1999, pp. 66-71.

[4] Zeng H., Fei D. Y., Fu C. T., Kraft K. A. Internet (WWW) based system of ultrasonic image processing tools for remote image analysis. *Computer Methods and Programs in Biomedicine*, 2003 Jul, 71(3), pp. 235-241.

[5] Serrano A. J., Soria E., Camps-Valls G., Martín J. D., Sepúlveda J. R., Magdalena R., Jiménez N. V. Web-based Clinical Decision Support System Using Neural Networks. *European Symposium on Intelligent Technologies, Hybrid Systems and their implementation on Smart Adaptive Systems EUNITE 2002*, Albufeira (Portugal), Sept, 2002, pp. 19-21.

[6] Norris A.C. Essentials of telemedicine and telecare. John Wiley & Sons Ltd., England, 2001, 177 p.

[7] Lavrac N., Keravnou E., Zupan B. Intelligent data analysis in medicine. In: *Encyclopedia of computer science and technology*, 2000, Volume 42, Supplement 27, Marcel Dekker Inc, pp. 113-157.

[8] Kuo W.-J., Chang R.-F., Chen D.-R., Lee Ch. Ch. Data mining with decision trees for diagnosis of breast tumor in medical ultrasonic images. *Breast Cancer Research and Treatment*, 2001, No. 66, pp. 51-57.

[9] Data Mining Tools See5 and C5.0, see *http://www.rulequest.com/see5-info.html*.

[10] Hasegawa T., Yamamoto S., Matsuno Y. Quantitative immunohistochemical evaluation of MIB-1 labeling index in adult soft-tissue sarcomas by computer-assisted image analysis. *Pathology International*, 2002, vol. 52, pp. 433–437.

[11] Ohkura Y., Furihata T., Kawamata H., Tabuchi M., Kubota K., Terano A., Sakai T. and Fujimori T. Evaluation of cell proliferation and apoptosis in Helicobacter pylori gastritis using an image analysis processor, *Gastric Cancer*, 2003, vol. 6, pp. 49–54.

[12] Matlab products, see *http://www.mathworks.com/products/webserver/*.

[13] Jegelevicius D., Lukosevicius A., Paunksnis A., Barzdziukas V. Application of Data Mining Technique for Diagnosis of Posterior Uveal Melanoma. *Informatica*, Institute of Mathematics and Informatics, Vilnius, 2002, Vol. 13, No 4, pp. 455-464.

[14] Sebeliauskienė D., Paunksnis A. Echographic differentiation of malignant intraocular tumors. *Ultragarsas*. Kaunas, Technologija, 2001, Vol.41, No.4, pp. 25-28.

[15] Seregard S. Posterior uveal melanoma. *Acta Ophthalmol Scand*,. 1996, Vol.74, 315–339.

[16] Vainoras A. Functional Model of Human Organism Reaction to Load – Evaluation of Sportsman Training Effect. *Eduaction. Physical Training. Sport.*, 2002, Vol. 3 (44), Lithuanian Academy of Physical Education, Kaunas, Lithuania

# Accessibility of Public Web Sites – the InHand Case Study

Elena JITARU[1], Ioana MOISIL[2], Adriana ALEXANDRU[1]
[1] *I.C.I. – National Institute for R&D in Informatics, Bucharest, Romania*
[2] *ULBS – "Lucian Blaga" University of Sibiu, Romania*

**Abstract.** Access to information and communication systems for PwD (Persons with Disabilities) is a priority both for the EU and candidate countries. This paper presents some results of the Romanian project called "InHand – Information Center for Persons with Disabilities)". The main goal of the project is to contribute to improving the quality of life and health status of this group of people. Our emphasis is on the benefits of universal design. By eliminating barriers that prevent people with disabilities from using Web sites, it is possible to make each site more useful for all visitors, not to mention ease of maintenance and cost-effectiveness

## Introduction

As government services and important public information become increasingly available online, ensuring access to public websites for all citizens becomes as important as ensuring access to public buildings [1]. In the context of citizens with special needs (disabled and elderly people), the challenge consists of ensuring the widest possible accessibility to information technologies in general as well as their compatibility with assistive technologies.

**Public sector Web sites** and their content in Member States and in the European Institutions **must be designed to be accessible** to ensure that citizens with disabilities can access information and take full advantage of the potential for e-government [1].

There are 37 million Europeans, i.e. some 10% of the entire population of the European Union, who suffer from one form of disability or another, and they stand to benefit directly from improved Web accessibility. Yet, accessibility concerns not only the disabled: elderly persons and people with intellectual disabilities may experience great difficulties in reading and understanding certain websites. Consequently, enhanced legibility will help not only people with disabilities, but also an additional sector of the population, estimated to represent some 30 to 40% of the total [2].

## 1. Definitions

**Accessibility** means providing flexibility to accommodate each user's needs and preferences. In an Internet context, accessibility is making computer technology and Internet resources useful to more people than would otherwise be the case. Internet accessibility is normally aimed at enabling participation of people with disabilities. Internet accessibility can also include consideration for people whose communication infrastructures or capabilities are not advanced or not in place [3].

**Web accessibility** involves the ability of a Web page to be read and understood, using adaptive technologies where necessary. The blind and visually impaired are the most affected by advances in the graphical nature of websites. Website developers can make Web pages both accessible and visually appealing by following good and simple Hypertext Markup Language (HTML) programming practices.

## 2. An Information Society for All

In December 1999, the European Commission launched an initiative entitled "eEurope - An Information Society for All", which proposed ambitious targets to bring the benefits of the Information Society within reach of all Europeans. The initial plan focused on ten priority areas, from education to transport and from healthcare to people with disabilities. One of the action plan's specific targets is to improve access to the Web for people with disabilities. Such people, as well as the elderly, often face a wide range of technical barriers in terms of their capacity to access the Internet. The accessibility challenges faced by these and other users of the Internet can, to a large extent, be solved by means of appropriate coding when constructing Web sites and content, and the application of some simple rules regarding layout and structures when designing Web pages. These techniques are, however, not widely known or applied by website designers and Web content providers.

The eEurope Action Plan 2002 proposed the adoption of the guidelines developed by the Web Accessibility Initiative (WAI) [4] as an initial step towards making European public Web sites and their content accessible to people with disabilities. By adopting the Guidelines, the Member States and European institutions give the target of Web accessibility broad recognition and support, through the use of a global de facto Web accessibility standard, represented by the work of the Web Accessibility Initiative. The guidelines are also recognized as a de facto global standard for the design of accessible Web sites.

Whereas the earlier eEurope 2002 Action Plan focused on extending Internet connectivity across Europe, eEurope 2005 will concentrate on translating this into improved economic productivity and better, more accessible services for all European citizens, underpinned by a secure, widely available broadband infrastructure. From 2004 onwards the list of indicators will also serve as the basis for Candidate Countries.

## 3. Romanian Action Plan Promoting Accessibility

The Information Society is an essential component of the political and economic programmes of development and a major condition for integration of Romania in the Euro-Atlantic structures. The transition to the Information Society is one of the strategic objectives of the Romanian government and one of the EU pre-adhering conditions. This society is created to the benefit of the citizen and it must provide access to information and knowledge. A series of actions are proposed in the "National Strategy for the New Economy and the Implementation of the Information Society" [5] in order to enable broad access to Information Society-specific services:

- special measures to adopt the standards for accessibility of information technology products ("Design for all"), in particular to improve the employability and social inclusion of people with special needs,
- a review of relevant legislation and standards to ensure conformity with the principles of accessibility,
- adoption of the Web Accessibility Initiative (WAI) guidelines for public websites,
- ensuring the establishment and network connection of national "Design-for-all" centers of excellence.

The Romanian Ministry of Communications and Information Technology has already developed a draft entitled "Regulations concerning the design of public administration websites", soon to be passed into law.

## 4. InHand – Information Center for Persons with Disabilities

### *4.1 General Presentation*

From the legal point of view, a disabled individual is, in accordance with Romanian regulations, a person "who exhibits a handicap as a result of various physical, sensory, psychic or mental disabilities which deny or limit that person's participation, under equal terms, in social life in relation to age, sex, social, material and cultural factors, and who should be carefully and specifically targeted for social integration".

In dealing with this problem, the Romanian government has the support of a technically specialized body – the National Authority for Persons with Handicaps. This body is supervised by the Ministry of Labour, Social Solidarity and Family. An additional 200+ NGOs have also been created, either by disabled people themselves or by people who have assumed the responsibility for taking special care of the former. Regrettably, communication between NGOs, the parliament and the government, essential for this domain, is evolving slowly and remains very poor. This is more acute in the case of data availability for keeping persons with disabilities informed.

It is well known that nothing else but data exchange and shared experience may determine successful concerted actions. That is why the idea of a website making the domain information largely available to those directly interested in it, and to those who are in charge of the domain, was incarnated in the InHand project. We call it "InHand" in hoped that we will be able to handle this problem, even with low financial support. Our expectations are that in time we will have the necessary support to develop Web-based applications on behalf of almost all categories of disabled people.

The aims of the InHand project are:

- to offer to the persons with special needs access to a wide range of information and societal resources and a means by which they can enter into social contact,
- to develop new Web-based applications for people with disabilities and the elderly, to enable them to participate more fully in social and economic life, eventually leading to an improvement of the quality of their life,
- to eliminate barriers to employment for workers who are disabled,
- to disseminate the "Design for all" standards for accessibility of information technology products.

### *4.2 Materials and Methods*

The InHand databases that are accessible via the Internet have been designed to back up the information delivery to persons with disabilities who ask for assistance. The databases store data on persons with disabilities who ask for assistance as well as data on organizations having the intention and the possibility to provide assistance for disabled or elderly people. Given the access to the databases via the Internet, the two categories (data users and data suppliers) get easily in touch with one another.

The InHand application was developed using HTML, XML and ASP (Active Server Pages) technologies. The InHand database was developed using Microsoft SQL Server 2000.

In many cases we have to choose between executing the script code on the client's machine, by browser interpretation, or on the Web server, using ASP. We have frequently used server scripts with the ASP technology in the InHand application, so the source code of the script is executed on the server and the user sees only the resultant HTML code.

We have used several methods for accessibility in the InHand application:

1. The Web site is resolution-independent and the pages extract or contract to fit the screen.
2. Font sizes are not fixed thus making it easier for the users to customize the screen to their liking.
3. Wherever possible, we have used Cascading Style Sheets (CSS) for presentation. In this way we have eliminated some elements which overload HTML pages, such as tags for font-face, font-size, color etc. By separating content from style, the InHand pages become simplified and more accessible.
4. Whenever we could not use CSS, we used layout tables.
5. Other techniques for accessibility used in the InHand application:
   - Pages can be read on monochrome screens. We used color to enrich the look for users who do not have visual disorders, but colors never affect the information.
   - The link texts were underlined so that assisting equipment can easily recognize them.
   - The contrast between text and background colors was carefully chosen.
   - Every image comes associated with alternative clear text. If the image is purely decorative, the ALT tag is empty.

We have developed two databases that contain:

- data about persons with disabilities (PwD-Electronic Record) and
- data about organizations (potential assistance providers), projects related to disability, laws and regulations, jobs and services offered to PwDs.

To collect the data about Persons with Disabilities a form known as the Electronic Record is distributed. The objectives pursued are the following: active identification of cases in which assistance is most needed, monitoring of the categories of beneficiaries, drafting of regulations pursuant to collected data analysis, offering new types of assistance. The PwD Electronic Record contains the following types of information:

- general data about PwD,
- living conditions,
- data concerning health and care (physical aspects (Figure 1), nursing (Figure 2), sociability etc.)

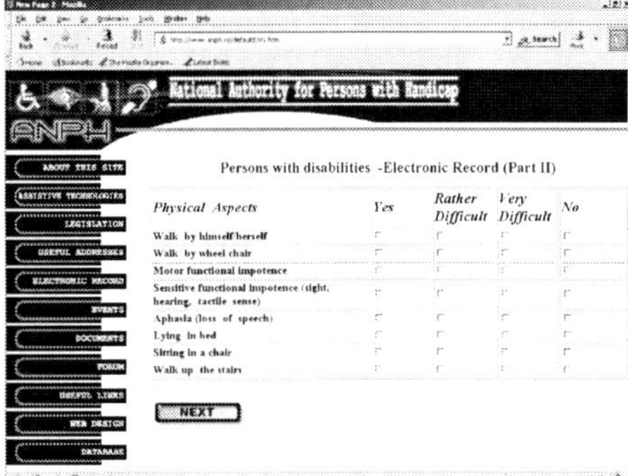


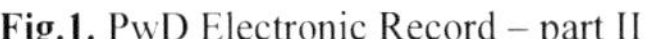
**Fig.1.** PwD Electronic Record – part II

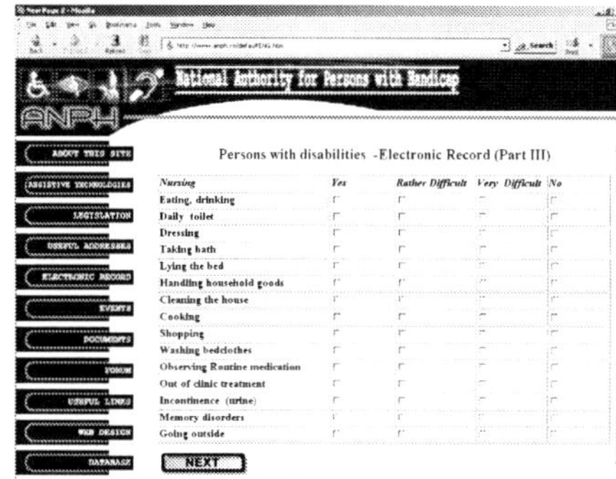


**Fig. 2.** PwD Electronic Record – part III

Records and information can be collected and incorporated continuously via the Internet, without extensive human resource requirements for re-entering information. Users have instant access to up-to-date information.

### 4.3 Results

A site presenting the InHand project has been launched, pursuant to the W3C Recommendation – Web Content Accessibility Guidelines. Focus is on the following aspects:

- to make our Web pages accessible to people with disabilities,
- to make the content comprehensible and navigable,
- to use clear and simple language,
- to provide navigation tools and orientation information in pages, maximizing accessibility and usability.

The information on the site is organized in the following main categories: about the site (destination; accessibility, site map, metainformation); assistive technologies (a guide to selection, principles and practice, resources); legislation; documents; electronic record; useful addresses (for vocational rehabilitation and integration, also including legal and medical advice); additional information (travel facilities for disabled persons, social security, hospitals and clinics offering recovery treatments); useful links; forums to exchange messages on any topics of interest (Figure 3).

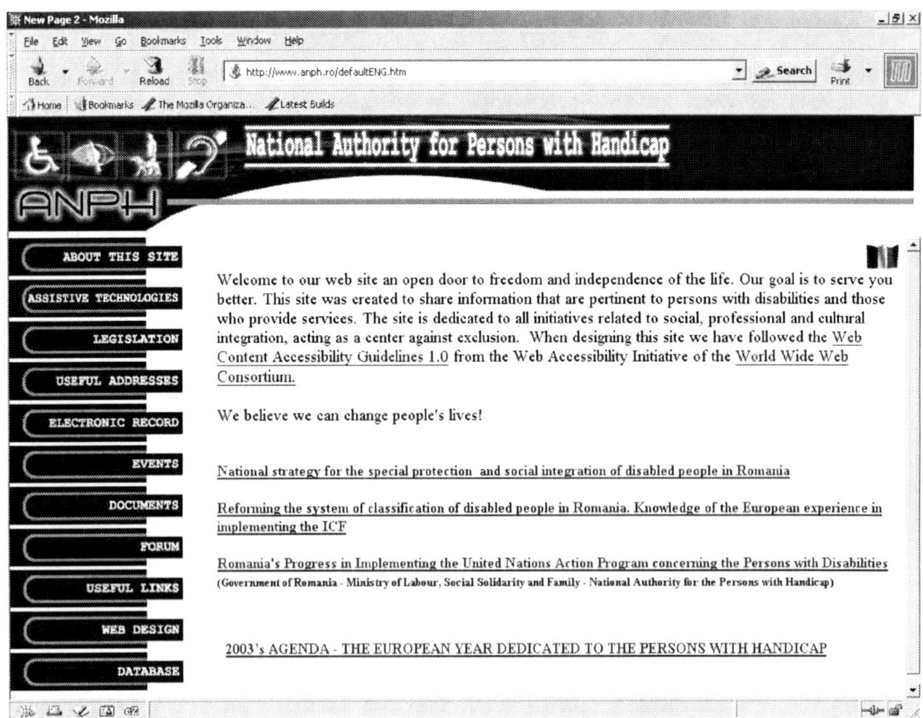


**Fig. 3.** InHand homepage

Great care was devoted to ensuring the accessibility of the site. If a site is not accessible, it will lose millions of visitors; not just those with disabilities, but also those who work with and otherwise support the accessibility community.

We analyzed the InHand Web site traffic using the WebTrends Log Analyzer, over a period of 14 months. The results show a linear increase in access to the InHand website.

### *4.4 Discussion*

We have tested the InHand site accessibility using some accessibility validation tools (Wave, Bobby) and with multiple browsers under a variety of conditions (Internet Explorer and Netscape under Windows and the Mozilla and Konqueror browsers under Unix). First end-user reports are positive.

We are also preparing a sound dissemination programme to make people aware of the existence of the site (mass-media, leaflets, other Web sites etc). We believe that the success of the application is directly determined by the access of the target population (here the PwDs) to the Internet.

### *4.5 Conclusions*

The InHand application is in accordance with the Web Accessibility Initiative (WAI) – Page Authoring Guidelines of the W3C (World Wide Web Consortium). The InHand project results meet the requirements of a largely-pristine area in Romania: keeping persons with disabilities informed. The InHand database is an attempt to bring together potential assistance beneficiaries and potential assistance providers.

## References

[1] eEurope 2002 – An Information Society For All, Action Plan prepared by the Council and the European Commission for the Feira European Council, 19-20 June 2000.

[2] The Economic and Social Committee of the EU has called for the Commission to issue a directive guaranteeing the accessibility of public web sites *http://www.disabilityeuropeancongress.org/english/news/new1.htm*

[3] Leo Valdes –Accessibility on the Internet – *http://www.un.org/esa/socdev/enable/index.html*

[4] W. Chisholm, G. Vanderheiden, I. Jacobs, Eds., Techniques for Web Content Accessibility Guidelines 1.0, *http://www.w3.org/TR/WAI-WEBCONTENT-TECHS/*

[5] National Strategy for the New Economy and the Implementation of the Information Society – MCTI *http://www.mcti.ro*

[6] Paciello, M.G., Paciello, M., Web Accessibility for People with Disabilities CMP books, New York, 2000.

[7] Stephanidis, C., Emiliani, P.L., "Connecting to the Information Society: a European perspective", Technology and Disability Journal, vol.10, pp.21-44, 1999.

[8] Jim Thatcher, Cynthia Waddell, "Constructing Accessible Web Sites", Glasshaus, 2003.

[9] Mueller, J., "Assistive Technology and Universal Design in the Workplace", Assistive Technology, vol.10, pp.37-43, 1998.

# Establishing an Internet-Based Paediatric Cancer Registration and Communication System for the Hungarian Paediatric Oncology Network

Gábor BORGULYA, Zsuzsanna JAKAB, Dezső SCHULER, Miklós GARAMI
*2nd Department of Paediatrics,*
*Semmelweis University of Budapest, Hungary*

**Abstract.** Cancer registration has developed in Europe over the last 50 years, and in the last decade intensive joint activities between the European Cancer Registries, in response to the need of pan-European harmonization of registration practices, have taken place. The Hungarian Paediatric Cancer Registry has been functioning as the database of the Hungarian Paediatric Oncology Network since 1971, aiming to follow the incidence and the treatment efficacy of malignant diseases.

The goals of this globally unique open source information system are the following: 1) to raise the quality of the registration system to the European level by developing an Internet-based registration and communication system, modernizing the database, establishing automatic statistical analyses and adding an Internet website, 2) to support clinical epidemiological studies that we conduct with international collaborators on detailed analyses of the characteristics of patients and their diseases, evaluation of new diagnostic and therapeutic methods, prevention programs, and long-term quality of life and side effects.

The benefits of the development of the Internet-based registration and communication system are as follows: a) introduction of an Internet-based case reporting system, b) modernization of the registry database according to international recommendations, c) automatic statistical summaries, encrypted mail systems, document repository, d) application of data security and privacy standards, e) establishment of a website and compilation of educational materials.

The overall objective of this scientific project is to contribute towards the improvement of cancer prevention and cancer care for the benefit of the public in general and of cancer patients in particular.

## 1. The Organizational Background

The Hungarian Paediatric Cancer Registry has been functioning as the database of the Hungarian Paediatric Oncology Network since 1971, aiming to follow the incidence and the treatment efficacy of malignant diseases. The Hungarian Paediatric Cancer Registry has a history of over 30 years of tradition and accumulated know-how. The registry has been audited by a review team of the International Agency for Research on Cancer. We practice population-based registration covering the whole country. High quality data on leukaemia incidence, and data on solid tumours have been gathered by the Hungarian Paediatric Oncology Network. We have close and productive contacts with clinicians, based on traditions and over 30 years of experience. A wide range of clinical information is accessible through the registry. Long-term follow-up has always been emphasized, therefore follow-up data are available from the earliest times. The registry operates with a fully motivated and qualified young staff. Recently, tender applications have been assembled for the funding of our projects, and moderate governmental support has been awarded for infrastructure improvements. The Ministry of Education and the Ministry of Information and Communication have announced our project as a leading initiative towards adopting the eEurope standard of the European Community.

We conduct clinical epidemiological studies with international collaborators (IARC – International Agency for Research on Cancer) through active data collection, detailed analysis of characteristics of patients and their diseases (SIOP – Société Internationale d'Oncologie Pédiatrique, BFM Berlin-Frankfurt-Münster Study Group), evaluation of new diagnostic and therapeutic methods, and their long-term follow-up. Therefore, we promote better understanding of tumorigenesis and improvements of treatment results.

We perform epidemiologic research to ensure the completeness of the data in the registry with active data collection and collaborating partners (National Cancer Registry, Hungarian Central Statistical Office, National Health Insurance). We analyze the incidence and possible causes (both retrospectively and prospectively), risk factors (spatially and temporally), and the efficacy of new therapeutic procedures. We actively follow up long-term survivors to assess their quality of life and long-term side effects.

## 2. The Difficulties of Paper-Based Cancer Registration

Since the early 1970's, the Hungarian Paediatric Oncology Network has been using a paper-based cancer registration system. Four kinds of registration forms were in use: an initial form for new leukaemia cases, an initial form for new solid tumour cases, a follow-up form for leukaemia cases and a follow-up form for solid tumour cases. All kinds of forms were filled in by physicians at treatment centres, towards the end of a year – usually using a typewriter or by hand. The forms were then sent to the registry by post, where they were verified and ordered into files. In 1982, computerized data storage commenced. As the computational power of personal computers grew and as better software for data analysis and visualisation appeared, the expectations towards the database increased as well. The coding system and the database structure have undergone three major overhauls and many smaller changes.

Filling in the forms with a typewriter and later typing the data into a computer is a waste of resources – at the same time there are no resources for recording detailed patient histories and disease courses.

The administrative burden on the reporting physicians was moderate in the earliest times: a relatively constant number of new patients were reported each year, together with the follow-up data of a few survivors. However, as the proportion of surviving patients increased due to the adoption of more successful treatments – more and more patients were followed up for longer and longer periods of time. Although the diversity of the collected follow-up data was reduced, by the end of the 1990's the quality of the follow-up data, one of the major strengths of the registry, was at risk. It became an everyday necessity for the registry staff to actively collect data.

Although the registry has always provided data for medical science and health research - often back to the reporting physicians themselves, they were still separated from the contents of the database by complicated access procedures.

The international studies aiming to improve cancer therapy, in which the Hungarian Paediatric Oncology Network participates, demand more and more detailed information on the progress of treatment, therapy toxicity and late effects. Genetic research also requires patients past their active therapy, i.e. it calls for long-term follow-up together with genetic information.

The explosion of data demand undermines the motivation of physicians to report, which leads to a deterioration of data quality. In turn, the registry staff has to make extreme efforts to fix missing and erroneous data. Although many physicians already have e-mail accounts, they cannot serve as a communication medium for verifying patient data, because the e-mails flow unencrypted on the Internet, making it impossible to send sensitive information.

The annual reporting scheme has the added disadvantage in that it is not possible for physicians to remember exactly the details of the treatment process of each patients treated since the previous report. Additionally, cases emerging during the last month of the year may still lack diagnostic information at the time of their submission to the registry. The former obstacle leads to the inconveniences in retrieving patient documentation, while the latter leads to missing data items which need to be actively resolved later on, by the registrar.

## 3. The Benefits of the Electronic System

The first goal of the system is to reintroduce reporting motivation to physicians. Bi-directional data flow has a key role: the data stored in the registry becomes instantly accessible to treatment centres, helping them in their everyday work, in research activities and in healthcare planning. Keeping the database up to date is in the interest of every physician in the network. A treatment centre can download all available data on its patients at any time.

Besides raw data on patients corresponding to the treatment centre, simple statistical summaries are available as well, which makes the system even more useful for treatment centres. Database queries converted into spreadsheets ready for importing into statistical software are also programmed.

The handling of missing and erroneous data becomes much simpler. Instead of a long process of posting forms, checking their contents and contacting the reporters for corrections, many checks are automatic and instantaneous, the errors can be corrected interactively. Entry time checking is possible for many logical relationships among data pieces, arising from the pathophysiology of tumours. The checking rules are based on the Child-Check rule set of the International Association for Research on Cancer extended with logistic relationships. Detection of missing values is possible at the time of data entry, and the reporter can be warned immediately.

A more sophisticated type of handling of missing and erroneous data is the scope of the warning system. The warning system is a simple rule-based expert system keeping track of the data flow during patient registration, diagnostics, treatment and follow-up. Some international studies, like the Acute Lymphoblastic Leukaemia Intercontinental-BFM 2002 protocol, involve complex data flow structures, including revised diagnostics and conditionally-repeated treatment elements. The warning system knows when and who to warn if data are inconsistent or missing. For instance, it warns the responsible physician if a long-term survivor has not shown up for a control examination or if the status or the results of an examination are not entered into the system. Other examples are laboratory tests returning results long after taking the specimen (post-deadline warnings), or non-routine examinations requested by a research study (pre-deadline, keep-in-mind warnings).

If the warning system cannot solve a particular data problem, it forwards that problem to the registrar or to national study coordinators. They can issue manual warnings that are later handled by the warning system, or they can use encrypted e-mail to communicate with the person responsible for the problematic data.

The use of hierarchical selection lists for data entry spares the registry developer a lot of work. The developer can concentrate on the ICD-O-3 coding, which requires more experience than a typical reporting physician possesses. Instantaneous conversion between disease morphology and localization coding systems also becomes possible.

These features of the system fill in the gaps at many network centres, where electronic heathcare scheduling is not internally supported.

As the data entry process is of a continuous nature, individually adjusted to the treatment process of the patient, there is no need to send half-filled forms due to pending laboratory tests – and there is no need to retrieve old patient files, because the warning system notifies the physician to enter data when it's still at hand. It is much easier to enter fresh data than months-old documentation.

## 4. Additional Features of the Electronic System for the Users

As the physicians will log in to the system almost daily, additional features, aiding them in everyday work, are also worth implementing.

### *4.1 Automatic Data Extraction for the Needs of International Studies*

The data format specified by the international data centres of international studies can be guaranteed by pre-programmed database queries and conversions. All that national study coordinators have to do is check the protocol-specific contents of the database, use secure e-mail for clarifications and use the protocol-wise data export function of the system.

### *4.2 Statistical Summaries*

Basic statistical summaries on the whole database are available to all the users of the system. As said before, the staff of a treatment centre can view and download detailed and aggregate data on their own patients. Nationwide data in aggregate form is available to anyone. The results of national statistics are regularly copied to the website for general publication.

### *4.3 Research-Related Database Queries*

With the electronic approval of the leaders of the network, requests for database queries can be sent to the server to gather data for research purposes. As these queries are subject to complex legal and ethical considerations, each transaction is logged with special verbosity.

### *4.4 Public Website Pursuant to the eHealth Code of Ethics*

In addition to the isolated virtual private computer network of the Hungarian Paediatric Oncology Network that hosts the cancer registration and warning systems, the project also provides a website for the general public. The intended audience comprises young patients and their parents, professionals, supporters, sponsors and casual visitors. It contains articles about the paediatric tumour types and their treatment results; the institutions and the scientific results of the network, the registry, statistical summaries and announcements – in a uniform structure and appearance.

The website adheres to the eHealth Code of Ethics of the Internet Health Coalition [1] and the Health On the Net Code of Conduct [2]. Although both of these rule sets are formulated in self-regulatory terminology, the website of the Hungarian Paediatric Oncology Network is audited by an independent enterprise.

The site can be visited at *http://www.gyermekonkologia.hu*. The site is under continuous development regarding both content and appearance.

### *4.5 Document Repository*

The members of the network can place all kinds of digital materials into the document repository and keep them ordered. These documents are accessible by all other members. Basic version management is available for documents in the repository and search is possible through metadata terms and inside document contents. The planned contents are international treatment protocol descriptions, ready-to-use presentations for the local media, useful documents and templates for everyday work, scientific results, application forms for events and multimedia presentations of instructive diagnostic results.

### *4.6 Encrypted e-mail System*

Physicians can send and receive encrypted e-mails using their USB encryption devices. The level of encoding will ensures the security of transmitted data for many years to come.

### *4.7 Mailing Lists*

Mailing lists are provided for physicians, leaders of the centres, stem cell transplantation board members, the staff involved in patient care throughout the network, research groups, physiotherapists and parents' associations. Some of these mailing lists work with encrypted traffic, which enables communicating sensitive patient data as well (e.g. minutes of stem cell transplantation board meetings).

### *4.8 Notice Board*

The notice board is integrated with the mailing lists, and periodically sends announcements to the users.

### *4.9 Address Book*

The address book stores the addresses, phone numbers etc. of physicians and leaders of the network, as well as collaborators. The address book is integrated with the mailing lists and a digest, containing filtered data, is periodically transferred to the contact section of the public website. Keeping the address book up-to-date is the duty of the warning system.

### *4.10 Internet Community*

The above features splice the physicians of the Hungarian Paediatric Oncology Network into an Internet community, using the modern communication modalities offered by the system on a daily basis.

The daily routine occasionally involves an urgent need to provide consistent explanations for patients, especially under the age of 18. Therefore, onsite access allows the doctor to provide these facilities for patients. Overall, the communication between the members of the paediatric oncology team is rapidly improving through the use of this new, advanced technology. Once the project completes, daily interactive communication will be established. Due to the above mentioned achievements we believe that our patients will receive better treatment and significantly improved rehabilitation opportunities.

## 5. Technical Features

### *5.1 Centralized Server-Client Structure*

The centralized server-client structure allows developments on the server side to become immediately available to all clients throughout the network.

### *5.2 Modern Database Structure*

The database of the National Paediatric Cancer Registry has been converted from its previous, obsolete structure to a flexible and extensible object-relational database structure. The format of the database reflects the pathophysiological characteristics of childhood cancers and the regulations and recommendations on handling personal data and metadata. If a new national or international scientific study emerges, the registry database can be easily extended to serve its needs.

### *5.3 Archiving*

Archiving of the registry database used to be manual and irregular. The new system secures valuable data regularly and almost automatically. If manual steps are necessary, the warning system issues warnings to the archiver. All manual steps are logged.

## 6. Information Technology Considerations

### *6.1 Software*

| | | |
|---|---|---|
| Application server | Debian Linux | Java-based Web application running in the JBoss framework. PostgreSQL object-relational database system. |
| Firewall server | Debian Linux | ZORP packet filtering |
| Public web-server | Debian Linux | ZOPE web application server |
| Clients | Windows XP Professional | Mozilla. Aladdin eToken driver |

### *6.2 Security*

The system is implemented to the highest security standards possible. User access to the database is secured by the following components:

- strict security settings on the Windows XP client (including windows security settings, firewall, anti-virus programs),
- client-side password authentication,
- the firewall refuses connections from unknown IP addresses,
- the server accepts known x.509 certificates,
- the certificates are stored on the users' Aladdin eToken USB keys, password-protected,
- database access is restricted both at the application and the database level,
- administrative access is restricted for both the server and client computers,
- the servers are physically secured.

## 7. Summary of Project Benefits

The Internet Based Paediatric Cancer Registration and Communication System for the Hungarian Paediatric Oncology Network is globally unique in the sense, that in the absence of uniform treatment principles and a nationwide computer system, Hungary is the first country in the region developing such a nationwide system.

The development is primarily based on open source software, and the source code of our product will be available too. Multilingualism is supported throughout the application and other aspects of internationalization were also kept in mind during planning, to ease the development of a future international version. We believe that open source code carries the promise of delivering an extensively tested, bug-free system.

Launching the new system will lead to instantaneous improvement of data quality in many data groups. The administrative burden of cancer reporting will diminish for the physicians in the network, and the number of errors and missing values to be corrected by the registry staff will radically decrease, too. The motivation to maintain the cancer registry at a high quality will grow on both sides.

Internet communication strengthens the community working for paediatric cancer patients by "shortening the distance" between distant parts of the country. This enables us to perform detailed spatial and temporal analyses of the diseases and their causes, based on a globally-unique open source information system. The modernization of the registry will improve both professional and economic conditions of medical care and the planning of prevention programs, through up-to-date information. The overall objective of this scientific project is to contribute to improvement of cancer prevention and cancer care for the benefit of the general public and of cancer patients in particular.

## References


[1] The eHealth Code of Ethics. *www.ehcca.com/presentations/HIPAA/mack-mon1.pdf*

[2] Health on the Net Code of Conduct *http://www.hon.ch/HONcode/Conduct.html*

[3] Hauser P., Jakab Zs., Láng O., Kondás O., Török Sz., Garami M., Bognár L. and Schuler D.: High Incidence of Brain Tumors of Childhood in Hungary Between 1989 and 2001. Medical and Pediatric Oncology, 41(6): 590-591, 2003.

[4] Pinter AB, Hock A, Kajtár P, Dober I. Long-term follow-up of cancer in neonates and infants: a national survey of 142 patients. Pediatr Surg Int 2003;19:233-239.

[5] Jakab Z, Balogh E, Kiss C, Olah E: Epidemiologic studies in a population based childhood cancer registry in North-East Hungary. Med Pediatr Oncol, 2002, 38, 338-344.

[6] Schuler D.: A gyermekonkológiai rehabilitáció helyzete. Rehabilitáció, 12(2): 8-9, 2002.

[7] Schuler D.: A gyermekonkológia helyzete hazánkban. Hippocrates, 4: 387-389, 2002.

[8] Török Sz., Borgulya G., Jakab Zs., Schuler D., Fekete Gy.: A gyermekkori leukaemiás megbetegedések epidemiológiájának vizsgálata hazánkban 1980 és 2000 közötti 21 évre vonatkozóan. Orvosi Hetilap, 143(48): 2675-2679, 2002.

[9] Török Sz., Borgulya G., Schuler D., A gyermekkori rosszindulatú daganatok gyakoriságának és túlélési mutatóinak változásai 1988 és 1997 között az Országos Gyermektumor Regiszter adatai alapján. Orvosi Hetilap, 142(23): 1211-1215, 2001.

[10] Babosa M., Garami M., Hauser P., Schuler D. és Szendrõi M.: A Ewing-sarcomás betegek tünetmentes túlélési esélyeinek értékelése a Gyermekonkológiai Szekció eredményei alapján. Magyar Onkológia, 44(4): 261-264, 2000.

[11] Balogh E, Kiss C, Jakab Z, Oláh É: Citogenetikai vizsgálatok jelentõsége gyermekkori myelodysplasiás syndromában. Gyermekgyógy, 2000, 51, 130-136.

[12] Kajtár P. A gyermekkori rákbetegségek ellátása Magyarországon. Gyógyszerészet 1999; 43:555-556

[13] Magyar Gyermekonkológiai Munkacsoport: A magyar Gyermekonkológiai Hálózat négy éve (1994-1997) Gyermekgyógyászat 2: 163-170, 1999

[14] Magyarosy Edina, Magyar Gyermekonkológiai Munkacsoport Az ALL-BFM 95 protokoll alkalmazása során a gyermekkori acut lymphoid leukemia kezelésében nyert tapasztalataink. Gyermekgyógyászat 50(5): 455-458, 1999

# Telemedical Database of Hodgkin's Disease

Piotr WALECKI[1], Krzysztof SARAPATA[1], Wojciech LASOŃ[1], Wiesław PYRCZAK[1], Irena ROTERMAN-KONIECZNA[1], Walentyna BALWIERZ[2]
[1]*Department of Bioinformatics and Telemedicine,*
*Medical College, Jagiellonian University,*
*ul. Kopernika 17, 31-501 Kraków, Poland*
[2]*Department of Oncology and Pediatric Hematology,*
*Polish-American Institute of Pediatrics,*
*Medical College, Jagiellonian University,*
*ul. Wielicka 265, 30-663 Kraków, Poland*

**Abstract.** The creation of a complex telemedical system oriented towards childhood Hodgkin's disease has been undertaken at the Department of Bioinformatics and Telemedicine of the Jagiellonian University Medical College in cooperation with the Department of Oncology and Pediatric Hematology of the Polish-American Institute of Pediatrics, JU MC. Data collecting, data processing and data transmission is aimed to aid and/or supervise surgical and drug treatment.

The Tele-Database of Childhood Hodgkin's Disease (TDCHD) is not a simple Internet database project. A few hundred data items are presented in each patient's record, covering the complete medical treatment period. Efficient management and proper data protection are necessary for a medical database. Therefore, the interface for entering data has been divided into several parts. Each part is subjected to separate editing and transfer. A double-layer debugging system has been applied in the program: the first pass occurs on the client side (programmed in JavaScript and XML), the second - on the server side (programmed in PHP). Strict authorization is requested for all participants. Clinical data collected according to management standards and information governance (data quality, security and confidentiality) is organized in a way that facilitates practical and scientific use.

## Introduction

Hodgkin's disease (HD) or Hodgkin's lymphoma is a type of a cancer of the lymphatic system. There are two main types of lymphoma: Hodgkin's lymphoma and Non-Hodgkin's lymphoma (NHL). Most lymphomas are of type NHL. Only about 1 in 5 lymphomas diagnosed belongs to the Hodgkin's category. The exact cause of this disease is not known: researchers have not yet discovered a risk factor with major influence, however there are several minor risk factors for Hodgkin's disease. Hodgkin's lymphoma is more common in people: a) with faulty or suppressed immunity, b) in particular age groups, c) who have been infected with the Epstein Barr virus and d) who have an identical twin diagnosed with Hodgkin's lymphoma, so a faulty gene may be at work. In fact, most people who develop Hodgkin's lymphoma do not share any obvious risk factors. Therefore, we require much more detailed information on a patient than in the case of other diseases. In our project, a few hundred data items in each patient's record cover the complete medical treatment period. Efficient management of such a variety of medical data requires a special database system.

The integration and coordination of healthcare in a country-wide or region-wide system contributes to optimization of therapeutic efforts. Internet makes database systems more uniform and readily available for online access. The improvement of medical services contributes to detailed monitoring of therapeutic treatment. Immediate access to a necessary specialist is possible for any patient with access to the system. Many major medical institutions develop their own Web-based database systems, but creating a well-designed complex computer system from scratch is very complicated. Some of the more technologically advanced medical institutions use stand-alone information storage systems, however such systems cannot communicate with each other. Yet, no problem precludes providing a standardized request for computer database searches or a standardized patient record. The actual difficulty is in the high operating costs, which force many institutions to limit the scope of accuracy of the medical data in their databases. There are, of course, fully developed databases implemented by various research projects; however databases for medical practices are currently limited to basic information on patients.

In this paper, was present a database project related to Hodgkin's disease (HD) in children. Our computer system is called the Tele-Database of Childhood Hodgkin's Disease (TDCHD). A Web-based database system should enable coordination between every healthcare institution in Poland treating lymphoma in children. A telemedical system was constructed at the Department of Bioinformatics and Telemedicine of the Jagiellonian University Medical College. Every medical procedure and method was consulted at the Department of Oncology and Pediatric Hematology of the Polish-American Institute of Pediatrics in Krakow. A standardized format will be essential for this mass integration of data. Demands involving physicians and medical researchers have been precisely described and the whole project arises from the area of cancer treatment.

## 1. Background

Our purpose was to design and create a convenient, reliable and comprehensive database, which could promote confidentiality and security of patient records, requests for data abstraction and other research requirements. An adequate diagnosis and a statistical interpretation of results depend on the quantity and quality of medical data. Large volumes of such data and more detailed descriptions require analysis by advanced computer systems, now available to the medical science community. Childhood Hodgkin's lymphoma (HD) is a fairly rare type of cancer, with less than 100 new cases in Poland every year. Therefore, we have proposed a horizontal structure – a small quantity of patients' records and a large quantity of data for one record. The chance of recovery and choice of treatment depend on detailed information about the type of symptoms and overall condition of the child. Also, a precise description of treatment history is very important for future prognoses.

A few hundred data items for one child call for a complex acquisition system. The TDCHD has a modular structure because data is captured in different time scales. The interface for entering data has been divided into several parts (see Fig. 1). When childhood HD is diagnosed, more tests can be performed. The stage of the disease is important for the treatment plan - this may be determined by physical examination, blood tests and different kinds of x-rays. Tests results can help find out whether the cancer has spread from where it had started to other parts of the body. Clinical staging and pathologic staging are useful during treatment and surgery. There are four stages of HD and each stage is further divided into categories A and B, based on whether the child has symptoms. Accurate descriptions aid surgical and drug treatment, however they are possible if only an appropriate database system exist. In TDCHD, we have applied Ann Arbor Staging and Cotwolds Staging.

## 2. System Architecture and Methods

### 2.1 Hardware

We decided upon the popular low-cost x86 PC architecture with at least 4 MB of RAM for TDCHD tests. However, the test architecture may prove insufficient for real work, therefore we have also prepared another server system, which uses AMD Opteron or Athlon 64FX 64-bit processors. That hardware platform is supported by the FreeBSD operating system (OS). The server was connected with a LAN and - via a router - with the Internet.

### 2.2 Software

#### 2.2.1 MySQL Relational Database Management System

We have used MySQL database server version 4.0.16 and Apache web server version 3.0 over the FreeBSD version 5.1 environment. MySQL is a non-proprietary cross-platform database management system. It consists of several software modules, including the MySQL server (**mysqld**), which manages the database, and the MySQL client (**mysql**) that provides the interface to the server, as well as various utilities.

The following tables were created in the TDCHD: a) user table (user passwords and privileges), b) patients' personal details table, and c) medical data tables. A combination of medical data tables covers all types of data items in the system. The medical-related tables will be used to store information such as the patient's medical history, medication, treatments, etc. This database organization enables extensible records, with the option of adding another table. Only the owner can perform operations with the objects in that database, and in order to allow other users to use it, privileges must be granted.

From the security perspective, the TDCHD and the Web server have been located on the same machine. This greatly eliminates any connectivity problems that might occur due to invalid configuration if they were placed on separate servers.

Configuration of the MySQL Server:

- server must be run from a different user account than **/root**,
- automatic backup of the databases,
- restricting access by making it impossible to connect from outside (*skip networking* option in file **my.conf**),
- creating users and passwords to application with limited access rights. Passwords are maintained in a separate file (**.php**) used to connect to the MySQL database. Passwords are written and supplied to the MySQL database in an encrypted fashion by use of `password()` or `MD5()` functions,
- making it impossible for users to edit the database on read-only access. Certain access rights are only given to **/root**,
- monitoring and logging events about the server in addition to client access events. MySQL logs client data such as client IP addresses, connection times and user keys.

#### 2.2.2 PHP Configuration

We have used PHP version 5 with SimpleXML and the XSLT extension, in conjunction with the MySQL database management system and the Apache Web server to generate dynamic Web forms. PHP was installed as an Apache module. When PHP is used as an Apache module it inherits Apache's user permissions (typically those of the "nobody" user). Escalating the Apache user's permissions to **/root** is extremely dangerous and may compromise the entire system, so using sudo, chroot, or otherwise running as root should not be considered by those who are not security professionals. PHP is subjected to security built into most server operating systems with respect to file and directory permissions. This allows the user to control which files in the filesystem may be read. Care should be taken with any public files to ensure that they are safe for reading by all users who have access to that filesystem. Apache can also configure parsing different file types through PHP, either with the **.htaccess** directive, or in the Apache configuration file itself. It is therefore important to avoid and detect misleading file extensions.

Using Register Globals. One feature of PHP that can be used to enhance security is configuring PHP with *register_globals=off*. By turning off the ability for any user-submitted variable to be injected into the PHP code, it is possible to reduce the amount of variable poisoning a potential attacker may inflict. They would then have to take the additional time to forge submissions and the internal variables are effectively isolated from user-submitted data.

User-submitted data: the greatest weakness in many PHP programs is not inherent in the language itself, but merely an issue of code not being written with security in mind. For this reason, users should always take the time to consider the implications of a given piece of code, to ascertain the possible damage if an unexpected variable is submitted to it.

Hiding PHP: in general, security by obscurity is one of the weakest forms of security. However, in some cases, every little bit of extra security is desirable. A few simple techniques can help hide PHP, possibly slowing down an attacker who is attempting to discover weaknesses in the system. By setting *expose_php=off* in the **php.ini** file, it is possible to reduce the amount of information available to them.

Staying up-to-date: PHP, like any other large system, is under constant scrutiny and improvement. Each new version will often include both major and minor changes to enhance and repair security flaws, configuration mishaps, and other issues that will affect the overall security and stability of the system. Like other system-level scripting languages and programs, the best approach is to update often, and maintain awareness of the latest versions and their changes.

### 2.3 Interface

A standardized digital form of storing patients' medical information system has been applied in the TDCHD. The form for entering data has been divided into several parts (see Fig. 1). We required a scalable and extensible cooperative information system, therefore programming has been performed in JavaScript and XML to take advantage of its portability onto different hardware & software platforms. Messaging protocols utilize the XML markup language. An XSLT processor can read an XML file along with an XSLT file and output a third file – HTML, which is readable by many browsers.

The software used has a significant potential for reducing both development and debugging time for new data. Every new data piece is syntactically and semantically verified. Syntactic verification uses regular expressions. This method allows one to compare data patterns, based on templates comprised of various field lengths and data types. Semantic verification is complicated from the programming perspective, because of the multitude of variables and causes to consider; hence it is often skipped. Authorization bases on the user's name and password. Any attempts ay breaking into the system will attract the attention of the administrator. We are using dedicated files to connect PHP with MySQL, so passwords and user names should be stored in secure locations on the server, always with the use of the `include()` function. All **.php** files should be analyzed and interpreted by a PHP interpreter, to avoid their contents being displayed in the Web browser, as **.php** files are script files containing source code, which should be kept secret.

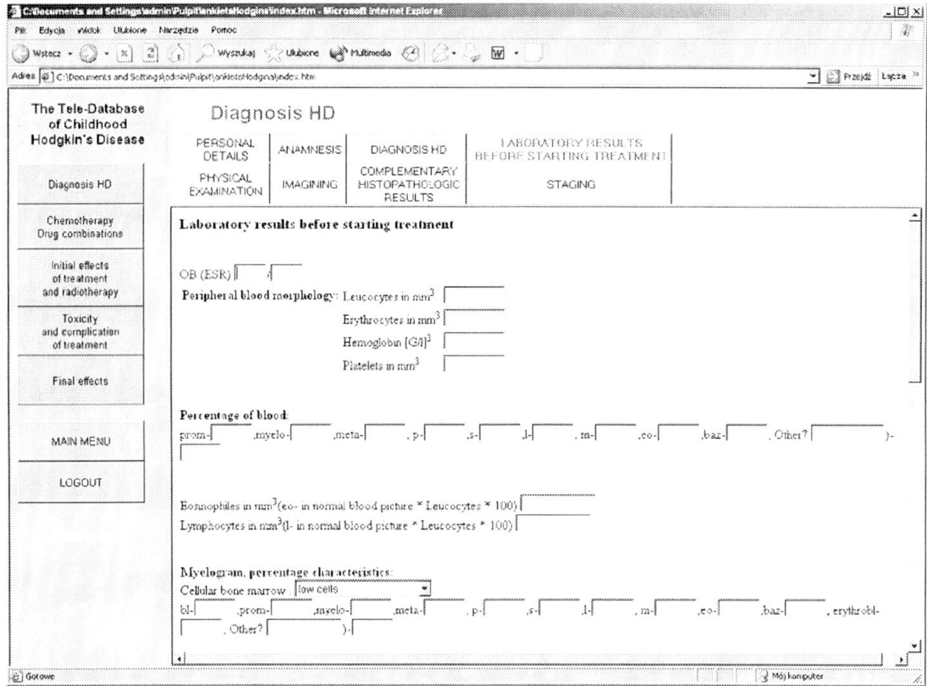


**Fig. 1.** Web interface between users and the database

## 2.4 *Security*

Multilevel security is needed for access control of various medical database applications. Every time the Web is involved, security must be considered. One of the inherent dangers involves unintentional programming bugs and user mistakes. Hackers can also attempt to break in via various methods and means by sniffing, hijacking of the system remotely, unauthorized access, modifying data, spoofing of any secure connection and social engineering. A highly sophisticated security-protection mechanism needs to be implemented in the system. Protection of the system can prevent data tampering by hackers and ensure data integrity.

To solve this problem, we need to realize the shortfalls of the system and counteract them. First, we need to secure the hardware (server) in a secure physical location. Second, we need to protect it from the outside through the use of hardware or software firewalls. One has to choose between host (multi service) and collocation or server and operator modes. At a minimum, the firewall has to be able to encrypt data using SSL (Secure Socket Layer), be able to authorize access for secure PHP application development and usage based on user names and passwords. It is also important to secure the database (MySQL) and the operating system itself.

All of the above mentioned criteria should be tested and retested to find any loopholes that can prove to be weak spots in the design and implementation of the project. When testing, we must understand, that there are endless possibilities for even the simplest of inputs. The input that we may receive may be totally wrong or intentionally malformed by someone who proves to be a disgruntled employee or a hacker with plenty of time on his hands. This is why it is best to look at the programming code from a logical perspective. This will aid in finding unexpected variables and data to help maintain its integrity. Once such findings occur, then they can be traced as to how data is modified, reduced, amplified or simply compromised.

### *2.4.1 Firewall*

A firewall is an essential security element in the TDCHD. It protects the system from the dangers of using the Internet. We have used an IP-Firewall "native" to the FreeBSD operating system. FreeBSD comes with a kernel packet filter, known as IPFW. Firewall configuration should take into consideration many aspects. One example could be to limit the IP address ranges to those originating in Poland. Of course, this assumes that only Polish users will have access to this system.

### *2.4.2 Encrypted Storage*

We have used Apache with OpenSSL. SSL/SSH protects data transfers from the client to the server. SSL is an on-the-wire protocol. In our system, **ssh** encrypts network connections between clients and the database server.

Configuration:

- organization of directories and files for the DocumentRoot hierarchy and creation of symbolic aliases (links),
- not exposing directories and files to clients,
- being able to start the server from user level "nobody",
- in case of lost connection and/or inactivity, having a timeout parameter,
- forced connection through port 443 (**https**) (in **httpd.conf** file *REDIRECTION*),
- limiting IP address ranges acceptable by the server to static IP addresses (not DHCP),
- SSL configuration using digital certificates from companies like Verisign to eliminate identity theft by false machines (spoofing).

## 3. Conclusion

The successful pilot application of the TDCHD contributes to propagation of telemedicine in clinical practice. Such global Web projects will help many people, patients and doctors alike, make better use of the information available to them. Attaining these goals will facilitate and improve advanced healthcare both for diagnosis and treatment. The TDCHD transforms the paper-based medical system into a Web-based real-time database system. Our system acts as a database-centered information of childhood Hodgkin's disease sharing services for doctors, medical researchers and medical institutions. We hope that healthcare institutions will adopt this system for their needs and our project will prove to be a useful tool in the field of medicine.

## References

[1] Bertino E., Fan J., Ferrari E., Hacid M.S., Elmagarmid A.K., Zhu X., A hierarchical access control model for video database system, *ACM Trans. on Info. Syst.*, vol.20, 2002

[2] Dolin R., Expressiveness and query complexity in an electronic health record data model. *Proc AMIA Annu Fall Symp*, 1996, 522-526

[3] Dolin R.H., Alschuler L., Behlen F., et al., HL7 document patient record architecture: an XML document architecture based on a shared information model. *Proc AMIA Symp*, 1999, 52-56

[4] Fayyad U., Uthurusamy R., Data mining and knowledge discovery in database, *Communication of ACM*, 39, 1996

[5] Lane D., Williams H.E., *Web Database Applications with PHP & MySQL*, O'Reilly & Associates 2002

[6] McDonald C.J., Overhage J.M., Tierney W.M., et al., The Regenstrief Medical Record System: a quarter century experience. *Int J Med Inf*, 1999, 54, 225-253

[7] Sarapata K., Walecki P., Pyrczak W., Lasoń W., Roterman I., Szybiński Z., Medical database of thyroid cancer, *E-he@lth in Common Europe*, IEEE Krakow 2003, 226-230

[8] Welling L., Thompson L., *PHP and MySQL Web Development*, SAMS 2003

[9] Zanstra P.E., Rector A.L., Ceusters W., de Vries Robbe P.F., Coding systems and classifications in healthcare: the link to the record. *Int J Med Inf*, 1998, 48, 103-9

[10] *http://www.cancer.gov/cancerinfo/types/hodgkinslymphoma/*

[11] *http://www.cancerhelp.org.uk/*

[12] *http://www.lymphomainfo.net/childhood/hodgkins.html*

[13] *http://www.meb.uni-bonn.de/cancernet/103043.html*

[14] *http://www.modssl.org/*

[15] *http://www.php.net/*

[16] *http://www.w3.org/*

# 2. Telemedicine Implementations

# New Developments in Digital Pathology: from Telepathology to Virtual Pathology Laboratory

Klaus KAYSER[1], Gian KAYSER[2], Dominik RADZISZOWSKI[3], Alexander OEHMANN [1]
[1] *UICC-TPCC, Institute of Pathology, Charite, Berlin, Germany*
[2] *Institute of Pathology, University of Freiburg, Freiburg, Germany*
[3] *AGH University of Science and Technology, Kraków, Poland*
*e-mail: klaus.kayser@charite.de*

**Abstract.** *Aims:* To analyse the present status and future development of computerized diagnostic pathology in terms of work-flow integrative telepathology and virtual laboratory.

*Present status:* Telepathology has left its childhood. The technical development of telepathology is mature, in contrast to that of virtual pathology. Two kinds of virtual pathology laboratories are emerging: a) those with distributed pathologists and distributed (>=1) laboratories associated to individual biopsy stations/surgical theatres, and b) distributed pathologists working in a centralized laboratory. Both are under technical development. Telepathology can be used for e-learning and e-training in pathology, as exemplarily demonstrated on *Digital Lung Pathology Pathology* (*www.pathology-online.org*).

*Features of virtual pathology*: A virtual pathology institution (mode a) accepts a complete case with the patient's history, clinical findings, and (pre-selected) images for first diagnosis. The diagnostic responsibility is that of a conventional institution. The internet serves as platform for information transfer, and an open server such as the iPATH (*http://telepath.patho.unibas.ch*) for coordination and performance of the diagnostic procedure. The size of images has to be limited, and usual different magnifications have to be used. A group of pathologists is "on duty", or selects one member for a predefined duty period. The diagnostic statement of the pathologist(s) on duty is retransmitted to the sender with full responsibility. First experiences of a virtual pathology institution group working with the iPATH server (Dr. L. Banach, Dr. G. Haroske, Dr. I. Hurwitz, Dr. K. Kayser, Dr. K.D. Kunze, Dr. M. Oberholzer,) working with a small hospital of the Salomon islands are promising. A centralized virtual pathology institution (mode b) depends upon the digitalisation of a complete slide, and the transfer of large sized images to different pathologists working in one institution. The technical performance of complete slide digitalisation is still under development and does not completely fulfil the requirements of a conventional pathology institution at present.

*Virtual pathology and e-learning:* At present, e-learning systems are "stand-alone" solutions distributed on CD or via internet. A characteristic example is the Digital Lung Pathology CD (*www.pathology-online.org*), which includes about 60 different rare and common lung diseases and internet access to scientific library systems (PubMed), distant measurement servers (EuroQuant), or electronic journals (Elec J Pathol Histol). A new and complete data base based upon this CD will combine e-learning and e-teaching with the actual workflow in a virtual pathology institution (mode a). The technological problems are solved and do not depend upon technical constraints such as slide scanning systems

*Perspectives:* Telepathology serves as promotor for a new landscape in diagnostic pathology, the so-called virtual pathology institution. Industrial and scientific efforts will probably allow an implementation of this technique within the next two years.

## Introduction

At the beginning, telepathology has been defined as "the work of a pathologist at a distance" [1,2]. In accordance with this definition at least two main applications can be distinguished: a) its use for primary diagnosis, and b) its use for secondary diagnosis [3-6]. The scope of primary diagnosis in telepathology is mainly covered by its application in frozen section services, and consecutively called on-line telepathology [1]. Specific remote control microscopes with fixed partners have been developed, working either on an individual or an open platform, i.e., the internet [7]. Whereas nearly all applications of on-line telepathology in frozen section services are related to a bilateral application (client – server configuration), the implementation of open standards to these systems offers, at least theoretically, the involvement of several pathologists located at different institutions in primary diagnosis services.

Similar to the history of on-line telepathology, the use of telepathology for secondary diagnosis started with point to point solutions [1]. However, already in the first trials of telepathology for second opinion services the necessity of an open platform has been realized [8-10]. The development of the world wide web as a common telecommunication standard, therefore, promoted the application of off-line telepathology to a large extent, and the internet served immediately for transfer of the client's request and the expert's answer [11]. Frequently, several experts are involved in reviewing a difficult case instead of consulting only one outstanding colleague [12]. Thus, again, the scenario of telepathology, as given by the above stated definition, has changed. Therefore, at present telepathology should be defined as an electronic, image related information transfer and classification in diagnostic pathology between 2…n partners, either on-line or off-line [13].

This extended definition includes, in addition, the possibility, that several clients (or information sources) might be involved in the process of diagnosis findings. The latter can be seen in image segmentation and measurement procedures, retrievals for logic evaluation of potential diagnosis, or adding clinical information from different data bases [14].

The use of the internet for consultation and primary diagnosis services has lead to the construction of specific servers, which replace the simple "letter-oriented" information transfer of e-mails with attached forms and still images. At present, three different server types have been installed, namely a) that of the Armed Forces Institute of Pathology (AFIP) *{http://www.afip.gov}*, b) that of the Institute of Pathology, University Basel (iPATH) *{http://www.telepath.patho.unibas.ch}*, and c) that of the Union contre le Cancre at the Institute of Pathology at the Charite, Berlin (UICC-TPCC) *{http://pathoweb.charite.de/UICC-TPCC/default.asp}*. The principal differences of these server in terms of structure and potential application have been discussed in detail elsewhere, and can be summarized as follows: The AFIP server possesses the highest diagnostic responsibility and most strict organization, that of the UICC-TPCC is equivalent to an intermediate realization of the mentioned teleconsultation services, and the iPATH is the most flexible system with the lowest diagnostic responsibility [15-21].

Based upon the recent development of telepathology systems, in this article we will describe the potential implementation of these systems into the daily workflow of a diagnostic pathology institution. The technical progress in digitising complete glass slides and implementation of artificial intelligence (AI) into these systems serve as additional parameters in judging and estimating the future "way of telepathology", which will probably lead to a new environment in pathology, the world of so-called digital pathology.

## 1. The Virtual Pathology Institution (VPI)

The outstanding majority of in telepathology trials results in diagnostic quality which is equal to or only to an insignificant lower level inferior to the conventional performance in frozen section service or in expert consultation [1,2]. For example, the only randomised frozen section service study on breast cancer describes nearly identical results of both the on-line telepathology or the conventional frozen section service [22-24]. Thus, telepathology is mature to be introduced into a pathology laboratory, which can be performed in two different ways: a) on distributed pathologists associated to different individual biopsy stations or surgical theatres, and b) on distributed pathologists working in only one pathology institution. The first scenario can be practically used for institutions working in developing countries or for surgical theatres without associated pathologists. It results in the assessment of a group of pathologists who diagnose only on an electronic display, and otherwise follow the conventional conditions of a pathology institution. These include the set up of a "duty plan", i.e., time schedules of the involved pathologists' availability to diagnose submitted cases, their individual responsibility, and an intra-institutional case discussion. The technical prerequisites for such a system are internet connections of each participating pathologists, and a system which handles the administration and management of the submitted cases and the diagnoses. This system has to be open and flexible. It has to administer the submitted cases, the availability of the pathologists, the information of the client, and an adequate documentation system. To our knowledge only one virtual pathology institution is working at present. It includes several well-known pioneers of telepathology (Dr. L. Bannach, Dr. G. Haroske, Dr. K. Kayser, Dr. K.D. Kunze, Dr. M. Oberholzer, and others) and uses the iPATH for administrative purposes. The cases are submitted from a small surgical institution which is not equipped with a local pathologist, namely, from the Honaria Hospital of the Salomon Island. More than one hundred cases have been analysed until now without major difficulties.

The second scenario, which focuses on different pathologists who are working in the same "umbrella institution" has not been implemented solely at a virtual basis to our knowledge. In contrast to the distributed VPI the local VPI might still be based upon conventional glass slides, from which selected still images at moderate and higher magnification are acquired and transferred to a combined image – case documentation system. Most of these systems are only extensions of the common pathology documentation systems, and have no or only minor principal advantages when compared to conventional pathology documentation systems. They might, however, additionally be associated with distinct measurement or diagnosis support systems, such as quantitative immunohistochemistry or neural networks. These extensions are of real clinical value. They need, however, an adequate artificial intelligence system (AI) to improve pathology diagnosis performance [26,27].

The final VPI as defined in the second scenario is based upon complete digitised glass slides (virtual slides). In principle, virtual slides posses several significant advantages in comparison to "normal" glass slides: Theoretically, these include easy documentation, storage, and retrieval, contemporary diagnosis of several pathologists, contemporary quality assurance and evaluation, fast performance of additional staining, or construction of large distributed VPIs. The general technological constraint is based upon the necessity to digitise a complete glass slide into a virtual slide. These virtual slides amount to several Giga Bytes in size, and are, thus, not easy and fast to handle at present. The parameters of the virtual slide technology, which is commercially available today, is listed in table 1.

**Table 1.** Features of commercially available slide scanners (based upon 3DHistech) and those needed for practical online use

| ***General features** (implemented)* | |
|---|---|
| input format | standard microscopic slides |
| scanning region | 20 * 50 mm |
| tissue finding | automatic |
| focus | automatic |

| ***Parameters*** | *available* | *needed* |
|---|---|---|
| scanning time/slide | appr. 5 min | < 10s |
| slide load/night | appr. 300 slides | >1000 slides |
| image size | appr. 3 – 4 GB | > 4 TB |
| network interface | < 1Gb/s | > 10 Gb/s |

As shown in table 1, the "practical necessity" is still a great distance away from the commercially available technology at present. A digitalisation of approximately 300 slides over night, and the use of digitised slides for implementation of a virtual slide data bank (image data bank) seem to be the only practical application until now.

In principle, a pixel resolution of 0.5 µm/pixel is required if a region of a complete glass slide should be scanned, and if all magnifications afterwards should be performed digitally. The best display available possesses 9 million pixels presented at a density of 200 pixels/inch. (IBM, flat screen T221). By a simple mathematical computation we can, therefore, display 0.1 mm to 1 inch on this screen, or, in other words, an area of 2 mm * 2 mm on the whole screen. This is the size of a normal biopsy. In addition, the areas of tissue arrays or fine needle punctions measure about 0.5 – 1 mm in diameter, and can, thus, scanned, computerized, and visualized as a whole. One need an array of approximately 16,000 pixels in order to display a complete biopsy on this screen without a patchwork procedure for digitalisation.

The technology, which is available at present, is, however, sufficient for additional practical use only if AI is implemented, too.

## 2. Introduction of AI

The technical development of image acquisition and storage induces image sizes which are difficult to handle, and even more difficult to transfer from the point of acquisition or storage to clients who are viewing or manipulating images. The image size of a complete glass slide measures several Giga Bytes. Image compression procedures might reduce the size by factor 10 however, do not result in an adequate size for normal application, such as viewing or performance of actions, which are based on viewing an image. The most appropriate solution can be seen in the application of artificial intelligence (AI), which takes into account the aim of the client. For example, if the client wants to perform relative measurements of image objects, the transmission of the objects might be sufficient instead of transmitting the whole image. If this is not possible due to segmentation problems, appropriate sampling might be another solution.

The prerequisite of AI application is to focus on the "aim of the user", i.e., the knowledge, what the user wants to do with the image. If this application has been defined, the original large sized image can be analysed in relation to these aims, and only the interesting compartments will be transferred, stored, or searched for the information wanted.

In practice, the simplest method is to perform an adequate sampling. Little has been published on "adequate sampling". Therefore, some basic aspects are presented here. As shown in table 2, in general, five different sampling techniques can be distinguished.

**Table 2.** Principles of different sampling techniques

| *Sampling procedure* | *Performance (pixel selection)* | *Application* |
|---|---|---|
| Random | Random start point | Stereology |
| Stratified | Object related start point | Diagnostics (cancer cell) |
| Passive (random or stratified) | Fixed segmentation procedure | Conventional stains |
| Active (random or stratified) | Local segmentation procedure | Immunohistochemistry |
| Functional | Evaluation of rare events | Molecular Pathology |

*Random sampling* is the most frequently performed sampling procedure. Its roots go back to the earliest days of stereology. A simple grid is superimposed to the image, and the hits of the grid points with segmented image points are counted. As the relationship between the grid starting points and the image points is random, this technique is a bias-free and easy to apply technique. It is used to calculate spatial and volume related fractions of the objects (volume fraction, surface/volume fraction, etc).

*Stratified sampling* requires a knowledge of object features which are searched for. Only those objects are taken into account, which fit into the predefined scale of the objects' scales. Stratified sampling is frequently used on cytology smears in search for rare events, i.e., cancer cells or cells with similar predefined features.

Both random and stratified sampling procedures can be further distinguished by the "relationship (function) of the "hits" between the grid points and the segmented image points. If this relationship is fixed, i.e., if the selection function $fs = \{1,0\}$, we have only points which hit and those, which do not. This relationship is fixed for the whole image. This procedure is called *passive sampling*, and is the most frequently used sampling technique.

*Active sampling* has to be performed, if the segmentation procedure requires a local function, for example, dependent upon the staining intensity. The selection function can then be described by $fs = \{g(x,y)\}$, whereas $0 < g(x,y) < 1$. In practice, this procedure leads to a secondary transformation of $g(x,y) \rightarrow \{0,1\}$ dependent upon additional features of the selected object. It is an appropriate technique to search for the best fitting segmentation threshold in immunohistochemical images, and can standardize variations in staining intensity or slide thickness.

*Functional sampling* tries to define the "biological significance" of segmented rare events, and to distinguish artefacts from those with real potential meaning. It is based upon syntactic structure analysis, i.e. an analysis of segmented rare objects in spatial relation to their environment, i.e., frequent objects with different features. Its is a useful technique for analysis of relationship between different (immunohistochemical) markers, such as proliferation (e. g. MIB-1) and expression of receptors (e. g. galectin-1, galectin-3), or for molecular pathology data [28].

The implementation of AI based upon the discussed sampling procedures induces new aspects of telepathology and the establishment of virtual laboratories. It can, for example, significantly diminish the time needed for primary diagnosis in telecytology [26].

## 3. E-Learning and e-Teaching in Pathology

AI seems to be, in addition, necessary when establishing a customer – oriented e-learning system in diagnostic pathology [29]. These systems have to meet a conclusive information agglutination in diagnostic medicine, based upon histological images. The "Digital Lung Pathology" CD gives a good example of the present status of the technique [30]. It presents a selection of about 60 rare and frequent lung diseases. It contains a regular structure based upon the experiences of the textbook "Analytical Lung Pathology" [31].

The electronic medium, however, permits a user-friendly presentation of all headlines related to an included lung disease, an easy fresh-up of the latest literature, and a suitable control of the user's diagnostic knowledge. Electronic zooming is possible on all included radiological and histological images, as well as rapid "jumps" to related diseases or information content by use of prepared links. The presented structure of any included disease are shown in Table 3.

**Table 3.** Disease structure of the Digital Lung Pathology CD *(www.pathology-online.org)*

| | |
|---|---|
| *Definition:* | |
| *Incidence/Epidemiology:* | *Clinical Presentation:* |
| *Prognosis:* | |
| *Endoscopy:* | *Images* |
| *Radiology:* | *Images* |
| *Pathology:* | *Gross* |
| *Histology:* | *Images* |
| *Image descriptors:* | |
| *Special stains:* | |
| *Genotype and cytogenetic analysis:* | |
| *Hallmarks of Diagnosis:* | *Differential Diagnosis:* |

## 4. Search for References (National Library)

The unique structure permits a user friendly information presentation and lookup. For each disease, at least four different histology images at different magnifications are included. The radiological images consist of normal chest X-rays and computed tomography images. To provide clinicians with adequate gross in vivo images, endoscopic images have been included as well.

The training scenario permits a test of the user's knowledge from two points of view: a) to assign a diagnosis to a given histological image (or a complete set of images), and b) to choose the correct image associated to a given diagnosis. The training procedures can be chosen from each "stage" of the CD independently from the selected disease or information source. Exemplarily, the training set up for disease recognition is given in Figure 1.

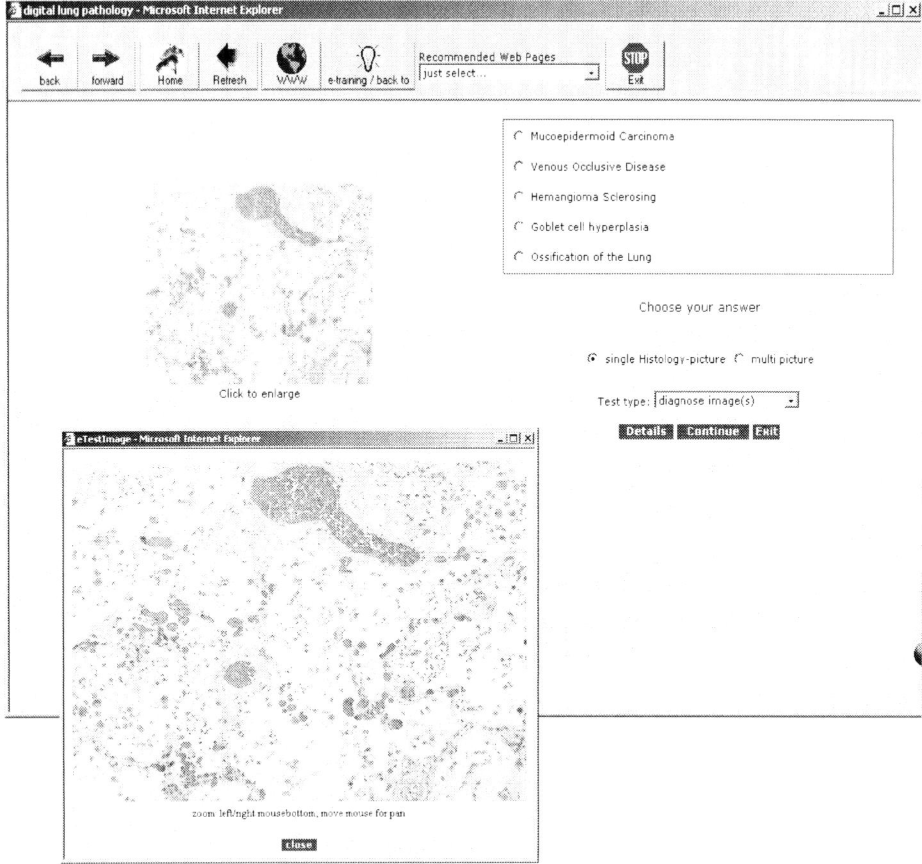


**Fig. 1.** E-training with "Digital Lung Pathology"

The thumbnail image can be enlarged, and the corresponding disease has to be selected from the presented five different choices. Another training presents a choice of five images, and the correct one has to be selected in accordance with the given disease. All choices of selection are randomly prepared in order to avoid a "memory" effect.

In addition to the disease presentation, several links are included, such as access to the Europath server, to the UICC-TPCC and iPATH servers, to the Electronic Journal of Pathology and Histology, and the home page of the International Academy of Telepathology (IAT).

All in all, the Digital Lung Pathology CD is a state-of-the-art-tool for e-learning and teaching. It offers simple expansion to be used as

- histopathological electronic textbook,
- open image data basis
- integrated training and knowledge test
- presentation with wireless internet access
- training set during the daily workflow
- integrative tool for virtual slide technology.

In the near future, these e-learning and e-training tools will become integrated into the daily work of a diagnostic pathologist, and will, in combination with the algorithms used for automated image analysis [32-35], permit contemporary disease classification, expanded learning, and – which is not discussed here – distribution of acquired knowledge, i.e. associated scientific publication.

**Acknowledgement.** The financial support of the International Academy of Telepathology, and IBM Germany is gratefully acknowledged.

## References

[1] Kayser K, Szymas J, Weinstein RW. Telepathology: Telecommunication, Electronic education and publication in Pathology, Springer, Berlin, Heidelberg, New York, 1999
[2] Weinstein R. S., et al. (2001) Telepathology overview: from concept to implementation. Hum Pathol 32: 1283-99
[3] Adachi H., et al. (1996) Frozen-section services by telepathology: experience of 100 cases in the San-in District, Japan. Pathol Int 46: 436-41.
[4] Dunn B.E., et al. (1999) Routine surgical telepathology in the Department of Veterans Affairs: experience-related improvements in pathologist performance in 2200 cases. Telemed J 5: 323-37.
[5] Dunn B.E., et al. (1997) Dynamic-robotic telepathology: Department of Veterans Affairs feasibility study. Hum Pathol 28: 8-12.
[6] Kayser K., Fritz P., Drlicek M., Rahn W. (1995) Expert consultation by use of telepathology the Heidelberg experiences. Anal Cell Pathol. 9, 53-60.
[7] Della Mea V., et al. (1996) Telepathology using Internet multimedia electronic mail: remote consultation on gastrointestinal pathology. J Telemed Telecare 2: 28-34.
[8] Kayser K., Fritz P., Drlicek M. (1995) Aspects of telepathology in routinary diagnostic work with specific emphasis on ISDN. Arch Anat Cytol Pathol. 43, 216-218.
[9] Weinstein R.S., Bloom K.J., Rozek L.S. (1987) Telepathology and the networking of pathology diagnostic services. Am J Clin Pathol 91 (4 Suppl): S39-S42.
[10] Kayser K., Beyer M., Blum S. Kayser G. (2000) Recent developments and present status of telepathology. Anal Cell Pathol 21: 101-6.
[11] Kayser K., Beyer M., Blum S. Kayser G. (2000) Telecommunication--a new tool for quality assurance and control in diagnostic pathology. Folia Neuropathol 38: 79-83.
[12] Weinstein R.S. (1986) Prospects of telepathology. Hum Pathol 27:99-101.
[13] Kayser K., (2002) Interdisciplinary telecommunication and expert teleconsultation in diagnostic pathology: present status and future prospects. J Telemed Telecare 8: 325-30.
[14] Kayser K., (1998) Telepathology, images, and multimedia archives. Adv Clin Path 2, 157.
[15] Williams BH, et al. (1998) A national treasure goes online: the Armed Forces Institute of Pathology. MD Comput 15:260-5
[16] Williams B.H., The AFIP center for telemedicine application - pathology for the twenty-first century. Telemedicine and Virtual Reality 1998; 3: 64-5
[17] Dietel M., Hufnagl P., TN Nguyen-Dobinsky (2000) The UICC telepathology consultation center - a global approach to improving consultation for pathologists in cancer diagnosis Cancer 89: 187-191.
[18] Brauchli K., et al. (2000) Teleppathology: design of a modular system. Anal Cell Pathol 21:193-199.
[19] Brauchli K., et al. (2002) Telemicroscopy by the Internet revisited. J Pathol 196: 238-243.
[20] Schrader, T. et. al. (2003) A user friendly Telepathology Service at the Internet – The Telepathology Consultation Center of the UICC Elec J Pathol Histol 9:031-007
[21] Kayser K., Kayser G., Schrader T., Hufnagl P., (2003) Recent developments and future aspects of telepathology in Europe (Zielinski K, Duplaga M, edts). Proceedings ehe@lth in Common Europe. PR Access, ISBN 83-915141-2-9, Krakow, pp 163-174.
[22] Weinstein R.S., Bloom K.J., Krupinski E., A.Rozek L.S. (1992) Human performance studies of the video microscopy component of a dynamic telepathology system. Zentralbl Pathol 138: 399-403.
[23] Nordrum I. et. al. (1991) Remote frozen section service, a telepathology project in northern Norway. Hum Pathol. 22, 514-518.
[24] Nordrum I, Eide TJ (1995) Remote frozen section service in Norway. Arch Anat Cytol Pathol. 43, 253-256.
[25] Nordrum I (1998) Real-time diagnoses in telepathology. Adv Clin. Path. 2, 127-131.

[26] Kayser K. Kayser G. Becker H.D. Herth F. (2000) Telediagnosis of transbronchial fine needle aspirations – a feasibility study. Anal Cell Pathol 21:207-12
[27] Anand S.S. et al. (1999) An evaluation of intelligent prognostic systems for colorectal cancer. Artif Intell Med 15:193-214.
[28] Kayser K., Hufnagl P., Kayser G., Zink S., (1999) Stratified sampling: Basic ideas and application in pathology Elec J Pathol Histol 5:994-08.
[29] Kayser K., Beyer M., Blum S., Kayser G. (2000) Telecommunication--a new tool for quality assurance and control in diagnostic pathology Folia Neuropathol 38:79-83.
[30] Kayser K., Oehmann A. (2003) Digital Lung Pathology. Rendevous Verlag Baden Baden. ISBN 3-936881-05-7
[31] Kayser K., Analytical lung pathology. Springer, Heidelberg, New York, 1992
[32] Bartels P.H., Weber J.E., Duckstein L. Machine learning in quantitative histopathology. Anal Quant Cytol Histol 10 (1988) 299-306.
[33] Bartels P.H., et al. (1989) Image understanding system for histopathology. Anal Cell Pathol 1:195-214.
[34] Bartels P.H., et al. (1999) Tissue architecture analysis in prostate cancer and its precursors: An innovative approach to computerized histometry. Eur Urol 35:484-491.
[35] Kayser G., et al. (2002) Towards an automated morphological classification of histological images of common lung carcinomas. Elec J Pathol Histol 8:022-03.

# New Trends in Diabetes Management: Mobile Telemedicine Closed-Loop System

M. Elena HERNANDO, Enrique J. GÓMEZ, Antonio GILI,
Mónica GÓMEZ, Gema GARCÍA and Francisco del POZO
*Grupo de Bioingeniería y Telemedicina, Universidad Politécnica de Madrid, ETSI Telecomunicación, 28040 Madrid, Spain*

**Abstract.** The rapid growth and development of information technologies over recent years, in the areas of mobile and wireless technologies is shaping a new technological scenario of telemedicine in diabetes. This telemedicine scenario can play an important role for further acceptance by diabetic patients of the existing continuous glucose monitoring systems and insulin pumps with the final goal of improving current therapeutic procedures. This paper describes a Personal Smart Assistant integrated in a multi-access telemedicine architecture for the implementation of a mobile telemedicine closed-loop system for diabetes management. The system is being evaluated within the European Union project named INCA ("Intelligent Control Assistant for Diabetes").

## Introduction

Over the last three decades, diabetes has been a major focus for biomedical engineering efforts to improve the diagnosis, monitoring and treatment of patients. The rapid growth and development of information technologies during recent years in the areas of mobile and wireless technologies is shaping a new technological scenario of telemedicine in diabetes, in which the traditional concepts of patient and medical units are blurred, undergoing a profound transformation to a new multi-access, mobile, universal and ubiquitous workspace concept for diabetes care.

Many different biomedical and information technologies, methods and approaches (such as biomedical sensors) have been developed, for continuous blood glucose monitoring, biomedical instrumentation, self-monitoring data collection and continuous insulin delivery. Mathematical modeling has also been used to better understand the physiological processes involved in metabolic control, and the application of information technologies, such as database management systems, data analysis and visualization tools, intelligent decision support techniques and telemedicine systems is on the rise [1], [2], [3].

The course of chronic diabetes care is a cyclic process that can be represented in a care model that involves the following actions: 1) ambulatory monitoring of blood glucose levels and other metabolic control variables (insulin, exercise, food, etc.); 2) assessment of metabolic control on the basis of data recorded and evaluation of the current treatment regimen; 3) planning of management actions whenever therapeutic goals are not achieved; and 4) therapy adjustment by the implementation of therapeutic actions (insulin dosage changes, meals, etc.) in order to maintain the required metabolic control of the diabetic patient.

At any stage of the care model described above, biomedical and information technologies can be applied to improve the diagnosis, monitoring and therapeutic actions taken by patients and doctors. The combination of insulin pumps and continuous glucose monitoring systems seems to be the best near-future solution to achieving good metabolic control for insulin-dependent diabetic people. Continuous glucose monitoring can detect glycemia patterns that cannot be discovered by means of few diary measurements alone [4]. The possibility to obtain a complete blood glucose profile allows for monitoring the suitability of an intensive therapy and can be used to fine-tune such a therapy. The old concept of "artificial pancreas" is finally turning into a reality, supported by the availability of said technologies and the integration of control systems able to close the loop, modifying pump parameters.

Although the intravenous route is ideal for control, the implementation of a closed-loop system to be used by patients during their daily life imposes the use of the subcutaneous (SC) route for insulin delivery and blood glucose measurement. However, glycemic control based on SC insulin infusion is complex, because of the delay in the absorption of the SC route. Several closed-loop control algorithms for subcutaneous infusion vs. subcutaneous sensing (SC-SC) setups have already been reported [5]. Control methods are based on several control strategies such as pole-assignment, self-tuning adaptive control and nonlinear predictive control.

One of the latest efforts to achieve a SC-SC close-loop control system based on a portable computer has been made within the EU-funded research project ADICOL: "Advance Insulin Infusion using a Control Loop" [6]. The project developed a minimally-invasive glucose sensor, measuring glucose levels in the subcutaneous tissue, and a glucose controller calculating an adequate insulin rate/dose to automatically administer the daily insulin dosage in a precise manner and in the required amount, using the information provided by the glucose sensor. A novel non-linear MPC with Bayesian learning [7] has also been developed to track the parameters of the glucoregulatory system and control the insulin pump with the aim to normalize, in a controlled way, hyperglycemia and to quickly recover from hypoglycemia.

Telemedicine is providing innovative solutions in the effective treatment of patients with diabetes [8]. Telecare services can provide people with the tools they need to take better control of their illness. The benefits of telemedicine over conventional care methods are mainly due to its ability to enhance physician-patient communication and also to increase the quality and quantity of information collected by patients, affording a better decisionmaking process for doctors and patients. Doctors are provided with the information and the tools needed to optimize the number of therapy adjustments and patients' education, which are the key points to achieve a positive impact in the patients' metabolic control.

The acceptance by patients with diabetes of the existing continuous glucose monitoring systems and insulin pumps could be extensively improved by the integration of these new technologies and therapeutic procedures within a telemedicine system. The goal to build a mobile telemedicine closed-loop system for diabetes management is currently under development within a new European Union project named INCA: "Intelligent Control Assistant for Diabetes" [9]. This project started in January 2003 and is creating a mobile intelligent Personal Smart Assistant (SA) for continuous monitoring of glucose and subcutaneous insulin infusions implemented in a portable device and integrated in a telemedicine system.

This paper focused on the description of the Personal Smart Assistant integrated in a telemedicine architecture for the implementation of a diabetes telemedical closed-loop system.

# 1. Methodology

## *1.1 Telemedicine-based Control Strategies*

Four control strategies have been defined in the INCA project that are being implemented following incremental clinical studies to minimize risk factors and to assure system feasibility in ambulatory environments (see Figure 1):

1. Patient control: the patient controls the insulin pump in an ambulatory environment and makes his/her own decisions about insulin therapy adjustments using the information provided by the glucometer and/or the continuous glucose sensor. The SA communicates with medical devices in a personal wireless network, to obtain the patient's monitoring data and the insulin delivered by the pump (basal profiles and bolus). Afterwards, the SA transmits data to the central server using the mobile GPRS network. Healthcare professionals can supervise the patient's therapeutic decisionmaking at any time by the use of Web telemedicine services.
2. Doctor control: after analysing patients' data, the doctor decides to modify the insulin therapy and uses the Web telemedicine service to define the new therapy, which is automatically transmitted to the patient's SA, notifying the patient and asking for his/her permission to re-program the insulin pump.
3. Control algorithms in the remote loop: whenever new data is received at the central server, it is automatically analyzed by closed-loop algorithms that calculate the required insulin therapy adjustments. Changes are transmitted to the patient's SA under doctors' supervision.
4. Control algorithms in the personal loop: closed-loop algorithms are implemented in the SA and provide real-time control of the insulin pump based on the glucose sensor data.

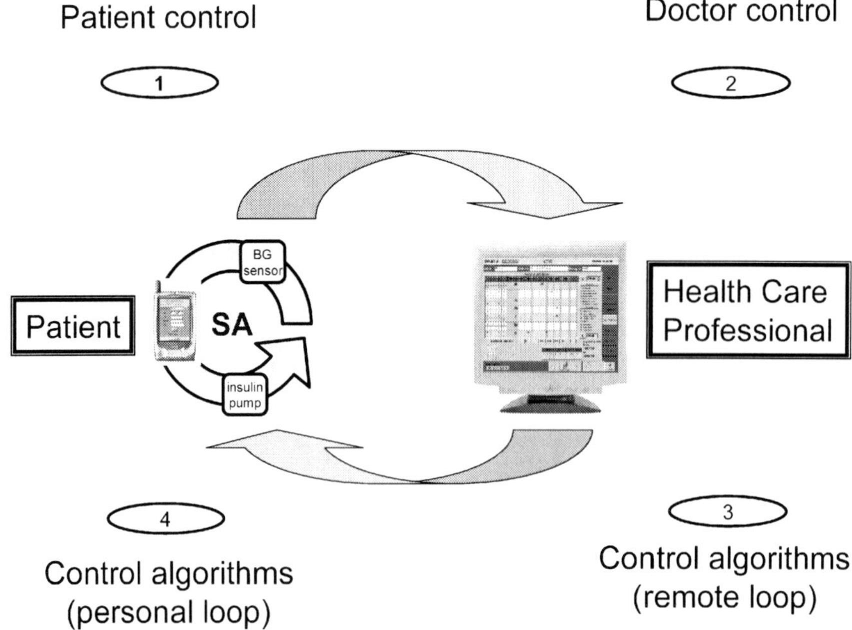


**Fig. 1.** The telemedicine-based control strategies

### *1.2 The Telemedicine MAS Architecture*

The telemedicine system in which the SA is integrated has to provide all the information needed for patient management and for decisionmaking through the provision of four main services: 1) Telemonitoring, which allows physicians to view the patient's self-monitoring data; 2) Telecare, which enables remote care of the patient (assessment of the patient's metabolic state, therapy modification, teleconsultations for patients and supervision of patients' decisions); 3) Remote information access, which permits both patients and doctors to access basic visit information, complete Electronic Health Records and stored messages; 4) Knowledge management tools, which supply doctors and patients with the knowledge they need when analyzing data and/or making diagnostic and management decisions, including automatic generation of intelligent alarms and notifications.

The implementation of the telemedicine system is based on a multi-access architecture (MAS) that considers a full range of non-expensive and widely accepted information technologies (Figure 2). The MAS architecture enables universal access to information through the use of basic technologies with wide penetration in the society (e.g. conventional telephone) combined with intermediate technologies, supported by computers or mobile phone terminals (e.g. Web, WebTV, SMS) and also combined with advanced and innovative technologies (e.g. PDAs, WAP and GPRS), whose use is limited to a smaller group of users due to their availability, costs or the required users' skills. The MAS allows to build a new environment of cooperation between patients and doctors in which, depending on their skills, their preferences or the scenario of use, users can access information through a set of integrated services with additional features for telecare and visit management, such as text and voice mailing, management of electronic patient records; automatic generation of reports, intelligent alarms, tele-education and intelligent knowledge management.

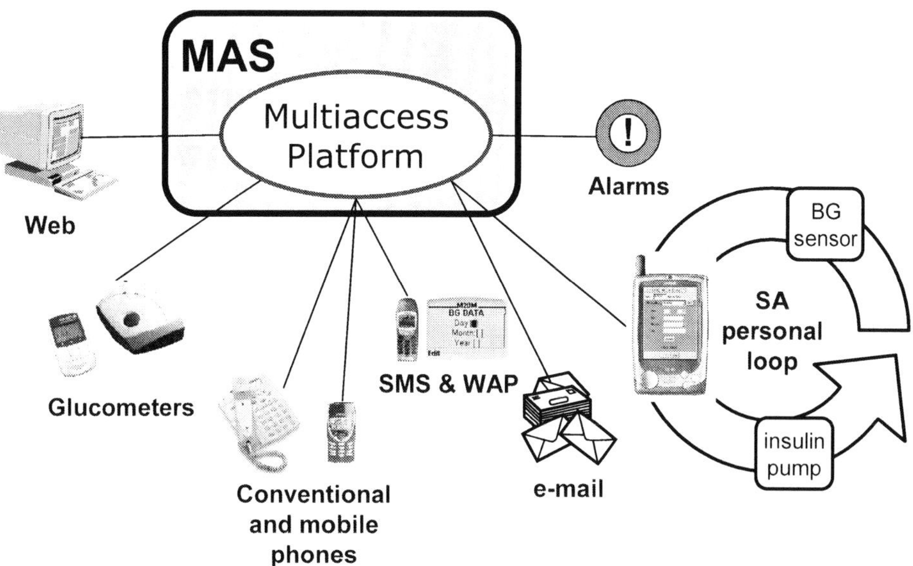


**Fig. 2.** Integration of the SA into the MAS architecture

The MAS comprises a set of "Communication Agents", that are in charge of communications with different user terminals in order to manage the dataflow and messaging/notification features. Additionally, the MAS architecture integrates "Application Server Agents" that are in charge of data analysis and automatic alarm generation. The Smart Assistant is integrated in the MAS architecture as an additional user terminal that interacts with a Communication Server Agent (called the SA Remote Agent) running on the central server (see Figure 2).

The MAS architecture has been evaluated with insulin-dependent diabetic patients during a one-year multicenter clinical trial in the M2DM project, funded by the European Commission [11].

### *1.3 Smart Assistant User-Centred Design*

The user interface is one of the most critical components that determine the ultimate success of an interactive system, since it is the main element responsible for system usability. A highly interactive system for clinical applications, such as a telemedicine system, requires a user interface that reuses user task knowledge and supports concurrent dialogues (where more than one dialogue flow can be handled at a time). Therefore, the design and development of a user interface for end-user applications is a difficult task that cannot be addressed without an appropriate, methodical approach.

The proposed methodology [12] follows a user-centered approach (medical/technical staff or patient) and relies on the definitions of all the cognitive domains for human-computer interaction in line with the "direct correspondence principle", that states that all objects and concepts of interest at any given time and for a particular user task should have graphical component counterparts represented in the user interface.

The main steps of the user-centred methodology are described in Figure 3 and can be summarized as follows:

1. User requirements capture, adapted to the development of interactive systems: this stage consists of a description of the context of use, where a questionnaire must be completed, with descriptions of system users, user tasks to be performed with the system and the physical, technical, and organizational environments in which the system is going to be used.
2. Task modeling (problem domain): problem domain modeling is based on hierarchical task analysis. It consists of a breakdown of tasks into simpler sub-tasks in order to identify the hierarchical structure, temporal relationships, and the real-world objects used to perform each task. The obtained task model represents the user's knowledge of the task domain.
3. System semantic domain design: on the semantic level of description, we define user interface metaphors to provide users with a coherent picture of the system, taking into account their previous knowledge described in the task model. Specifically, the metaphor consists of an assignment of tasks to system semantic objects, which will be presented by the user interface. The general dialogue structure with the system semantic objects is also designed, in line with the temporal relationships between tasks (described in the task model).
4. User interface development (syntactic and articulation domains development): a graphical representation and a style of interaction are designed for all of the system's semantic objects, without modifying the dialogue's general structure. The necessary user interface prototypes are developed using a "User Interface Management System" (UIMS), and complying with design guidelines and standards.

This four-step methodology must be seen as an iterative process: after each step is completed, its outcome evaluation can enable further refinement of the previous step. The iterative process becomes more relevant in the last stage, in which evaluation with real user participation normally produces a redesign of the user interface.

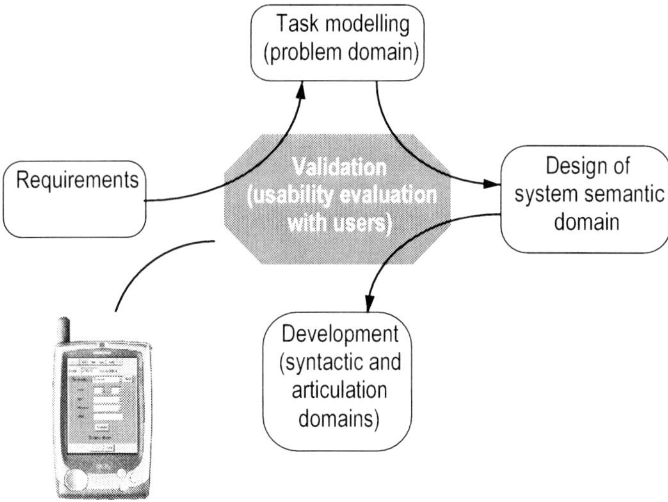


**Fig. 3.** SA user-centered design methodology

Technology reliability is another critical issue for human-device interaction, because the technologies and the applications must be reliable enough to assure that the number of failures encountered is as low as possible. Users should not be "beta testers" of the technology but testers of the new clinical process.

The final aim of the enhancement of human-device interaction is to lower the technical and behavioural knowledge barriers that could prevent the success of a highly-complex telemedicine system, such as the one described in this paper.

## 2. The Personal Smart Assistant

The Personal Smart Assistant (SA) provides an augmented information self-management environment that communicates with the patient's devices through a personal wireless network (local loop) and through a mobile Wide Area Network for providing telemonitoring, telecare and remote information services (remote loop).

The user terminal that supports the SA is a commercial PDA, provided with wireless communication facilities, such as infrared, Bluetooth and GPRS. The SA can work as a standalone system, supported by its own local application and database, and integrate an "electronic logbook" that allows patients to perform the following data management tasks:

- management of monitoring data, obtained both from medical devices (pump, glucometer and continuous glucose monitors), and directly from patients (diet data and additional events affecting blood glucose profiles such as illness, menstruation, etc). Patients cannot modify data coming from the devices, but they can augment them with extra information that is not automatically recorded;

- visualization of graphics and statistics of past monitoring data;
- consultation of the patient's active therapy in terms of basal profiles, bolus and prescribed diet.

Additionally, the SA behaves as a virtual interface to the medical devices operating in the Personal Area Network. This virtual interface allows patients to visualize and modify the configuration of their devices and to upload monitoring data without any physical interaction. The patient's Personal Area Network integrates the SA and the patient's medical devices, communicated through local wireless technologies that do not require the availability of any public network.

Figure 4 shows the integration of an insulin pump into the Personal Area Network and the interaction between the patient and the SA to control the medical device through the Pump Virtual Interface: 1) The SA periodically obtains the information recorded by the pump (insulin delivery, error events, start-stop events, cartridge replacement, etc); 2) The patient interacts with the SA to visualize the logbook and to decide upon insulin therapy adjustments; 3) The patient can remotely control medical devices through the SA user interface; 4) The patient interacts with the SA to update the information from/to the central database.

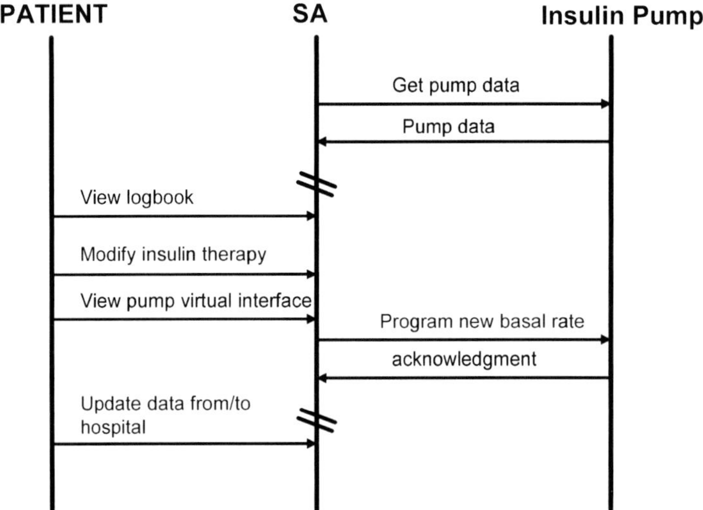


**Fig. 4.** The SA Personal Area Network

The use of always-on networks such as GPRS makes it possible to perform communications transparently to users, periodically downloading the SA data from medical devices and transferring the new data to the central server. Communications can also be activated on demand. There are two possible scenarios for remote on-demand communications: 1) to force bi-directional data exchange between the central server and the SA at any moment, and 2) to remotely control the medical devices through the SA. Remote control can be demanded by physicians, through interaction with the professionals' Web interface.

Figure 5 shows a simplified example of the interaction diagram for scenarios of control loop strategy number 2 presented in Figure 2: 1) The SA periodically obtains the information recorded by the pump and transmits it to the central database; 2) The physician analyzes monitoring data from the patient using the Web application, and decides upon an insulin therapy modification (control strategy); 3) The insulin pump is remotely re-programmed with the new basal rate. Patient's consent could be solicited, with a message displayed by the PDA.

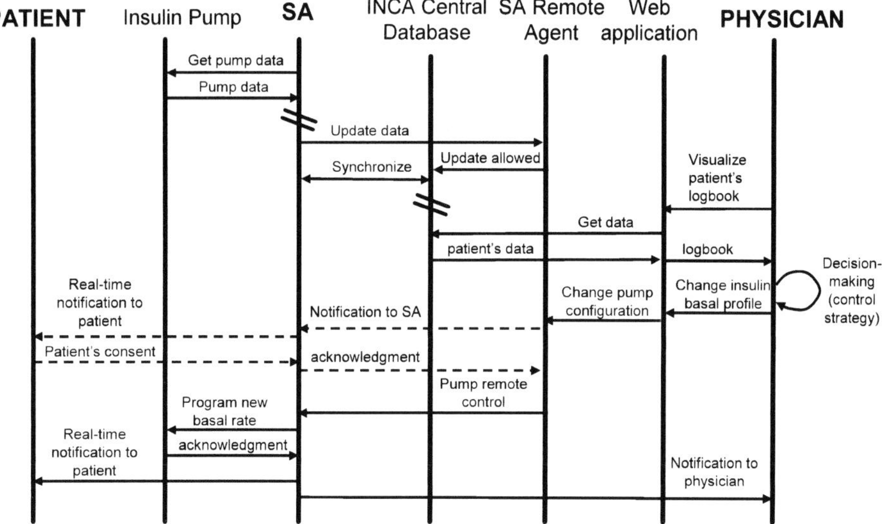


**Fig. 5.** Interaction diagram of the physician's control scenario

The implementation of remote control-loop strategies requires bi-directional real-time communications to allow remote interaction with the patient's medical devices from the hospital. The patients' Smart Assistants need to behave as distributed agents, able to process requests and also to act under remote requests originated by physicians. Each SA Agent interacts with the SA Remote Agent running on the central server.

Distributed objects are implemented with the CORBA standard (Common Object Request Broker Architecture) and communicate using the IIOP protocol (Internet Inter-ORB Protocol) [13]. Public interfaces are described with IDL (Interface Definition Language). There are other possibilities of implementing distributed objects, such as RMI [14] and DCOM [15], but one of the advantages of using CORBA is that it is platform-independent, so different programming languages and operating systems can be used to develop and store the objects.

The SA Agent is implemented with the Java 2 Platform Micro Edition (J2ME) and the CDC Personal Profile. It integrates two distributed objects that behave as the client and the server and can use communication modules that implement local and remote communication loops. The SA agent runs on a PDA with the Windows PocketPC operating system.

The SA Remote Agent is implemented with the Java 2 Platform Enterprise Edition (J2EE). It also integrates two distributed objects: the server object can be called both from the Web application and from the SA Agent. The SA Remote Agent runs on a PC server with the Windows operating system.

## 3. Conclusions

Over the last decades, the development of an artificial pancreas has been a huge challenge in the application of biomedical technologies to diabetes therapy. The evolution of continuous glucose monitoring and insulin pumps technologies is creating a very promising situation for the near future. However, current reliability constraints of continuous glucose sensors, the non-linearity of the glucoregulatory system and the inherent complexity of the design of a glucose controller for a SC-SC setup are still some of the problems to be faced before obtaining a portable artificial pancreas.

This paper presents research work aimed at developing a mobile telemedicine closed-loop system for diabetes management. Its main component is a Personal Smart Assistant integrated into a telemedicine multi-access system. The ambulatory use of this type of control-loop systems requires their integration into telemedicine services, to enable not only the monitoring of the Smart Assistant performance, but also interventions (by a physician) to modify the patients' medical device settings.

The implementation of telemedical closed-loop control strategies requires prior development of distributed objects able to perform always-on bi-directional real-time communications. The complexity of the system increases when those agents have to be implemented in portable devices (PDAs), with significant constrains in terms of memory and computing power. This work shows how Java and CORBA technologies can be used to build portable solutions for distributed mobile objects. Additionally, Java and CORBA allow building systems that can be easily ported and adapted to most of the existing or future platforms, in keeping with the rapid evolution of mobile phone and PDA markets.

The mobile telemedicine closed-loop system will be evaluated in two feasibility pilot studies carried out within the European Union INCA project. The reliability of portable systems will be one of the most important issues to take into account when implementing the closed-loop system in clinical practice. Possible interruptions of radio-frequency connections could also cause undesired delays in the performance of automatic control strategies. The outcome of the INCA feasibility studies will allow testing the reliability of the technologies, identifying the incidence of hazard situations for the patient, and their potential impact on the management of diabetes with insulin pump therapy.

The augmented availability of continuous glucose sensors, insulin pumps, mobile computing technologies and telemedicine services is bringing closer to reality the "Holy Grail" in diabetes care: a feasible and reliable closed-loop glucose control system, integrated into a telemedicine system, as the best current solution to achieve a good metabolic control for insulin-dependent diabetes mellitus patients.

**Acknowledgments.** The authors wish to acknowledge the valuable work of the researchers of the Grupo de Bioingeniería y Telemedicina of UPM, especially of Angel García, Verónica Torralba, Silvia Lafuente and Javier Perdices. Likewise, the authors would like to express their gratitude to all partners of the INCA Project, especially to Dr. Mercedes Rigla, E. Brugués and Dr. A. de Leiva (Fundación Diabem, Hospital Sant Pau of Barcelona), as well as to Dr. Thomas Vering, Ivo Hutzli, Caroline Patte and Michael Haeberli (Disetronic-Roche). This research work has been partially funded by the EU Project INCA (IST-2001-37632) and the Spanish Research Projects MCYT Middlecare (TIC2002-02129) and Red Telemedicina (G03/117).

## References

[1] S. Andreassen, E.J. Gómez and E.R. Carson, Computers in Diabetes 2000, *Comput. Meth. Prog. Biomed*, 69 (2002) 93-95.

[2] E. Colloff, The Promise of Technology in the Management of the Patient with Diabetes, *Diabetes Technology & Therapeutics*, 2 (1) (2000) 91-99.

[3] D.C. Klonoff, Welcome to Diabetes Technology & Therapeutics, *Diabetes Technology & Therapeutics*, 1, (1) (1999) 1-2.

[4] B.W. Bode, T.M. Gross, K.R. Thornton and J. Mastrototaro, Continuous glucose monitoring used to adjust diabetes therapy improves glycosylated hemoglobin: a pilot study, *Diabetes Research and Clinical Practice*, 46 (1999) 183-190.

[5] R. Bellazzi, G. Nucci and C. Cobelli, The Subcutaneous Route to Insulin-Dependent Diabetes Therapy, *IEEE Eng. Med. Biol. Magazine*, 20 (1) (2001) 54-64.

[6] ADICOL Project, Disetronic, *http://www.disetronic-usa.com/releases/adicol.htm*.

[7] R. Hovorka, Closing the Loop with Portable Systems, Seminar on "Technical, biological and bio-technical approaches of the diabetes treatment", *Diabetes Technology & Therapeutics*, 5(5) (2003) 873-874.

[8] E.J. Gómez, M.E. Hernando, A. Garcia, F. Del Pozo, R. Corcoy, E. Brugués, J. Cermeño and A. De Leiva A., Telemedicine as a tool for intensive management of diabetes: the DIABTel experience, *Comput. Meth. Prog. Biomed.*, 69 (2002) 163-177.

[9] INCA Project, Internet site address *http://www.ist-inca.org/*.

[10] M. E. Hernando, E.J. Gómez, A. Garcia A. y F. del Pozo, A multi-access server for the virtual management of diabetes, *Proceedings ESEM 99 – Fifth conference of the European Society for Engineering and Medicine*- (ISBN: 84-95185-29-6), (1999) 309-310.

[11] R. Bellazzi, M. Arcelloni, G. Bensa, H. Blankenfeld, E. Brugués, E. Carson, C. Cobelli, D. Cramp, G. d'Annunzio, P. De Cata , A. de Leiva, T. Deutsc, P. Fratino, C. Gazzaruso, A. Garcìa, T. Gergely, E. Gómez, F. Harvey, P. Ferrari, E. Hernando, M.K. Boulos, C. Larizza, H. Ludekke, A. Maran, G. Nucci, C. Pennati, S. Ramat, A.Roudsari, M. Rigla, M. Stefanelli. "Design, methods and evaluation directions of a multi-access service for the management of diabetes mellitus patients." *Diabetes Technology & Therapeutics*, 5 (4) (2003) 621-629.

[12] E.J. Gómez, J.A. Quiles, M.F. Sanz, F. Del Pozo, A User-Centered Co-operative Information System for Medical Imaging Diagnosis, *Journal of the American Society for Information Science* 49 (1998) 810-816.

[13] CORBA technology – Object Management Group *http://www.corba.org*.

[14] DCOM White Papers, Microsoft. *http://www.microsoft.com/com/wpaper/default.asp#DCOMpapers*

[15] RMI Trail, Ann Wollrath and Jim Waldo, *http://java.sun.com/docs/books/tutorial/rmi/index.html*

# Migration Aspects of Telemedical Software Architectures

Jacek CAŁA, Łukasz CZEKIERDA, Krzysztof ZIELIŃSKI
*AGH-University of Science and Technology*
*al. Mickiewicza 30, 30-059 Cracow, Poland*

**Abstract.** Many existing medical systems are good candidates for improvement via incremental migration. Incremental software improvement is, however, much more difficult if the system consists of independent functional modules built with different technologies. The goal of this paper is to present architecture migration aspects of contemporary telemedical systems. The paper discusses two approaches: the Software Architecture Analysis Method, and the Architecture Tradeoff Analysis Method in the context of migration of the medical teleconsultation system Konsul. The system, designed and implemented under KCT activity, is being successfully employed in day-to-day activities at the John Paul II Hospital in Krakow despite many existing drawbacks in its internal architecture.

The paper presents the SAAM method of analysis of legacy systems. Two architectures are proposed as a result of this analysis – one based on the migration of the existing architecture, the other built according to the state-of-the-art Service Oriented Architecture.

Konsul II, implementing the migration approach, has already been developed whereas Konsul III is in the design phase. The paper concludes with remarks about migration of telemedical systems

## Introduction

Software architectures and styles of computer system programming change continuously. The important questions in this are: how to modernize existing systems to keep up with new trends? How to assure cooperation between new and legacy components?

Medical systems are good candidates for discussion about architectural migrations. They are usually mission-critical applications, with high requirements regarding security and availability. Therefore, they demand efficient software architectures.

The goal of this paper is to present architectural migration aspects of contemporary telemedical systems. Migration should be preceded by a detailed analysis of existing and designed systems. A good way to assess existing software is to use a software architecture evaluation process. The Software Architecture Analysis Method (SAAM) [1], [3] and the Architecture Tradeoff Analysis Method (ATAM) [2], [3] were designed specifically for this purpose.

The software analysis process presented in this paper has been illustrated by an example using the cardiology teleconsultation system Konsul. The system, designed and implemented under a Krakow Center for Telemedicine and Preventive Medicine activity, is successfully exploited in day-to-day operations at the John Paul II Hospital in Krakow despite many existing drawbacks in its internal architecture. As a result of assessment according to the SAAM method, two versions of the Konsul system have been proposed – one incrementally increasing its functionality and the other being a complete rebuild of the system in a new state-of-the-art Service-Oriented Architecture.

The scope of the paper is as follows: first, in section 2, SOA as the most advanced software paradigm for software architectures is introduced. Section 3 discusses software analysis methods and the migration process of software architectures. In section 4, a general classification of Internet-based telemedical systems is presented. Section 5 is devoted to SAAM practical usage, where the migration process of the Konsul system is described. The paper ends with conclusions.

## 1. Service-Oriented Architecture

The modern design approach recommends building systems according to a service-oriented architecture (SOA). In this style, the main functional components of the software are packaged as separate service implementations providing simple and well-known interfaces for use by other architectural components. Isolating the specifics of a service implementation behind a well-known interface is the key to achieving an incremental migration strategy. SOA is an architectural style that formally separates services into two categories: services which *are* the functionality that a system can provide, and service consumers which *need* that functionality. This separation is accomplished by a mechanism known as a service contract, which is coupled with a mechanism allowing providers to publish contracts and consumers to locate the contracts that provide the service they desire.

The functional components being developed should be supported by special, already-existing, so-called infrastructure components, which provide a set of common services needed by the service implementations of functional components. The reusable entities can, among others, supply the programmer with remote communications between components (e.g. CORBA, J2EE, Web Services, COM/DCOM, JMX), data and event logging, security mechanisms, thread management and user interfaces. The exploitation of the rich spectrum of available services guaranties considerable speed-up in system development and increases code reusability [7].

Characteristics of SOA can be summarized in the following items:

- services have well-defined interfaces (contract) and policies,
- services usually represent a business function or domain,
- services have a modular design,
- services are loosely coupled,
- services are discoverable and support introspection,
- location of services is transparent to the client,
- services are transport- and platform-independent.

It should be emphasized that SOA should not be equated with Web services, which are only a specialization of SOA to fit the Internet implementation.

## 2. Software Analysis Methods and Migration Process

Architectures of nontrivial systems are complex and involve many design tradeoffs. A proper architecture is the key ingredient of business or technological success.

There exists several formal methods for analyzing software architectures, which allow determining if the goal is achievable *before* great effort is invested into development and implementation of the system, and when any discovered problems can be solved at relatively low cost and in a seamless manner.

Analysis methods should be also applied to legacy systems. This frequently occurs when a legacy system requires major modifications or porting, when it is expected to integrate with other systems, or when it needs other significant upgrades. The result of the software architecture assessment is a decision on how (or even whether) to implement a migration or functional enhancement of the architecture. In this context, a crucial issue is the difference between migrating the existing software and its enhancing. The basic distinction says that *migration* involves proactively moving towards a new software architecture, while *enhancements* are typically made within the constraints of the existing legacy software architecture.

The incremental migration strategy is designed to reduce engineering investment. It requires a mapping from the legacy software components to a new set of components. Such mapping is rarely one-to-one. Typically, some existing components must be split and/or combined. In addition, migration usually involves a move to new software infrastructure technologies.

The Architecture Tradeoff Analysis Method (ATAM) is a technique of evaluating software architectures developed and refined at the Software Engineering Institute of the Carnegie Mellon University. The purpose of the ATAM is to assess the consequences of architectural decisions in light of quality attribute requirements such as performance, availability, security, and modifiability [2]. Attributes are understood in a very general way; ATAM does not need to either produce detailed analysis of any measurable quality attribute of a system (e.g. latency, mean time to failure, etc.) or attempt to precisely predict quality attribute behavior – which is impossible at an early design stage. Instead, ATAM focuses on recording *risks*, *sensitivity points* and *tradeoff points* found during the analysis. These important terms will be described in a more detailed way [2].

- **Risks** are architecturally important decisions:
  - that have not been made – e.g. the architecture team has not decided what scheduling discipline they will use, or has not decided whether they will use a relational or object-oriented database, or
  - that have been made but whose consequences are not fully understood – e.g. the architecture team has decided to include an operating system portability layer, but is not sure what functions need to go into this layer.
- **Sensitivity points** are parameters in the architecture to which some measurable quality attribute response is highly correlated. For example, it might be determined that overall throughput in the system is highly correlated to the throughput of one particular communication channel, and availability in the system is highly correlated to the reliability of that same communication channel.
- A **tradeoff point** is found in the architecture when a parameter of an architectural construct is host to more than one sensitivity point where the measurable quality attributes are affected differently by changing that parameter. For example, if increasing the speed of the communication channel mentioned above improves throughput but reduces its reliability, then the speed of that channel is a tradeoff point.

The other method, also developed at the Carnegie Mellon University is the Software Architecture Analysis Method (SAAM) – a predecessor of the ATAM approach. ATAM focuses mainly on evaluating new architectures being designed, while the SAAM technique is usually used to assess existing software architectures – whether it is feasible to perform desired modifications and at what cost. The SAAM approach concentrates, among others, on extensibility, subsetability and portability of software. In short, the evaluation process consists of the following steps [3], [4]:

- **identifying stakeholders** i.e. persons or institutions who use, develop or maintain the system,
- **developing scenarios** representing possible future changes to the system; enumerated scenarios are then prioritized,
- **describing candidate architecture(s)** allowing the implementation of said scenarios,

- **evaluating scenarios** i.e. identifying components, data connections, control connections and interfaces which should be added, modified or deleted,
- **revealing interactions** i.e. summarizing interactions between evaluated scenarios and components, and then estimating the costs of migration.

SAAM, although less comprehensive than ATAM, is simpler and generally easier to learn with respect to efficient analysis. Furthermore, the analysis itself costs less in terms of time and budget. The final decision on which methodology to use should depend mainly on the scale of the system – larger systems require more sophisticated assessment methods.

## 3. Software Architectures of Medical Systems

Medicine, similarly to other domains affecting our lives, benefits from electronic exchange of information. Such exchange can support better organization of medical data and improve healthcare, especially when distance separates participants – e.g. doctors and patients or doctors themselves. Generally, the Internet health industry can be divided into three segments [6]:

1. **Content, services, and community.** This category covers health portals, i.e. organized medical sites that contain information connected with the functioning of medical centers as well as provide expert advice to a wide range of recipients. Medical portals can act in a number of ways. They can improve the healthcare service level for patients allowing them e.g. to make appointments at hospitals or outpatient clinics [9]. More advanced systems can provide users with personalized information and services facilitating access to their medical documents or interaction with medical personnel or equipment tracking their health condition.
2. **Connectivity and communications.** The second application of the Internet in medicine is in increasing the efficiency of healthcare operations. Internet-capable applications are able to electronically deliver medical records, claims submissions, referrals, eligibility verification, lab reports, prescriptions and other clinical and administrative data. Online teleconsultations between medical centers either in the well-known Web-based style or with the ability to conduct collaborative interactive work on shared medical data [8] can not only considerably decrease costs but also provide great educational opportunities.
3. **E-commerce.** The e-commerce segment of the Internet health industry generates the greatest opportunity for revenue. Pharmaceutical companies have recognized the value of this alternative marketing and distribution channel. Health-related e-commerce also encompasses other products, including health insurance and business-to-business services.

According to the above classification, the Konsul system (also referred as Konsul I) belongs to the 'Connectivity and communication' category. The system has been developed as a simple tool for radiology teleconsultations. Several hospitals from southern Poland occasionally direct difficult cases to the Krakow John Paul II Hospital in order to consult with specialists. Previously, this was done by burning and sending CDs with patient examinations or by transferring data via computer networks using general-purpose tools. As the solution was cumbersome, error-prone and consumed a lot of time and money, hospital technical staff decided to deploy a simple consultation environment facilitating such a process.

The architectural model of the Konsul system is very simple and consists of three main components running in a client-server schema. Each component has been shortly described below and their coupling is presented in Figure 1.

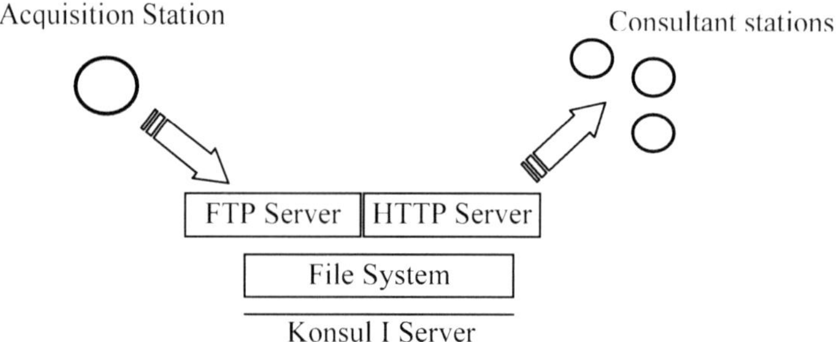


**Fig. 1.** The Architecture of the Konsul I system

- **Acquisition station** runs the FPImage tool, one of many existing DICOM viewers, which can, among others, convert DICOM images to various common data formats. The main advantage of FPImage, compared to other similar tools, is the built-in simple proprietary script language which allows users to customize the application behavior by writing their own programs. The language facilitates processing of loaded DICOM images, invoking operating system scripts and also contains an embedded FTP client. One of scripts supplied with the FPImage distribution converts DICOM files to AVI or JPEG formats, links the converted files to pre-generated HTML pages and sends them to a selected FTP server. Making cosmetic changes in the script has enabled us to use it for data acquisition.
- **Konsul system server** consists of an FTP server and an HTTP server. Patient examinations, sent via FTP, are stored in a filesystem, providing the interface used by the HTTP server. Finally, the HTTP server allows users to access data using Web browsers. As a security mechanism, an ordinary login/password method is used.
- **Consultant station** of the Konsul I system is an ordinary Web browser. Doctors consulting the delivered cases use it to download files to their personal computers. Occasionally, phone conversations with the ordering hospital are established to provide consulting specialists with additional information regarding the discussed case. The computer used for consultations is expected to have only a graphical Web browser and an AVI player installed – a requirement satisfied by nearly all of today's PC computer systems.

The FPImage application has been installed at peripheral hospitals and the FTP/HTTP server runs at the John Paul II hospital. The consultations soon became very popular, taking place even several times a day. It turned out that the system, initially treated a pilot implementation without attention to security, efficiency, ease of use, or user interfaces, now requires modifications and improvements. Below we present the results of an analysis performed according to the SAAM approach. The ATAM method seems to be too sophisticated for such a small system and thus has not been used.

## 4. SAAM Analysis of the Konsul I System

The following sections provide a detailed analysis of the architecture of the Konsul system according to the SAAM technique. As a result of the analysis, new architectures have been proposed.

### *4.1 SAAM Step 1 – Identify and Assemble Stakeholders*

Stakeholders are selected people responsible for using, maintaining and developing the system. They participate in subsequent steps of architecture analysis and evaluation. In the case of Konsul system, stakeholders are acquisition station users, doctors consulting the examinations, hospital personnel maintaining the system and developers.

### *4.2 SAAM Step 2 – Develop and Prioritize Scenarios*

In step 2 of the evaluation process, a detailed analysis of the system drawbacks has been performed. The most important points (referred to as *scenarios*) are depicted and commented below in the order of decreasing importance.

[S1] **No DICOM support.** Despite the fact that FPImage can handle DICOM files, the application is currently used only to convert the images into general-purpose formats. This is due to two main reasons. First, DICOMs are usually greater in size than compressed AVI/JPEG files, which may be burdensome in the case of slow network connections. Second, popular Web browsers do not provide generic support for the DICOM format and hence require a plugin.

[S2] **No security.** Neither FTP nor HTTP are secure. To provide a sufficient level of security of medical information, it is necessary to apply VPN or other security mechanisms. The scenario has been raised by all stakeholders.

[S3] **No additional information.** Lack of additional information describing patient cases is becoming more and more inconvenient as the number of consulted cases grows.

[S4] **No possibility for storing diagnosis.** Access to examinations is available only through static Web pages, which does not allow the consulting doctor to store any results of diagnoses. The scenario has been raised by the consultation specialists.

[S5] **Difficult concurrent access.** Web pages are generated entirely on the acquisition station and it is the client application which decides on the directory in which the data is to be stored. Consequently, the system is client-heavy, making it very difficult to enable users to run FPImage on more than one computer at a hospital. The scenario has been raised by the acquisition station users.

[S6] **Difficult system updates.** Sometimes it is necessary to make single corrections in HTML pages' appearance or functionality. This requires not only sending modified scripts to all acquisition stations but also making changes in stored examinations. The scenario has been raised by the system developers.

[S7] **Unstable work of FPImage.** Several crashes of FPImage have occurred. This scenario has been raised by the acquisition station users.

[S8] **No server-side features.** Examinations to be consulted are stored on the server in static directories and there is no easy way to indicate actions triggered by e.g. incoming data pieces. It is also not possible to prioritize the cases e.g. by an emergency state.

[S9] **No support for interaction.** The only possibility to exchange data during the consultation is through external tools, such as phone calls.

[S10] **No efficient search mechanism.** When the number of examinations stored on the server increases, it becomes more and more difficult to cope with the volume of data since the structure of directories is flat and examinations are available through lists. There is also no possibility to easily archive some older examinations and retrieve them if necessary.

[S11] **No support for various user interfaces.** It could sometimes be necessary to use the application on systems different than ordinary PCs – e.g. tablets or handhelds with a variety of display sizes. Web page appearance and presented images (in particular DICOMs or lossy compressed images) should be suited to such needs.

### *4.3 SAAM Step 3 – Describe Candidate Architecture(s)*

During the architectural analysis, two following approaches were proposed:
[A1] preserving the existing architecture of the Konsul system with all its advantages and disadvantages described above,
[A2] proposing a new architecture which best fits the scenarios described in step 2.

Preserving the existing architecture would lead to change of selected modules in order to match the presented requirements. Unfortunately, it is not possible to fulfill all of them easily, e.g. providing multi-user access would entail changing the interface between the FTP server and the acquisition client station, and, additionally, some minor changes in the Web server. Similarly, conformance of the user interface to different end-user devices could be implemented using e.g. XML technology, but this would imply different preprocessing of medical documentation in the acquisition station as well as exchanging ordinary Web server for some kind of application server supporting XML technology.

On the other side, the new architecture may benefit from using n-tier application architecture models, such as in J2EE or similar technologies which propose some well known frameworks and design patterns for creation of modern Web systems according to the SOA paradigm. Figure 2 depicts, the most common, 3-tier architecture of the server side.

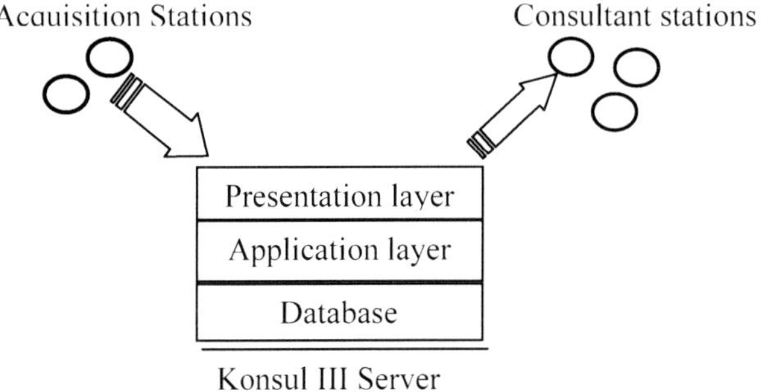


**Fig. 2.** General Architecture of the Konsul III System

The advantages of this architecture [A2] can be summarized as follows:

- an application is managed in a centralized way, making it easier to maintain current and implement new versions of the application,
- centralized management of data makes it easier to maintain its integration,
- the client side of the n-tier architecture is 'thin' i.e. it merely requires a \web browser,
- thin client architecture may easily support multi-user access to the system, different kinds of terminal devices as well as customization of user interface, making it very attractive for end users,
- the architecture provides well-known mechanisms to support security (e.g. through SSL and HTTPS protocols) for access to the Web server,
- this approach allows the client to read, update, and remove data on the server immediately, which greatly improves data integration and facilitates communication processes between clients.

It is worth noticing that changing the architecture of the system also alters the contents of data transferred between acquisition stations and the server. The advantage of Konsul I system is the conversion of DICOM images to one of general-purpose formats, performed by the acquisition stations just before data are sent to the server. This operation reduces the size of the data being sent, diminishing transfer costs. It is most important for small peripheral medical centers, with low budgets and low-bandwidth connections to the Internet. Of course, changing the format at the acquisition station implies that no user accessing the image can obtain the original DICOM image, regardless of their connection's bandwidth. Conversely, the new architecture, according to scenario [S11], requires the acquisition station to sent far larger DICOM images, but it also allows consultant stations to access them in any available format supported by the server.

### 4.4 *SAAM Step 4 – Classify Scenarios as Direct and Indirect*

The SAAM approach proposes dividing scenarios specified in step 2 into two categories: direct and indirect. Direct scenarios don't require modifications in the existing system and are usually easy to implement, while indirect scenarios require much more thorough changes.

Although it is, in principle, possible to implement almost all scenarios specified above by improving the existing architecture, such a solution seems to be burdensome and makes the resulting system extremely error-prone and hard to maintain.

Only scenario [S7] has been classified as direct, but because of the lack of organizational abilities, it must be left unimplemented. All the other scenarios are classified as indirect and are evaluated according to the SAAM analysis process in the following section.

### 4.5 *SAAM Step 5 – Perform Scenario Evaluation*

This step identifies changes and estimates the effort needed to modify the system in order to realize each scenario developed in step 2. The process of evaluation depends on the chosen architecture, hence for each particular scenario two descriptions will be presented in table 1.

**Table 1.** Evaluation of scenarios [S1]–[S11]

| | | **[A1] – Legacy architecture** | **[A2] – New architecture** |
|---|---|---|---|
| [S1] – No DICOM support | Affected components: | • acquisition station: modifying FPImage scripts for DICOM transfer support,<br>• Web server: Web control displaying DICOM images | • presentation layer: components processing/converting DICOM images,<br>• presentation layer: Web control displaying DICOM images |
| | Estimated effort: | • unstable work of FPImage makes it hard to estimate effort of modification of the scripts,<br>• using LEAD Tools[1] library for DICOM images processing – 1-2 person-months | • using LEAD Tools library for DICOM images processing for building application server components: 3-4 person-months<br>• Web control: same as in [A1] |
| [S2] – No security | Affected components: | • acquisition station: modifying FPImage scripts to support change of FTP server part of Konsul system,<br>• Web server: protecting access to the server using HTTPS protocol, supplying appropriate certificates for each consultant station | • supplying security subsystem throughout all components and layers of the server |
| | Estimated effort: | • a common way of ensuring security between the Web server and the Web browser – below 1 person-month | • all layers should be aware of the security subsystem, hence a lot of effort is needed |

[1] LEAD Tools Medical Toolkit is a commercial library for processing the DICOM file format.

| | | **[A1] – Legacy architecture** | **[A2] – New architecture** |
|---|---|---|---|
| [S3] – No additional information | Affected components: | • acquisition station: modifying FPImage scripts for uploading additional information,<br>• tool for gathering patient data | • application and presentation layer: data access components. |
| | Estimated effort: | • about 1 person-month | • it is a part of core functionality, hence it requires a lot of effort to develop. |
| | Remarks: | | read/write access to the system is its main functionality and includes: storing and retrieving diagnosis, DICOM files and other documentation. |
| [S4] – No possibility for storing diagnosis | Affected components: | • Web server: providing interface through CGI, PHP or servlets | same as [S3] |
| | Estimated effort: | • about 1-2 person-months | same as [S3] |
| | Remarks: | investing in development using outdated technologies seems to be impractical | |
| [S5] – Difficult concurrent access | Affected components: | • all excluding consultant clients | • application layer: components responsible for maintenance of session between server and client |
| | Estimated effort: | • complete rebuild of the system | • not much effort: below 1 person-month |
| | Remarks: | this is one of the main drawbacks of the architecture – providing concurrent access for users from one peripheral center implies a total redesign of the system due to the interface between the FTP and HTTP servers | it is a paradigm of the 'thin client' architecture |
| [S6] – Difficult system updates | Affected components: | • tool for automatic resending updated versions of the application to acquisition stations | • none |
| | Estimated effort: | • about 1-2 person-months | • not applicable |
| | Remarks: | this is one of the main drawbacks of the architecture – every modification in the system functionality requires resending improved versions to all acquisition stations | an immanent feature of the 'thin client' architecture is easy system update and modification; there is no need for any special component or tool |
| **[S7] – Unstable work of FPImage –** Direct scenario | | | |
| [S8] – No server-side features | Affected components: | • [option] FTP server: components providing event notification on data upload,<br>• [option] Web server: CGI or PHP scripts or servlets providing event notification on data upload | • application layer: event notification service,<br>• presentation layer: components providing access to the information about data modifications |
| | Estimated effort: | • below 1 person-month | • moderate: effort 2-3 person-months |
| | Remarks: | one of the above is needed to provide server-side notification on data upload; both of them seem to be inconvenient for development | |
| [S9] – No support for interaction | Affected components: | • additional tool for interactive communication loosely coupled to Konsul | • system for interactive communication tightly coupled to the server |
| | Estimated effort: | • not applicable | • a lot of effort due to sophisticated requirements, see [8] |

| | | | |
|---|---|---|---|
| | Remarks: | the most natural way to support interaction between consulting clients is to provide an additional tool such as Microsoft NetMeeting, Robust Audio Tool or any other | as in [8], providing interactive communication between consulting clients can be a convenient way for performing medical teleconsultations. Additionally, supporting it with a data access system like Konsul may be very valuable. |

| | | [A1] – Legacy architecture | [A2] – New architecture |
|---|---|---|---|
| [S10] – No efficient search mechanism | Affected components: | • Web server: CGI or PHP scripts or servlets providing search mechanisms | • application layer: searching engine components,<br>• presentation layer: components for presentation and filtering search results |
| | Estimated effort: | • little effort: below 1 person-month | • little effort: 1 person-month |
| | Remarks: | there are tools enabling website searches, but investing in development using outdated technologies seems to be impractical | there are components enabling website searches |
| [S11] – No support for various user interfaces | Affected components: | • none | • presentation layer: components for defining user and display profiles |
| | Estimated effort: | • not applicable | • moderate effort 2-3 person-months |
| | Remarks: | it is almost impossible to provide support for various user interfaces due to improper architecture; look at [S6] | common method making use of the XML technology |

## 4.6 SAAM Step 6 – Reveal Scenario Interactions

The goal of this step is to reveal relations between scenarios and components. A scenario affecting a number of components could indicate high coupling among components and may prove detrimental to the architecture. Whereas, if a component is affected by many scenarios, this could indicate a need to redesign the component [4]. As the presented system is small in size, it is practical to measure whether a component is referred to only by one or two scenarios and whether each scenario refers to no more than two components.

The evaluation of scenario interactions concerns two different architectures [A1] and [A2] and therefore is presented in two following tables:

**Table 2.** Scenario Interactions for Architecture [A1]

| [A1] – Legacy architecture | |
|---|---|
| **Component** | **Changes** |
| Acquisition station | [S1], [S2], [S3], [S4] |
| Web server | [S2], [S4], [S5], [S8], [S10] |
| Web control for DICOM processing | [S1] |
| Tool for gathering patient data | [S3] |
| Resending tool | [S6] |
| FTP server | [S8] |
| Tool for interactive communication | [S9] |

**Table 3.** Scenario Interactions for Architecture [A2]

| [A2] – New architecture | |
|---|---|
| **Component** | **Changes** |
| DICOM processing components | [S1] |
| Web control for DICOM processing | [S1] |
| Security subsystem | [S2] |
| Data access components | [S3], [S4] |
| Session maintenance components | [S5] |
| Event notification service | [S8] |
| Interactive communication system | [S9] |
| Searching engine components | [S10] |
| User interface profiling | [S11] |

Results of analysis confirm the earlier remarks about architecture [A1]. The main components, i.e. **acquisition station** and **Web server** require a redesign, as they are subject to change according to numerous scenarios: 4 and 5 respectively. Other components should be modified according to step 5. Moreover, scenarios [S1], [S2], [S3] and [S8] refer to more than one component. This excessive coupling of the components triggers a cascade of changes if any of the components should conform to the scenario.

On the other hand, architecture [A2] is properly divided on many loosely coupled components. In this case, **data access components** are the subject of change by two scenarios but this is a good indication, as scenario [S3] is a variant of scenario [S4]. Similarly, scenario [S1] affects **DICOM processing** and **Web control for DICOM processing** but it is justified, as those components are at the same (presentation) layer and are variants of the same functionality.

### *4.7 SAAM step 7 – Generate Overall Evaluation*

The SAAM analysis resulted in two different architectures: the legacy one [A1] and the new one [A2]. Preserving the legacy architecture clearly requires a redesign of the **acquisition station** and **Web server** components. Unfortunately, the redesign implies a complete rebuild of the whole system, which would take about 6–9 person-months. Moreover, the rebuilt system would resemble architecture [A2], but would be developed using outdated technologies. The other solution, architecture [A2], has a proper structure and passes SAAM analysis very well, but requires a lot of effort to implement (about 1.5 person-years).

Thus, to fulfill the stakeholders' expectations as well as time constraints, a tradeoff is proposed which assumes rapid implementation of Konsul II on the basis of the legacy architecture and, at the same time, development of the Konsul III system based on architecture [A2]. This approach is shown in figure 3 as the *new + enhance old* migration strategy [5]. The figure shows schematically the relation of the cumulative effort in time depending on various migration strategies. As may be seen, the overall costs of the tradeoff in short-term perspective would be greater than mere migration to Konsul II i.e. *slow migration* or building a new Konsul III system (*fast migration*) but are justified by achieving the most important goals (scenarios [S1], [S2] and [S3]) quickly and can be expected to pay off in the long run.

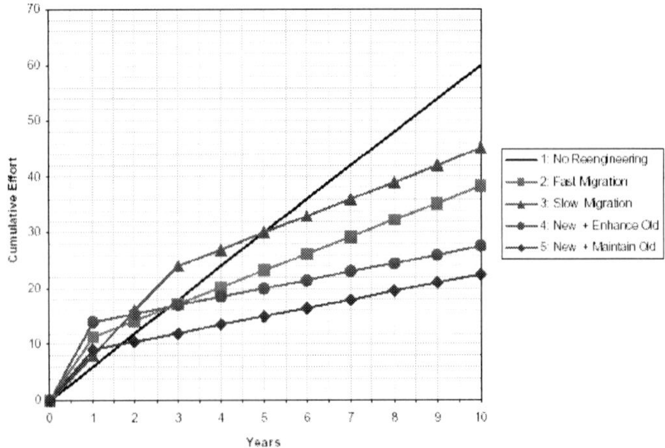


**Fig. 3.** Relation between cumulative effort in time depending on the strategy of migration

Obviously, such a general estimate as the one shown in Figure 3 should be treated very carefully due to different sizes of systems, needs of stakeholders or quality of legacy systems. Nevertheless, it shows certain tendencies and clarifies relations between the strategies.

The best long-term strategy (*new + maintain old*) has not been chosen due to transient nature of the pilot version of the implemented Konsul I system. In such a case, costs of maintenance and further data conversion grow rapidly.

## 5. Conclusions

Thanks to SAAM analysis, the effort required to modernize the Konsul system has been estimated, allowing developers to consciously take up intensive, albeit limited, tasks to develop and implement the Konsul II system as a transient application. Concurrently, Konsul III is being developed in a less time-critical fashion, since the most important expectations have been already satisfied. Thanks to such an approach, Konsul III as a quite large project can be developed in a long-term perspective, and built according to state-of-the-art architecture, easily extensible in the future. Konsul III is going to be a data starage subsystem of the TeleDICOM environment, designed for collaborative and interactive work on shared medical documents, as described in [8].

The analyzed Konsul system is a telemedical application, so particular attention has been paid to its security and providing diagnostic quality of images. While designing Konsul III – due to the expected growth of the system up to middle scale – scalability aspects have also been taken under consideration.

This paper only concentrates on one specific application, but we believe it can be helpful for people involved in software architecture migration in other areas as well.

## References


[1] R. Kazman, L. Bass, G. Abowd, M. Webb, *SAAM: A Method for Analyzing the Properties of Software Architectures*, Carnegie Mellon University

[2] R. Kazman, M. Klein, P. Clements, *ATAM: Method for Architecture Evaluation*, Technical Report, Carnegie Mellon University, August 2000

[3] R. Kazman, *Architecture Analysis – The SAAM-ATAM*, Carnegie Mellon University, 2000

[4] J.I. Hong, *Analysis of AOCS Framework*, Group for User Interface Research, University of California, Berkeley, USA

[5] W.A. Lobb, *Incrementally Migrating Semiconductor Equipment to a New Software Architecture*, Foliage Software Systems, March 2003

[6] S. McGeady, *The Internet as Disruptive Force in Healthcare*, Internet Technologies in Healthcare, Industry Report, 1999

[7] M. S. Pallos, *Service-Oriented Architecture: A primer*, eAI Journal, December 2001

[8] Ł. Czekierda, J. Cała, *TeleDICOM – environment for collaborative medical consultations*, Proceedings of International Conference on E-health in Common Europe, Kraków, Poland, June 2003.

[9] B. Kwolek, D. Radziszowski, P. Rzepa, *Transparent Public Access to Medical Services*, Proceedings of International Conference on E-health in Common Europe, Kraków, Poland, June 2003

# The Impact of Teleconsultations at a Referential Centre on the Management of Pulmonary Patients

Mariusz DUPLAGA[1], Jerzy SOJA[1], Jacek CAŁA[2], Mikołaj LESZCZUK[3], Dariusz WĄSOWSKI [1], Krzysztof SŁADEK [1], Krzysztof ZIELIŃSKI [2]

[1] *Department of Medicine, Jagiellonian University Medical College, Skawińska Str. 8, 31-066 Kraków, Poland, e-mail: mmduplag@cyf-kr.edu.pl*

[2] *Department of Computer Science, AGH University of Science and Technology, Mickiewicza Str. 30, 30-059 Kraków, Poland*

[3] *Department of Telecommunication, AGH University of Science and Technology, Mickiewicza Str. 30, 30-059 Kraków, Poland*

**Abstract.** Teleconsultation services at referential centres are an important area of telemedicine development. The implementation of such scenarios brings high-level competencies to peripheral hospitals through telecommunication links. Pulmonary teleconsultations were one of the key aspects of Krakow Centre of Telemedicine (KCT) activities conducted in 2002-2003. The role of the referential centre for respiratory medicine was played by the Division of Interventional Pulmonology, Jagiellonian University Medical College. Peripheral centres were pulmonary wards situated in local hospitals or policlinics located 20-80 km from Krakow. These hospitals were equipped with PC-based telemedical workstations and ISDN lines (256 kbps). Dedicated software (Telenegatoscope) was used for real-time discussions among physicians on medical images (X-rays, CTs) sent from peripheral centres to the referential centre. Images inserted in light boxes were cropped at peripheral centres with a high-resolution digital camera.

During the pilot phase, about 40 pulmonary patients were referred via telemedical links to the University Hospital. The frequency of soliciting a second opinion at the referential centre was analyzed for each main type of disease. Top positions are currently occupied by diagnoses of lung cancer, pleural fluid of unknown origin, asbestosis and tuberculosis. About 70% of the patients referred for virtual consultation were admitted for further diagnostics and treatment in an ambulatory or inpatient mode at the Division of Interventional Pulmonology. The review of teleconsultations results indicates that teleconferencing contacts, even if conducted through relatively limited bandwidth, may bring considerable benefits to patients requiring complex diagnostic and sophisticated, procedures available at the referential university hospital.

## Introduction

The process of developing telemedical services seems to be considerably influenced by external factors related to the status of the healthcare system in specific countries, the existence of organizational links between partners participating in telemedical contacts as well as the readiness of medical and managerial personnel to support such connections [1]. The Krakow Centre of Telemedicine has been designated as a Centre of Excellence in an attempt to establish pilot telemedical implementations in the Malopolska region, located in the southern part of Poland. The issue of telemedicine development remains a popular political buzzword in Poland, however not many initiatives are actually supported by the local or central authorities. The Centre has been established as a result of an initiative supported by medical and technical university partners interested in the progress in health telematics in this region [2]. Pulmonary medicine has become one of the priority areas for the activities undertaken by the Centre. Focusing on this medical speciality was due to several circumstances. First of all, the occurrence of malignant neoplams of the respiratory system is high in Poland due to high prevalence of smoking habits in the population. Furthermore, there are endemic areas of exposure to asbestos in the Malopolska region, covering mostly the locations of former industrial facilities using asbestos for production of construction elements. Currently, even if these factories are no longer active, the ecological devastation of the environment and exposure of local population to asbestos is tremendous. Second, the issue of limiting the occurrence of tuberculosis is pressing, particularly in the light of high incidence of multi-drug resistant tuberculosis in former Soviet Union countries and large numbers of people crossing the eastern border of Poland for economic reasons. Finally, most of the medical centres participating in the establishment of KCT are focused on the diagnostics and treatment of chest disorders.

The status of the healthcare system in Poland, more than 10 years after radical changes in the economy, is still unclear. The reform initiated in 1999 was focused on limiting unnecessary costs in healthcare institutions. Since that time, health professionals have remained under increasing pressure to decrease the duration of patient hospitalizations as well as to reduce their number. In this situation, smooth communications between local medical institutions, hospitals and policlinics and higher referential facilities at the University Hospital have become vital for competent dealing with complex, challenging cases. Furthermore, the distribution of advanced medical equipment is uneven in Poland and medical centres located in small or peripheral towns face essential problems with access to such procedures as computer tomography or magnetic resonance imaging. This is another important factor supporting the use of telemedical-type communications.

## 1. Development of a Telemedical Scenario for Pulmonary Medicine

### *1.1 The Framework of Activities Performed at the Krakow Centre of Telemedicine*

The Krakow Centre of Telemedicine was initially established as a Centre of Excellence within the SCI-TECH II project, carried out under the PHARE programme. It resulted from an initiative to proceed with pilot telemedical projects in southern Poland, maintained by medical and technical university partners in Krakow [3]. These partners represented the Jagiellonian University Medical College and the AGH University of Science and Technology. The activities of the centre were focused – from the beginning – on development of teleconsultation scenarios related to chest medicine as well as testing various telecommunications links for medical data transmission. An important part of these activities, performed at the Centre, was related to the establishment of a medical digital video library containing digitized procedures in the area of chest medicine, e.g. videothoracoscopies or bronchofiberoscopies. The medical digital video library was prepared as a tool supporting the development of multimedia patient records as well as a source of teleeducation activities addressed to medical students and physicians undergoing training in specialities related to chest medicine [4].

Teleconsultation scenarios were based mainly on communication between peripheral and referential centres or between invasive diagnostics labs and surgical departments. The activities performed within the Centre resulted in the implementation of several modes of teleconsultations, both in relation to their type (offline or real-time) and telecommunication links used for the transmission (broadband fiber-optic connections, ISDN lines, public telephony lines).

### *1.2 Pulmonary Teleconsultation Scenario – Organizational and Formal Requirements*

The teleconsultation scenarios developed in the Malopolska region were based on existing organizational links between local medical centres and the University Department. The University Hospital Departments focused on interventional pulmonology, maintaining vivid organizational connections with pulmonary departments at local hospitals situated outside Krakow. The scope of diagnostics and therapeutic options is usually quite limited in smaller peripheral or satellite hospitals, so they rely on close co-operation with the University Hospital or other metropolitan area hospitals. The selection of appropriate patients for interventional pulmonology procedures performed at the Department of Interventional Pulmonology was an important part of the teleconsultations performed during the pilot period. The procedures available at the University Department included videothoracoscopy, rigid bronchoscopy and bronchofiberoscopy combined with various methods of sampling (transbronchial needle aspiration performed under endobronchial ultrasonography guidance, transbronchial lung biopsy, broncho-alveolar lavage), bronchial stenting and imaging techniques (high-resolution computed tomography, spiral computed tomography, SPECT, NMR).

Through cooperation with the Krakow Centre of Telemedicine, peripheral hospitals were equipped with telemedical workstations enabling the exchange of data, images and personnel interaction, using existing telecommunication links in the most cost-effective way, adjusting for the organizational and formal requirements resulting from ongoing changes of the healthcare system financing mechanisms.

Several years of healthcare reforms have brought about a more active approach of health professionals and hospital managers to the use of new technologies for care deliver, although the reimbursement for telemedical services remains an unsolved issue in the current healthcare framework. Pulmonary teleconsultations developed by KCT could be perceived as a substitute for on-site consultations at referential centres, however, the healthcare funding system is not currently open to new options regarding intra-disciplinary services.

### *1.3 Telemedical Workstation*

The pilot scenarios developed within the activities of the Krakow Centre of Telemedicine were supposed to be replicated in other medical fields and centres. As health providers face substantial financial problems due to unclear healthcare regulations and ongoing reforms of the system adding to the failure of medical services reimbursement, the cost-effectiveness of the telemedical application proposed by the Krakow Centre of Telemedicine becomes one of the primary objectives. The use of off-the-shelf telemedical products offered by leading suppliers of Western European and American markets is not possible, as their prices would considerably exceed the resources available to Polish hospitals. This resulted in a maximum cost-effective strategy employed within the specification of the telemedical workstation to be used by peripheral/local medical facilities and the University Department. It encompasses a standard, off-the-shelf personal computer (the minimum requirements at the time of initial pilot implementations were: Pentium II 233 MHz or Pentium 200 MMX, 32 MB RAM, 21 MB of free hard disk space, two full-size PCI slots, a CD-ROM and a 3.5" FDD, a Direct-X-compliant VGA board with 8 MB RAM, a Sound Blaster 16-bit board compatible with speakers, Windows 95, Windows 98, Windows 2000 or Windows

NT 4.0, or above). The telemedical workstation was also equipped with multimedia peripherals: a digital camera for cropping still images (e.g. X-rays in a light box), a camcorder, an Internet camera and a beamer. The application supporting the transmission and real-time discussions on the exchanged digital images (Telenegatoscope) was developed and installed in teleconsultation workstations by computer scientists from the AGH University of Science and Technology, to avoid the relatively high costs of commercial products, whilst offering analogous functionality. Its concept resembles the "whiteboard" tools available in teleconferencing applications, however it also offers functions specific to medical teleconferences, as it enables the exchange of still images (X-rays, CT slides, ink drawings, textual data). The image acquired in the centre on one side of the teleconferencing connection is automatically sent to other side. Real-time discussions on specific images among professionals present on both sides of the teleconferencing transmission was enhanced with such options of the Telenegatoscope as online pointer synchronization on both sides, online marking and region of interest presentation, and multi-image support. The transmission of video and voice between teleconferencing sites was carried out with the use of a free application e.g. MS NetMeeting.

### *1.4 Telecommunication Links*

Most hospitals located in smaller cities in the Małopolska region do not have access to broadband fiber-optic connections. The cost-effective approach in this situation included the use of ISDN lines (Proszowice, Oswiecim) or PSTN (Medical Centre in Szczucin) to connect peripheral units with referential centres remaining within the Metropolitan Area Network in Krakow. The hospitals situated in Proszowice and Oswiecim were connected with the Metropolitan Area Network in Krakow through two ISDN lines (2 x BRA). The active device between the computer network (IP) and the ISDN network was a ZyXel Prestige 480 router with one Ethernet 10/100 Mbit/s interface along with two ISDN interfaces. At both peripheral locations, PC and ISDN routers were installed. Both external units were connected to the Academic Computer Centre CYFRONET through an ISDN network, where transmission was routed through an IP network established within the MAN to a referential centre located in Krakow. Such an approach resulted in the installation of routers only in peripheral medical centres and the Academic Computer Centre CYFRONET. The routers installed at the hospitals in Proszowice and Oswiecim were able to connect only with the router located at the Academic Computer Centre CYFRONET and only to the network designated for telemedical communications. The rules governing connecting and disconnecting, accompanied by security options, were enforced through appropriate router settings related to password-dependent user logging.

### *1.5 The Schedule of Teleconsultations*

Teleconsultations between the Respiratory Medicine Department of the University Hospital and pulmonology wards at hospitals located in Proszowice and Oswiecim were carried out every two weeks, or more frequently if an adequate number of cases could be accumulated. Teleconsultations with the Medical Centre in Szczucin, which is the epicentre of an area with a high prevalence of asbestos-related diseases in the Malopolska region, were performed less frequently, usually once a month. The time spent on presentations did not typically exceed 25 minutes per case and 90 minutes for one teleconsultation session.

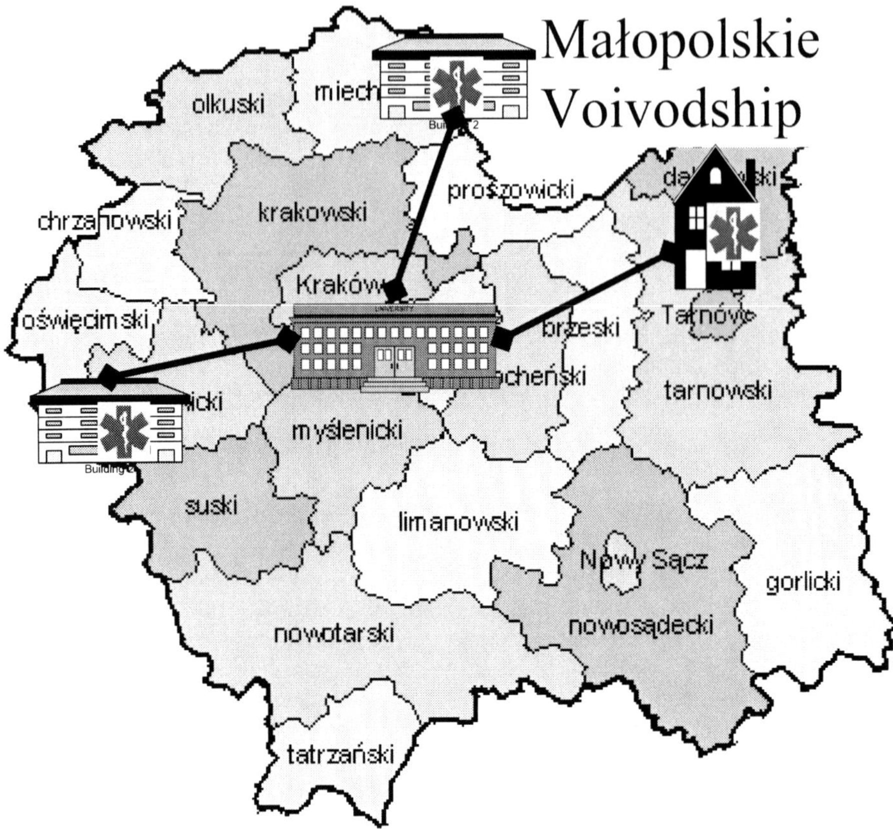


**Fig. 1.** The map of the Malopolskie region (voivodship) and relative location of peripheral medical centres and the University Hospital department participating in pulmonary teleconsultations

### *1.6 Patients*

The choice of cases for teleconsultations was dependent on the decisions of health professionals employed at each peripheral centre. The main criteria supporting the use of the teleconsultations scenario in specific cases included their complexity, lack of diagnostic options at the peripheral centre, lack of therapeutic options at the peripheral location or discussions regarding possible diagnostic and therapeutic modes.

## 2. Outcomes of Pulmonary Teleconsultations in the Pilot Period

In the pilot phase (between April 2003 and September 2003), 41 patients were referred from three peripheral locations in Proszowice, Oswiecim and Szczucin to the University Department of Interventional Pulmonology in Krakow. The range of medical problems presented during teleconsultations is shown in Table 1. The most common problems were related to a suspected malignant lung or pleural process, occult forms of tuberculosis or suspected atypical mycobacterial infection, asbestosis as well as inquiries to perform an extended diagnosis of persistent pleural fluid.

**Table 1.** The distribution of medical problems among the cases presented during teleconsultations between the peripheral sites and the referential centre.

| Initial diagnosis at the peripheral centre | % of cases |
|---|---|
| Lung or pleural neoplasm: pulmonary infiltration, pulmonary metastases with unknown primary focus | 22,0% |
| Pleural fluid – recurrent, of unknown origin | 14,5% |
| Asbestosis | 12,1% |
| Suspicion of tuberculosis without bacteriological confirmation, atypical mycobacterial infection | 9,8% |
| Recurrent episodes of haemoptysis | 9,8% |
| Chronic respiratory failure | 9,8% |
| Pulmonary embolism | 9,8% |
| Mediastinal tumor or enlarged lymph nodes | 7,3% |
| Disseminated pulmonary lesions | 4,9% |

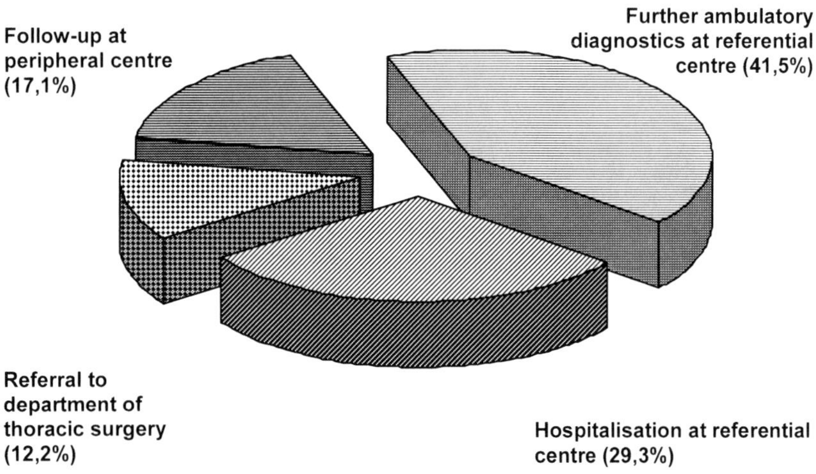


**Fig. 2.** A pie chart showing the outcomes of pulmonary teleconsultations carried out within the pilot activities of the Krakow Centre of Telemedicine

The direct impact of teleconsultations on diagnostics and treatment of patients in terms of organizational aspects is shown in Figure 2. From all patients referred for teleconsultation, 41.5% were selected for further diagnostic procedures performed in an ambulatory mode, in the diagnostic labs of the referential centre (e.g. bronchofiberoscopy with endobronchial ultrasonography, accompanied with transbronchial needle aspiration or transbronchial lung biopsy, computed tomography enabling the diagnosis of pulmonary embolus). Furthermore, 29.3% patients were admitted to the Department of Interventional

Pulmonology for videothoracoscopy procedures or extended diagnostic work-ups. Of all cases presented to the referential centre, 12.3% were further referred to thoracic surgery departments located in Krakow and Zakopane for operational, diagnostic or therapeutic procedures. Only 17.1% of cases remained in diagnostic, treatment or ambulatory control at the peripheral centres.

## 3. Discussion

The outcomes of pulmonary teleconsultations carried out during the pilot phase reveal good understanding of the appropriate use of a telemedical framework by medical personnel in the context of cooperation between peripheral and referential centres. From all patients presented during teleconsultation sessions more than 70% were accepted for hospitalization or further diagnostics on an ambulatory basis at the University Departments. This seems to confirm the appropriate selection of cases for teleconsultations by physicians employed at peripheral centres.

In Poland, access to advanced diagnostic and therapeutic procedures in medical centres (hospitals, policlinis) located some distance from main metropolitan areas is generally limited. The efficiency of specialized diagnostics depends heavily on smooth cooperation between peripheral medical units and referential centres. Experience from other areas shows the usefulness of telemedical applications for the improvement of access to more sophisticated medical procedures for patients from peripheral or rural regions [5] [6].

The value of pooled multidisciplinary competencies is another important aspect explored in telemedical implementations [7]. Referential centres, especially those based at the University Hospitals, are usually able to assemble a multidisciplinary team in place during teleconsultations, to establish a consistent diagnostic and therapeutic approach in cases requiring integrated care or a multifaceted view of the medical problem.

IT tools supporting pulmonary teleconsultations performed in the range of the Krakow Centre of Telemedicine activities were relatively simple and inexpensive. The use of a cost-effective approach assuring appropriate quality of transmission and safety of physicians' decisions is perceived as key factor influencing the promotion of telemedical applications in developing countries. However, even a simple and inexpensive information infrastructure may be effectively used for enhancement of communications among health professionals [8], [9].

The attitude of health professionals to the use of telemedical systems in medical practice is not homogenous. The role of "leaders" interested in the use of the tools offered by telematics is vital for the success of the implementation process in specific medical environments. The level of acceptance depends strongly on the existing working contacts between medical units and health professionals, who in a natural way, adopt the IT infrastructure as an extension of other, pre-existing channels of communication. A substantial obstacle to telemedical contacts between professionals on different referential levels is the fear of revealing existing practices at smaller centres. Younger physicians are usually more open to such communications, as they perceive it as an opportunity to continue their medical education.

Teleconsultation scenarios in pulmonary medicine have been developed not only as a substitute for existing organizational links between medical institutions, but also as an attempt at improving pulmonary care. The improvement of care is related to enhanced access to invasive/operational procedures for patients from peripheral or rural areas and better allocation of resources (optimized use of health personnel time, lowering the transportation costs, optimization of diagnostics and therapy through contacts with referential centres, etc.) [10].

The legal status of telemedical services is still unclear in many countries. However, the use of a telemedical infrastructure for communications among health professionals does not seem to be as legally controversial (according to Polish legislation) as electronic communications between patients and physicians [11]. Obviously, existing regulations do not follow the changes occurring in the approach to health services delivery resulting from the new models of care and the use of modern technologies. Formal recognition of telemedical services would be an essential argument for the development of efficient reimbursement mechanisms.

## 4. Conclusions

The deep economic transformation initiated in Poland in the early 90s does not translate directly into improvements of the status of the healthcare system. Numerous medical institutions experience substantial problems in adjusting to new management challenges and requirements brought by consecutive reforms of the healthcare system. Teleconsultation scenarios developed under the auspices of the Krakow Centre of Telemedicine are an attempt at demonstrating a new approach to health services delivery through the use of IT tools. Telemedical applications may be particularly valuable in priority healthcare areas, such as oncological care or chronic disease management. Pulmonologists deal with several types of medical problems essential from the perspective of public health. These problems include the screening and early diagnostics of lung cancer, treatment of patients with multi-drug tuberculosis, long-term care delivered to patients with chronic obturative disease (bronchial asthma, COPD) or assuring appropriate care to a population with high prevalence of asbestos-related respiratory disorders. The outcomes of teleconsultations carried out in the pilot phase has revealed that this type of communications among health professionals representing medical units on different referential levels may have considerable influence of the quality of pulmonary care.

## References

[1] Duplaga M., Radziszowski D., Dul M., Nawrocki P., Zieliński K.: Technical and Non-technical Factors Influencing the Process of Teleconsultation Services Development Carried Out in the Krakow Centre for Telemedicine. Tromso Telemedicine Conference, Tromso, Norwegia, Proc. TTC 2003

[2] Duplaga M.: Developing Supportive Environment for e-Health in Conditions of Economy Transformation" e-He@lth in Common Europe 2003 Kraków, pp. 251-260

[3] Zieliński K.: Krakow Center of Telemedicine – Developing the Platform for Regional Telemedical Networks" Ed.: K. Zielinski, M. Duplaga. Proc. of 1 Int. Conf. on e-He@lth in Common Europe 2003 Kraków, pp. 19-27

[4] Duplaga M., Dańda J., Juszkiewicz K., Leszczuk M., Łoziak K., Papir Z., Sikora M., Szczepański D., Watza R.:Digital Video Library for Presentation of Thoracic Medicine Resources. Telemed J e-Health 2003; 9(Suppl 1): S39-40.

[5] Agha Z., Schapira R.M., Varkey B., Frahm J.A., Dunn D.E.: Telemedicine for delivery of pulmonary outpatient care to a rural site: a cost analysis. J General Intern Med. 2000; 15(1): 97

[6] Pacht E.R., Turner J.W., Gailiun M., Violi L.A., Ralston D., Mekhjinan H.S., StJohn R.C.: Effectivenesss of telemedicine in outpatient pulmonary clinic. Telemed J 1998; 4: 287-293

[7] Davison A.g., Eraut C.D., Khan N., Haque S., Tanqueray A., Trask C.W., Lamont A., Uppal R., Sharma A.: Telemedicine for lung cancer: A new multidisciplinary approach. Thorax 1999; 54(3): 73

[8] Larson A., Lynch D.A., Zeligman B.: Accuracy of diagnosis of subtle chest disease and subtle fractures with a teleradiology system. Am J Roentgenol 1998; 170: 19-22

[9] Xu Z., Yamauchi K., Ikeda M., Yang S., Hasegawa Y.: Evaluation of a PC-Based teleconferencing system for reading chest radiographs. J Telemed Telecare 1999; 5: 1222-1225

[10] Duplaga M.: Could telemedical systems improve the quality of health care. Proc. Conf. Information and quality in healthcare. Kraków, April 9-11 2003, pp. 103

[11] Budyn M., Duplaga M.: Legal aspects of telemedical systems development. Part I. Health and Management 2002; IV(2): 45-52

# Web Access to Data in a Mobile ECG Monitoring System[1]

Jimena RODRIGUEZ, Lacramioara DRANCA, Alfredo GOÑI
and Arantza ILLARRAMENDI
*University of the Basque Country (UPV/EHU). LSI Department.*
*Donostia-San Sebastián, Spain*
*http://siul02.si.ehu.es*

**Abstract.** Cardiovascular diseases and, in particular, diseases related to arrhythmias are a problem that affects a significant percentage of the population, being one of the major causes of death in Europe. New advances in the fields of PDAs, mobile phones, wireless communications and vital parameter sensors have permitted the development of revolutionary medical monitoring systems, which strikingly improve the lifestyle of patients. However, not all those monitoring systems provide patients with real assistance – anywhere and at any time. We have developed a system that goes a step further than the previous approaches, being designed to capture, record and, as a distinctive feature, locally analyze the ECG signals in a PDA carried by the patient. In that sense, the system has a decision support module based on decision tree methods that can detect, with high precision, any arrhythmias that the user may be suffering. Alarms can then be activated in time to alert a medical center in order to provide the proper medical assistance. One of our aims when building the system has been to optimize limited and expensive resources like PDA memory size and wireless communication costs. Moreover, accessibility is also an important feature of the system that has been achieved by the development of web services to query the data computed in the PDA. In this way, authorized personnel (physicians and relatives) can easily obtain access to that data.

## Introduction

Traditionally, Holter recording has been used during normal patient activity to record the cardiological signal called the electrocardiogram (ECG). A Holter is a small, mobile and light device that records – during a period of 24 or 48 hours – ECG signals which are later analyzed at the hospital [1]. Although this solution carries the advantage of enabling patients to continue living a normal life at their homes, it also presents a serious drawback: if the patient suffers from a serious rhythm irregularity, the Holter only makes a recording of it for later diagnosis, but it does not react to it in real time.

Innovations in the fields of PDAs, mobile phones, wireless communications and vital parameter sensors have permitted the development of revolutionary medical monitoring systems, which strikingly improve the lifestyle of patients, offering them security even outside the hospital. In this regard we can mention, for example, modern mobile phones e.g the Vitaphone [2] which, in case of an emergency, can record the signals through metal electrodes situated on its back and transmit them to the cardiac monitoring center situated at the hospital. There are other commercial monitoring systems that use PDAs to store ECG signals, e.g. Ventracor [3] and Cardio Control [4]. For these systems, additional features

[1] This work was mainly supported by the University of the Basque Country, and the Diputación Foral de Gipuzkoa (co-supported by the European Union)

like GSM/GPRS transmission to an analyzing unit are also being developed. These systems continuously send ECGs to a health center through a wireless communication network, enabling the signals to be analyzed.

In the monitoring research area, several research projects stand out, such as: @Home [5], TeleMediCare [6], or PhMon [7], whose aims are to build platforms for real time monitoring. Those systems perform some local real-time monitoring in computers *near* the patient, in order to detect some anomalies and send alarms to a control center or a hospital. However, we have not been able to find precise descriptions of what kind of ECG analysis is performed exactly in any of these local computers.

In spite of the advantages the above mentioned systems provide in relation to holters, they still present problems related to the fact that a complete ECG analysis is not performed in the place where the signal is acquired. Therefore, there is a loss of efficiency in the use of the wireless network because normal ECGs are also sent (and wireless communications imply a high cost); and when the wireless network is not available (e.g. in a tunnel, in an elevator, etc.), there might be some loss of the ECG signal, with the corresponding risk of not detecting some anomalies.

Our proposal, the MOLEC[2] system, is a solution that allows continuous ECG monitoring of patients outside the hospital, in their normal lives by locally analyzing the ECG signal in a PDA carried by the patient and by quickly communicating possible emergencies to an alarm center. Moreover, it provides physicians with all the necessary information for fast and correct diagnostics and it also gives authorized relatives information about the current health state of the patient.

The main goal of this paper has been to investigate that last part of the system: the possibilities of accessing PDA data through the web. In order to do that we have defined a set of web services, implemented them in different components of the MOLEC system and obtained some performance measures with the aim of choosing the best architectural alternative to deploy the web services.

The next section of the paper is devoted to explaining the global architecture of MOLEC (section 1). Afterwards, we detail the MOLEC's patient tool (section 2) and MOLEC's surveillance server (section 3) with the additional web services that they provide. Next, considerations relating to performance and availability of web services are discussed (section 4) and, finally, some conclusions are presented.

## 1. Global Architecture of MOLEC

The main components of the proposed architecture appear in Figure 1. The *MOLEC Monitor* is a standard PDA (handheld computer) that acquires signals sent by ECG sensors carried by the users. The *MOLEC Monitor* is not only capable of storing the ECG signal like Holter does, but it is in fact an embedded real-time system that captures, processes, detects, analyzes and communicates possible dangerous abnormalities to an alarm center through the network from anywhere and at any time. It also maintains a small, database (referred to as local database) with references to compressed signal files and details of abnormal ECG events so the physicians can find out valuable information regarding recent cardiac activity of the patient.

---

[2] MOLEC stands of "Monitorización On-Line de Enfermos del Corazón" (On-Line Monitoring of Herat Patients)

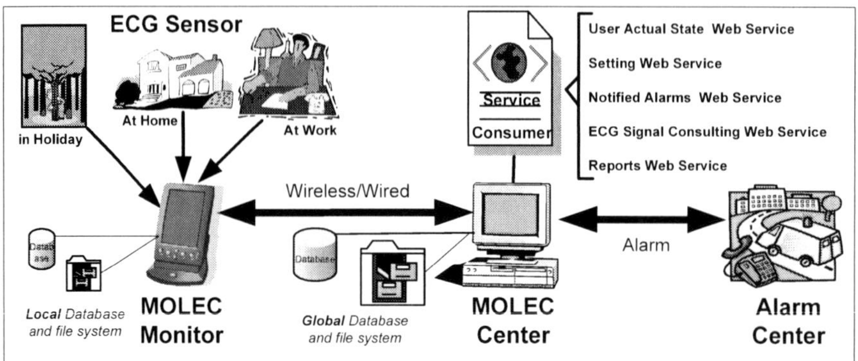


**Fig. 1.** Architecture of MOLEC

The *MOLEC Center* is the system part that manages communications with all the PDA monitors and updates the MOLEC Center's database (referred to as global database) with new information that it receives from each of them. Moreover it acts as an intermediary between a PDA and the alarm center (when alarm events are detected) and provides various types of information about the monitored users through specialized web services. The *Alarm Center* receives all the risk alarms detected by the PDA, in order to react and immediately provide proper medical assistance.

## 2. MOLEC Monitor

The MOLEC Monitor has a modular implementation where each module corresponds to a distinct task that the PDA performs. A brief description of each module is provided below (for more details refer to [8] and [9]).

The *ECG Signal Acquisition Module* manages communication between the PDA and the ECG sensors in order to receive the ECG signal and convert it into a signal understandable by the entire system. Thus it acts as a mediator between the PDA and the ECG sensors so that the system may be adapted to any type of ECG sensors.

The *Data Preprocessing Module* analyzes the ECG signal in order to detect the beats and their typical segments (wave events). Arrhythmia detection requires prior identification of the presence or absence of some wave events: the points where P, QRS and T waves start and finish, as well as their peaks. For the implementation of this module we have used the ECGPUWAVE tool [10] that extracts the wave events of an ECG signal, and we have built an automaton that divides the signal into a sequence of beats.

The *Decision Support Module* is the module in charge of arrhythmia detection. Two main steps take place during this analysis: identification of beat types and classification of the arrhythmias. In order to classify the beats we have used a method based on decision trees. The learned functions are represented by a set of *if-then* rules to improve human readability. Those rules have been extracted, codified in a programming language and tested. The validation of the previously-generated rules takes place using the hold-out validation mechanism. In order to classify the rhythms, we have used a combination of cardiologic and inferring rules. Cardiologic rules were obtained through the translation of the arrhythmia descriptions found in specialized cardiologic literature and in parallel, we have obtained inferring rules by using techniques based on decision trees. Subsequently, we combined them and chose the best rules to detect each rhythm. Further details on this process can be found in [8].

The *Interface Module* is responsible for signal visualization and analysis results display. Figure 2 shows a picture of real-time analysis in the PDA. It provides a friendly interface that draws the ECG signal as soon as the current beat and rhythm types are obtained online by the Decision Support Module.

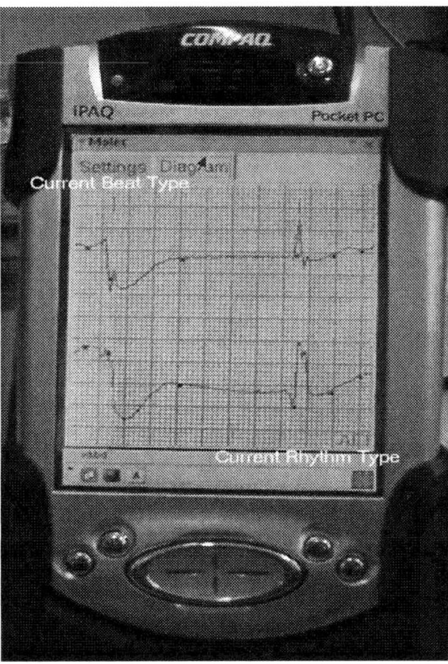


**Fig. 2.** ECG visualization in MOLEC Monitor

The *Alarm Manager Module* receives the current heart rhythm detected by the decision support module and decides whether to generate an alarm and to send the corresponding ECG signal. Not all arrhythmias should be sent in real time to cardiologists for immediate responses: we only need to send those, that are considered dangerous. With the help of some cardiologists, we have identified two groups, one for high-risk arrhythmias, that is, arrhythmias that should be communicated to the alarm center as soon as they are detected by the system, and another one, for moderate-risk arrhythmias and normal rhythms that are stored but not immediately communicated.

The *Communication Module* manages all communication between the MOLEC Monitor and the MOLEC Center using web services that each of them implements.

The goal of the *Data Manager Module* is to efficiently manage the restricted memory resources available in the PDA, at least when compared to the great capacity of ECG sensors to generate data.

We have chosen the compressed XML file format to locally store ECG signals. XML files offer an appropriate method to store the ECG signals together with the detected annotations. They also permit easy exchange of the data and support a very good compression ratio. In this way the amount of data is significantly reduced which is important, not only due to the limited memory of the PDA, but also for reducing communication costs. These files are managed through a local database that stores references to all of them, thus permitting quick retrieval of any signal. An example of an XML file that contains the information of an ECG signal appears in Figure 3.

```
<?xml version="1.0"?>
<signal>
    <header>
        <patient>207</patient>
        <frequency>360</frequency>
        <no_samples>1054</no_samples>
        <gain>200</gain>
        <channels>1</channels>
        <baseline>1024</baseline>
    </header>
    <data>
        <samples annotation="V">
            <channels0 rel="1061">0 </channels0>
        </samples>
        <samples>
            <channels0 rel="1061">0 -3 2 4 6 7 7 5 7 8 9 12 12 22 23 27 28 26 23
            </channels0>
        </samples>
    </data>
</signal>
```

**Fig. 3.** XML representation of an ECG signal fragment with annotations

In case of a detection of anomalous beat and rhythm, the relevant information is also stored in the local database. Thus, the physician can query it and obtain information about the evolution of the monitored user. At this point, we assume that physicians only make queries about abnormal beats and rhythms.

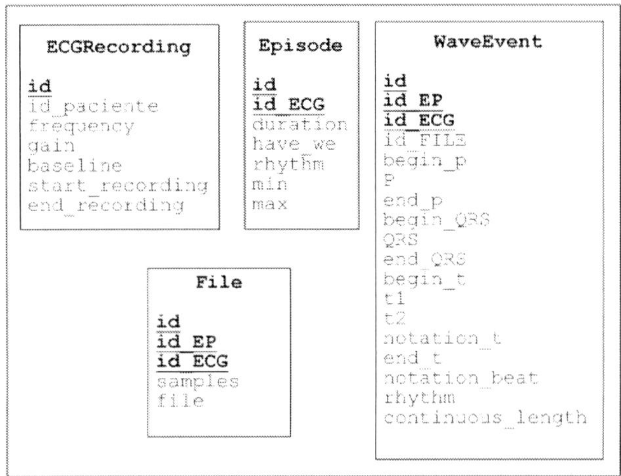


**Fig. 4.** Database of the MOLEC Monitor

Figure 4 presents the structure of the database used. The ECGRecording table identifies continuous monitoring intervals. The Episode table stores information on the different rhythm changes that the monitored user suffers during each monitoring interval. The WaveEvent table registers information about anomalous beats. Finally, the File table maintains the references to all signal files located in the PDA.

The possibility to query the database is offered by the system through a set of web services as explained in the next section.

## 3. MOLEC Center

The main tasks that are carried out at the MOLEC Center are the following: 1) to manage communication with all PDA Monitors; 2) to forward alarm messages that PDA Monitors send, and 3) to offer information about the monitored users through *web services*. Web services allow the actors who query the system to quickly obtain actualized reports from information processed in the PDA through a simple web page. These reports vary, depending, on the one hand, on the required detail level and, on the other hand, on the access level to the system. We have chosen web services to expose the functionality of MOLEC because they make use of standard technologies that reduce heterogeneity and facilitate application integration [11]. These web services supplied by the system are described below.

### *3.1 Reports Web Service*

Specialized literature [12] associates the functionality of holters with a set of reports, which enable physicians to analyze data easily and quickly. Commercial products also offer various kinds of reports. The MOLEC system supplies a set of reports, which include the information that the previous reports provide. The reports are offered through the Reports Web Service in order to answer queries commonly asked by physicians. Moreover, they offer the possibility of obtaining *updated* information about the cardiac activity of the monitored user in *real time* through a simple web page.

Three are kind of reports offered by MOLEC:

1. The *Arrhythmia Identification* report shows the different rhythm types that the user suffers during a monitoring period and the number of episodes involved for each rhythm with the corresponding duration as well as minimum and maximum frequency.
2. The *ST Segments Evolution* report informs about the behavior of the T wave, which is relevant when detecting isquemic episodes. We identify six different morphologies for the T wave and inform about the occurrence number of each of them.
3. The *Abnormal Beats Detail* report informs about the abnormal beats discovered in the ECG signal. This report is the most complex and costly one. The queries formulated to supply this kind of report depend on the origin of the beats that can be ventricular (corresponding to beat types V, !, E and e) or supraventricular (corresponding to beat types S, F, a and J) and offer details on the beat types involved, on whether they are isolated or not, and if not - on the number of consecutive beats. An example of this type of query is presented below for a ventricular origin (V, !, E or e) of the beat and performed for patient number 207 of the MIT-BIH [13].

**Table 1.** Detail of abnormal ventricular beats

```
SELECT w.rhythm, w.notation_beat, w.continuous_ length, count(*)
FROM ECGRecording e, Episode p, WaveEvent w
WHERE e.id_patient = 207 and e.id = p.id_ECG and
            p.id = w.id_EP and (w.notation_beat = "V" OR
            w.notation_beat = "E" OR w.notation_beat = "!" OR
            w.notation_beat = "e" ) and end_recording is null
GROUP BY w.id_EP, w.continuous_ length
```

The resulting columns show the rhythm and beat type and the length of a continuous sequence and the number of its occurrences. Note that this query involves an actual monitoring sequence (as the end_recording is null).

### *3.2 User Current State Web Service*

The aim of this web service is to inform about the current state of the monitored user at the current moment (whatever the user's location). It offers information about the user's current rhythm, cardiac frequency and the rhythm duration. This kind of service is mostly intended for relatives. One possible extension of this could consist of sending the latest changes in the monitored user state to the family using SMS messages.

### *3.3 Notified Alarms Web Service*

This web service supplies information about the problems that the user may have experienced during a certain monitoring period. More exactly, it informs of the alarms that the system has communicated to the Alarm Center, including the type and duration of each episode and the moment when they took place.

### *3.4 ECG Signal Consulting Web Service*

The ECG Signal Consulting Web Service permits authorized agents to obtain parts of the ECG signal registered from a certain patient for printing and extra analysis. The response latency for this service depends on whether the signal in question has already been transferred from the PDA to the MOLEC Center (e.g. with an alarm message) or not. This type of request could increase wireless communication costs with the MOLEC Monitor if the requested signal part is still in the PDA. Nevertheless it is expected that physicians will only ask for a signal segment still placed into the PDA if they consider it relevant to a fast diagnosis, after analyzing the previous reports that MOLEC offers.

### *3.5 Setting Web Service*

This service gives the physician the capability of setting a set of parameters for a monitored user. In this way, the service responds to several needs, such as: diagnosis verification, medicine dosage adjustment or alarm notification policy setting.

For example, in the case of the alarm notification policy setting, physicians could customize the standard alarm cases set for a monitored user. They could increase this set by adding new alarm cases to be acted upon or, on the contrary, to consider that some alarm cases occur fairly often for that particular user and should be communicated only if they exceed a certain duration.

## 4. Web Services in MOLEC System: Access Performance and Availability

The web services mentioned previously are provided by the MOLEC System in order to allow authorized actors to obtain information processed in the MOLEC Monitor independently of its location. Issues like response latency and communication costs are taken into account in order to define a proper communication and web service allocation policy so that the system can supply promptly and at any time the widest spectrum of information possible, in response to the formulated queries. In this sense we have tested two types of approaches: PDA-oriented vs. PC-oriented web services, using as test case the reports web service presented above.

### *4.1 Two Approaches: PDA-oriented vs. PC-oriented Web Services*

In the *first approach,* the reports web service is offered by the PDA (see figure 5) where the XML-RPC Server is located. This approach implies that the PDA receives the service request, processes the SQL query over the local database and sends the answer back to the Service Consumer to be displayed.

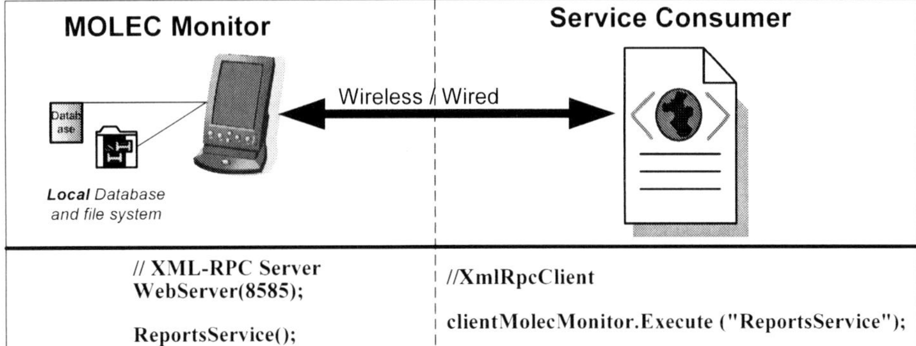


**Fig. 5.** Web Service Report invoked in the PDA

In the *second approach* the web service report is offered by the MOLEC Center (see figure 6) where an XML-RPC server is located. In this case, the MOLEC Center would be the one that responds to requests solicited by external actors. Thus it invokes a transfer database web service offered by the PDA in question, updating the global database, and processes the SQL query over this database.

The performance aspects of this approach are influenced by the volume of data to be transferred from the PDA to the MOLEC Center. We have considered several scenarios of data distribution at the moment of the request: 1) the entire database placed in the PDA; 2) 90% of the database already transferred to the MOLEC Center; 3) half of the database already at the MOLEC Center.

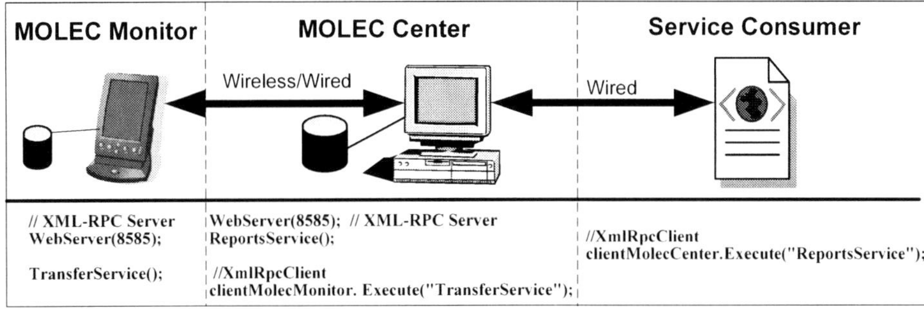


**Fig. 6.** Web Service Report invoked at the MOLEC Center

Before presenting the performance results for each approach, we have to mention the technologies used for the tests. Previous figures show that services offered by both approaches use the XML-RPC. It is a lightweight solution (compared with standard web services – WSDL and SOAP), that we found easy to deploy in our system, and that allows monitoring and the simultaneous remote invocation in the PDA. The PDA used for these tests was an IPAQ 3970 with Linux OS and SQlite, an embeddable SQL database engine.

### 4.2 Test Results without Monitoring

The latency of the responses for different types of queries when PDA monitoring was stopped is reflected in Figure 7.

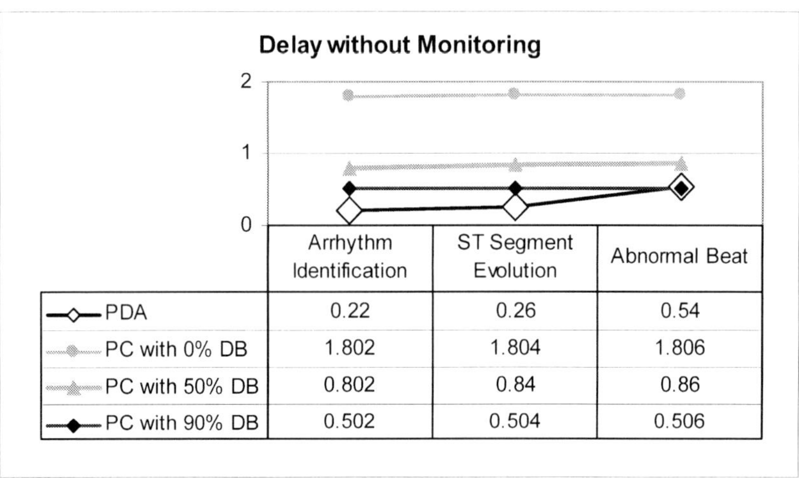


| | Arrhythm Identification | ST Segment Evolution | Abnormal Beat |
|---|---|---|---|
| PDA | 0.22 | 0.26 | 0.54 |
| PC with 0% DB | 1.802 | 1.804 | 1.806 |
| PC with 50% DB | 0.802 | 0.84 | 0.86 |
| PC with 90% DB | 0.502 | 0.504 | 0.506 |

**Fig. 7.** Query response delay using a database that contains ½ hour monitoring data and with no monitoring by the PDA

It can be seen that, without performing the monitoring process, the delay of the query response when the SQL query is performed in the PDA and the case of a PC with 90% of the database are similar. In the other two cases, the delay obtained increases proportionally with the amount of information that has to be transferred. Obviously, these results may vary according to the available bandwidth. For the tests we have used Bluetooth which offers a bandwidth of up to 1Mb/sec which is an intermediary value between those offered by GPRS and UMTS.

### 4.3 Test Results with Monitoring

The response latency can increase drastically when monitoring is performed in parallel by the PDA or when the database size increases. Moreover, the way each method affects the monitoring process also has to be considered. The results for the same set of tests but with the PDA performing the monitoring process can be observed in Figure 8.

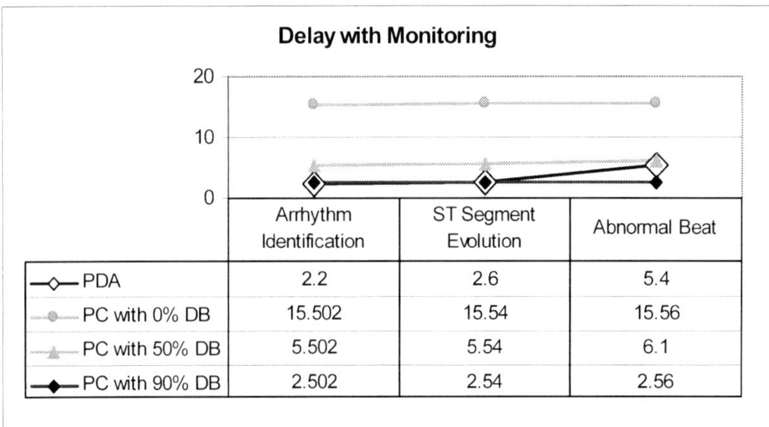


| | Arrhythm Identification | ST Segment Evolution | Abnormal Beat |
|---|---|---|---|
| PDA | 2.2 | 2.6 | 5.4 |
| PC with 0% DB | 15.502 | 15.54 | 15.56 |
| PC with 50% DB | 5.502 | 5.54 | 6.1 |
| PC with 90% DB | 2.502 | 2.54 | 2.56 |

**Fig. 8.** Query response delay for ½ hour monitoring database

In this case it is clear that the monitoring process affects each query response. The delays are appreciably greater than in the previous scenario, when monitoring was not being performed.

### *4.4 Comparison between the PDA and PC Alternatives, with Monitoring*

With respect to the PDA-oriented web services case, the previously-considered example gives acceptable results when monitoring is on, however, we have also tested larger databases and verified that response delays increase. In particular, for the abnormal beat report, we have observed delays of up to 30 seconds for databases that contain information from eight hours of monitoring, and the monitoring process itself is affected considerably. With regard to the availability of the service, if the wireless communication is not available at that moment, the external actor querying the system would receive no response.

The best solution, according to the delays obtained in the previous tests, seems to be to deploy the web services at the MOLEC Center and to have the greater part of the database there. This solution has additional advantages in case of further consecutive requests because no additional information would be necessary to be transferred from the PDA. In this way, response time would decrease to values on the order of milliseconds. Moreover, the transfer data service gives the possibility of removing some data from the PDA database once it is sent, optimizing the use of the limited PDA memory. With regard to the availability of the service, it is guaranteed because the MOLEC Center can always offer at least a partial response, even if the transfer of data from the PDA is not possible at any given moment.

Nevertheless, if we compare the two alternatives from the point of view of communication costs, the PDA-oriented web services case seems to be more economical because only a response to a query is sent through the wireless network, while in the PC-oriented web services case, all the information from the PDA database is sent. In the first case, communication costs increase with the number of queries made to the system, while in the second case the costs are static (depending only on the amount of abnormal episodes that the monitored user suffers). If the physicians use the web services often, then the second approach (web services at the MOLEC Center) would require lower communication costs.

Therefore, at this moment, although it would be technically possible to answer SQL queries required by the web service from the PDA, the involved delays, service availability and the impact on the monitoring process performance of the PDA makes this option impractical. Our proposal consists on locating most of the web services that the system offers close to external actors at the Monitoring Center and on limiting the web services that the PDA provides according to its processing capabilities and wireless communication availability. This solution assumes not only the presence of a transfer database web service in the PDA but also a policy of updating the global database with the latest data from the PDA (e.g. when the PDA database reaches a predetermined volume or when an alarm occurs[3]). One exception could be made for the Setting and User's Current State Services that are more connected with PDA processing and, additionally, less costly (with regard to both communications and processing costs).

## 5. Conclusions

Monitoring systems, that provide assistance anywhere and at anytime, are of great interest nowadays, particularly for people who suffer from arrhythmias. The use of small but powerful computers (like PDAs) with wireless interfaces permits us to define architectures where local, real-time ECG monitoring is performed.

Moreover, the accessibility of the information generated by this kind of monitoring is guaranteed by a web service integration approach. In this way, physicians and relatives can quickly obtain relevant information on the cardiac activity of the monitored user.

A set of web services has been defined, implemented and several tests have been performed in order to decide upon the best localization of web services in our architecture.

Although, at this moment, it would be technically possible to deploy all the web services at the PDA, it is better to deploy some of them on an intermediary element (like our MOLEC Center) in order to obtain better performance and better availability, as well as to avoid degrading the monitoring process at the PDA.

## References

[1] Despopoulos, A, Silbernagl, S. 1994, Texto y Atlas de fisiología. ISBN: 84-8174-040-3.

[2] Daja, N., Relgin, I., Reljin B., 2001. Telemonitoring in Cardiology –ECG transmission by Mobile Phone. Annals of the Academy of Studenica 4, 2001.

[3] Ventracor Limited. 2003 *http://www.ventracor.co*

[4] Cardio Control.2003. *www.cardiocontrol.com/cardio.htm*

[5] Dimitri Konstansas Val Jones, Rainer Hersog. 2003. MobiHealth- innovative 2.5/3G mobile services and applications for healthcare. Workshop on Standardization in E-Health. Geneva, Italy.

[6] Sachpazidis 2002. @Home: A modular telemedicine system. Mobile Computing in Medicine. Workshop on mobile computing. Germany, 2002.

[7] Kunze, C., Gromann, U., Stork, W., Müller-Glaser, K.D.,2002. Application of Ubiquitous Computing in Personal Health Monitoring Systems. 36. annual meeting of the German Society for Biomedical Eng.

[8] Rodríguez, J., Goñi A., Illarramendi, A. 2003. Classifying ECG in an On-Line Monitoring System. Submitted for Publication to IEEE Transactions on Information Technology in Biomedicine. In revision process.

[9] Rodríguez, J., Dranca L., Goñi A., Illarramendi, A wireless Application that Monitors ECG signals on-line: Architecture and performance. ICEIS: 6th International Conference on Enterprise Information Systems. April 2004.

[3] More intelligent conditions could be added here – for example, when the PDA is connected to a fixed network, or to a non-expensive network, like WLAN or Bluetooth.

[10] Jané, P., Blasi, A., García, J., Laguna, P. 1997. Evaluation of an Automatic Threshold Based Detector of Waveform Limits in Holter ECG with the QT database". Computers in Cardiology, vol. 24, pp. 295-298.

[11] G. Alonso, F. Casati, H. Kuno, V. Machiraju, "Web Services: Concepts, Architecture and Applications". ISBN 3-540-44008-9.

[12] Farreras and Rozman, "Medicina interna". 13th Edition. CD-ROM Edition. Section 3. Cardiologia pag 395 – 523, October, 2001.

[13] MIT-BIH Database Distribution. 2003, *http://ecg.mit.edu*

# Remote Continuous Cardiac Arrhythmias Detection and Monitoring

Haiying ZHOU[1], Kun Mean HOU[1], Jean PONSONNAILLE[2], Laurent GINESTE [1], Julien COUDON[1], Gil de SOUSA[1], Christophe de VAULX [1], Jian-Jin LI[1], Pierre CHAINAIS[1], Romuald AUFRÈRE[1], Abdelaziz AMAMRA[1] and Jean-Pierre CHANET[1]

[1]*Laboratoire LIMOS UMR 6158 CNRS, ISIMA, UBP Clermont-Ferrand II, France*
[2]*CHU de Clermont-Ferrand, Université d'Auvergne, France*

**Abstract.** The current techniques used to diagnose cardiac arrhythmias such as Holter, Rtest and telemetry systems are partially efficient because they are limited either in time or in space. In this paper, a platform dedicated to the real-time remote continuous cardiac arrhythmias detection and monitoring is proposed. Such a platform allows to improve the accuracy and the efficiency of the diagnostic of ventricular tachycardia among the high-risk patients and enables the implantation of ICD to prevent sudden death. The new method allows the patient to lead a normal life while being remotely monitored in real-time by an ambulatory wireless ECG sensor. When a cardiac arrhythmia is detected a message including a sequence of ECG signals and the patient's images (indoors only) is sent to a remote surveillance server. According to the gravity of the symptom, the cardiologist can intervene in real time or later. The system has been evaluated on some ten patients with regard to heartbeat and cardiac rhythm disturbance. The real-time results are similar to those offered by HP telemetry systems.

**Keywords:** Telemedicine, real-time remote continuous cardiac arrhythmias detection, wireless ECG sensor network, remote monitoring server.

## Introduction

Thanks to the rapid developments of pathological research and clinical technologies, most heart diseases can be effectively treated and prevented in the modern society. Nevertheless, this can't change the fact that heart disease is still the world's number one killer. It is responsible for one in every three deaths, which is an estimated seven million deaths around the world each year [15].

Most of these are sudden cardiac deaths following a heart attack. Sudden death is defined as death arising less than one hour after the first symptoms felt by the patient. It concerns about 50,000 persons per year in France. 90% of sudden deaths are due essentially to cardiac arrhythmias: 20% are caused by heart block or pause (bradycardia) and 80% are caused by ventricular fibrillation (VF), frequently initiated by ventricular tachycardia (VT). The principal aetiology of sudden death in adults is due to myocardial infarction. Among the group of patients suffering from coronary pathologies and chronic ischemia, the risk of death is particularly high.

This "massive heart attack" is generally considered as an unpredictable and unpreventable event. In spite of the effectiveness of the post-heart-attack treatment, the patients die because the heart attack usually occurs suddenly, without a shred of a warning. Recent studies have shown that there are common significant cardiovascular abnormal symptoms such as palpitations, faints, chest pain, shortness of breath etc, before the sudden appearance of lethal heart arrhythmia. If these symptoms can be detected and diagnosed early enough, there is time to prevent the occurrence of a heart attack. Therefore, to reduce the number of disabilities and deaths caused by heart attack, it is necessary to install an effective method for early detection and early treatment.

The most effective preventive therapy of sudden death due to cardiac arrhythmias is the implantation of an implantable cardioverter-defibrillator (ICD). ICD is used to apply a strong electrical shock to the heart. By adjusting the cardiac rhythm to an orderly and effective status, this device helps treat cardiac disorders such as ventricular fibrillation, ventricular tachycardia, atrial fibrillation, and atrial flutter. Unfortunately, its high cost is the main factor impeding wide adoption of ICD. Moreover, it is an invasive technique requiring a major surgery with potential complications. The complications that a physician may encounter during surgery involve venous access, lead placement, intravascular thrombosis/fibrosis, and the generator itself [16].

Currently, ICD is mainly applied to high-risk patients who have cardiac arrhythmia, especially VT or VF, when the risk is accurately identified. Nevertheless, recent surveys have shown that sudden cardiac death occurs not only in people who have had heart attacks (myocardial infarction) in the past, but also among young people who are entirely well up until the moment of their death [17]. Therefore, we need an effective personal diagnosis system which can continuously monitor cardiac status. This system should be cost-effective, risk-free and easy to use in daily life.

The ECG (Electrocardiograph) is the most commonly performed cardiac test, because it is a useful screening tool for a variety of cardiac abnormalities; the test is simple to perform, risk-free and inexpensive. From ECG tracing, the following information can be determined [18]:

- heart rate,
- heart rhythm,
- conduction abnormalities: abnormalities in the way the electrical impulse spreads across the heart,
- coronary artery disease,
- heart muscle abnormality etc.

The Holter technique is also frequently used to record 24h or 48h worth of ECG signals. The recorded ECG signals are analyzed by dedicated software and a report is produced to be interpreted by the cardiologist, but this proves largely insufficient for long-term predictions because critical cardiac arrhythmias do not necessarily occur during the 24h or 48h of monitoring time [19]. Another technique, called RTEST allows the patient to monitor the record of a sequence of ECG signals [11]. The recorded ECG signals may be sent to a remote server or analyzed later. One of the drawbacks of the RTEST technique is that most of the time the patient does not feel palpitation or VT. In fact, some cardiac rhythm disturbances are just asymptomatic. A new generation of RTEST devices may be configured by the physician to record ECG signals automatically. Thus, these two techniques are limited in time (4 weeks for RTEST) and prove only somewhat efficient. Furthermore, telemetry cardiac arrhythmia detection systems (for example Agilent) are expensive and limited in space because they can typically only be installed at hospital cardiology departments.

Hence, it is very important to propose a new method improving the efficiency and the accuracy of cardiac arrhythmia diagnostic; one which would not be limited in time and in space. Furthermore, the comfort of the patient has to be taken into account by allowing the patient to live normally and stay at home. All cardiac rhythm disturbances should be recorded and analysed continuously and automatically in real time and, according to the gravity of the detected symptoms, emergency messages should be sent to a remote server. The cardiologist can then confirm or reject the emergency message by analysing the sequence of ECG signals included in the message. If necessary, he can also remotely analyse (in real time) the patient's ECG signals.

In fact, we believe that such a platform is able to improve the result of prediction and diagnostics for the patients suffering from cardiac arrhythmias, because it is not limited in time and in space. Moreover, the patients can feel more at ease and more secure at their homes. When a high-risk patient is definitely identified, ICD should be proposed. Finally, the platform is able to monitor a large number of patients at home.

This paper is organized as follows: in section 1 key system elements and operation modes of the platform are described. Section 2 presents the key operations realized by the platform. Finally, in section 3, performance tests and evolution as well as conclusions and notes on ongoing work are presented.

## 1. Overview of the Platform

Our main objective is the development of a platform adapted to telemedicine applications especially to real-time remote continuous cardiac arrhythmia detection and monitoring. The platform integrates the advanced wireless telecommunication technology such as WiFi, Bluetooth, GSM and UMTS and the distributed embedded real-time intelligent sensors communicating over the Internet.

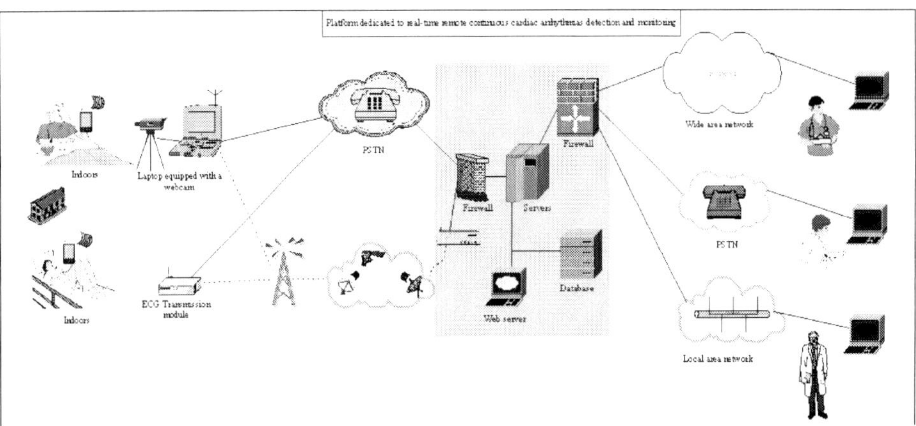


**Fig. 1.** A platform dedicated to real-time remote continuous cardiac arrhythmia detection and monitoring

### 1.1 Platform Elements

The platform structure shown in Figure 1 comprises two parts: a local system and a remote system, which contains four main configurable elements. The local system has a wireless ECG sensor (WES) and a local server, and the remote system includes a remote server and a remote surveillance system (diagnosis and visualization).

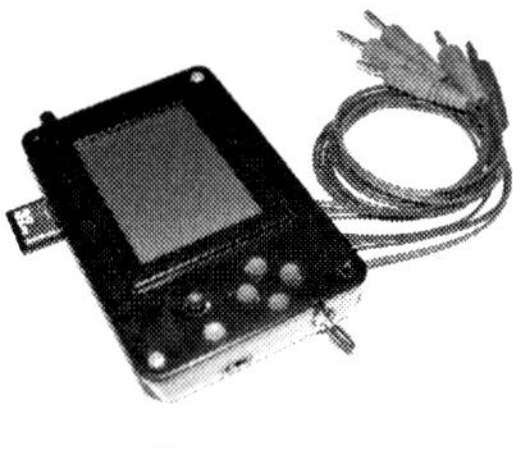

a.

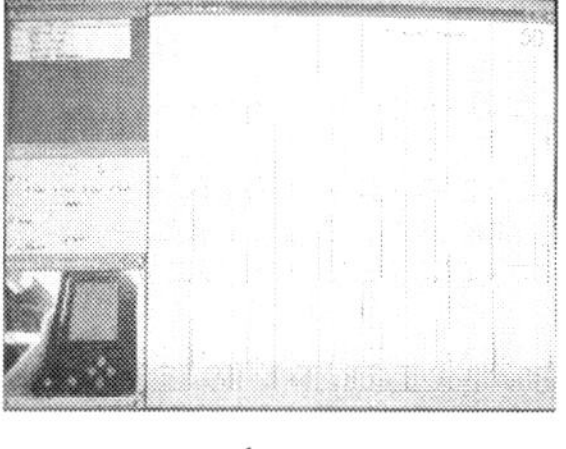

b.

**Fig. 2.** a) Wireless ECG Sensor, b) Remote surveillance server

### *1.1.1 WES*

To minimize cost we use energy-efficient compact wireless ECG sensors (WES) responding to the latest AHA recommendations [6]; additionally, the embedded basic technologies such as a distributed real-time fault tolerant microkernel [3, 4], dedicated hardware and firmware [12] and a TCP/IP protocol stack [1, 4] are implemented in the WES.

The wireless ECG sensor prototype (figure 2a) is a real-time wireless embedded portable sensor (size=70*100mm) based on the Texas Instruments ultra-low-power MSP430 microcontroller [13], corresponding to the recommendations of AHA [6]. The sensor, without a wireless adapter, consumes only 10mA of power. The key features of the WES are:

- Gain: 1000
- CMMR(min): 120dB
- Bandwidth: 0.05Hz to 125Hz
- Programmable sample frequency more than 500Hz
- Analogue to digital converter: 12 bits
- Leakage current: 10μA.

The WES makes it possible to capture 4 lead ECG signals sampled at 500Hz in real time (the sample frequency is reprogrammable). These sample signals are sent to the local server over a wireless medium such as WiFi or Bluetooth. In offline mode, ECG signals can be stored in flash memory of the WES. The duration of the ECG records depends on the capacity of the flash memory card, the sample frequency and the number of ECG leads. The two latter parameters may be configured by the user. For example, a 128M flash memory card can store 24h of continuous 4-lead ECG signals sampled at 500Hz. In this way, the WES works as a Holter or an RTEST.

### *1.1.2 Local Server*

The local access server that may be implemented by a standard PC or a mobile phone or a dedicated network access medium. It provides two network medium access services: wireless connection with the WES by a wireless medium (WiFi or Bluetooth), and network connection with the remote system by multi-support network access media.

The different access media that patients can use include: modem, broadband, wireless and satellite connections. The network bandwidth of the access mediums fluctuates over time because it is affected by various disturbance factors [20]. Therefore, the remote system must be adaptable to meet various network access medium bandwidths and local server performance. Hence, in accordance with the network access medium and local server resources, a local peer can be configured to provide real-time ECG signals and patient's image transmission as well as diagnosis. Otherwise, if the local server is a mobile phone, only short high-level alarm messages can be sent to the remote server. Thus, the local server may be configured to support 4 different operation modes (section 3).

For 4-lead ECG signals sampled at 500Hz, a 5-second frame contains 20,000 bytes of ECG signal data (4 leads x 500Hz x 5s x 2 bytes). The fluctuation of a 56Kbps modem bandwidth does not allow real-time continuous transmission of ECG data. Therefore, it is important to minimize the amount of data transmission to reduce network traffic load. A lossless ECG signal compression algorithm is implemented by taking into account the resolution of the ADC (Analogue to Digital Converter) of the WES and the type of ECG signals. Compression ratio can reach 50~60%, so only 8000~10,000 bytes of data are transmitted. Furthermore, if ECG signal diagnosis is performed by the local server, only 25% of ECG signals raw data (2000~2500 bytes per each 5-second frame) are really transmitted to the remote server for display. In fact, ECG signals sampled at 125Hz are acceptable for visualisation.

Depending on the network traffic, the patient's images captured from a webcam connected to the local server are used to confirm the emergency state and remote diagnosis. In fact, in spite of the advancement of techniques used to detect cardiac arrhythmias, currently the accuracy of the results is still only around 90% [5, 7, 8, 9, 10]. Consequently, 10% of emergency messages are false and it will be hard to manage first aid. Therefore, for real-time remote assistance and surveillance, patient images are absolutely essential.

### *1.1.3 Remote Server*

The remote server provides network connections and patient database management. Thus the remote server is composed of three servers: a PPP server, a WAP server and a database server. The PPP server allows the patient to connect to the remote server through a traditional Public Switched Telephone Network (PSTN). The PPP server supports various PSTN medium bandwidths: 56Kbps (standard modem), 512Kbps and 1Mbps (ADSL). The WAP provides a seamless network connection over a wireless mobile communication network and tunes automatically to the available medium bandwidth: GSM (9,6Kbps) or GPRS (115Kbps). Moreover, in case of a limited area, such as a department of a hospital, the local servers and the remote server may be configured to communicate through an Ethernet LAN.

The database server stores patients' ECG signals sequences, ECG diagnostic reports, images and profiles, as well as account information. Thus, at all times, the physician can visualize the status of a patient and remotely reconfigure the function mode of the local system.

### *1.1.4 Remote Surveillance System*

The remote surveillance system contains a visualization surveillance platform and a background real-time communication system.

In order to improve the efficiency of data transmission, an adaptive communication protocol with acknowledgment is implemented over the UDP protocol (User Datagram Protocol offering non-guaranteed datagram delivery) to deliver ECG signals. As stated previously, ECG signals are compressed before transmission to the remote system (each frame is a window of 5 seconds of ECG signals). The received ECG signals are be decompressed and stored in the data frame list, and then displayed after a 25~30 second delay (5~6 data frames). Data buffering and delay are necessary to guarantee real-time, continuous display of ECG signals.

Furthermore, compared with image data used to confirm diagnosis results, ECG data has a higher transmission priority level. Thus, if the network traffic is heavy, the remote server will request the patient peer (local server) to stop or reduce image transmission.

Finally, in order to guarantee the security of data transmission, a private 64-bit key is used to perform encryption and decryption of all of the patient's data.

The interactive visualization surveillance platform (Fig. 2b) allows the system to display continuous ECG signals sequences and patients' images, to respond to various alarm messages, and to support real-time or online diagnosis. The 4-lead ECG signals and their diagnoses results can be recorded in local data files in the WFBD format [14]. It is to be noted that the interactive visualization system provides the same GUI as modern commercial devices (Agilent telemetry system, ELA etc.)

### *1.2 Operation Modes*

The platform enables 4 operation modes in order to adapt to different application environments and requirements. The operation mode is decided upon by the physician, after taking into account the patient's physical status and network medium access bandwidth. The key features of the 4 operation modes are as follows:

1. **Level 1:** Real-time *continuous ECG signal*. For the sake of remote real-time display and diagnosis, the data - including continuous ECG signal acquisition and its detection report - will be sent in real time to the remote system. This operation mode is the highest alarm level, which enables real-time online diagnostics. This mode is not suitable for monitoring a large number of patients due to the limitations placed on network bandwidth, system resources and human resources but it is necessary to monitor high-risk patients. In practice, each physician can survey approximately 4 patients. To assure reliable cardiac arrhythmia diagnosis, patient images may be required.
2. **Level 2:** *ECG signal sequence*. In order to satisfy remote real-time multi-patient detection and monitoring, the WES is configured to automatically send a sequence of ECG signals (pre- and post- abnormality) to the remote system when a cardiac arrhythmia event defined by the cardiologist is detected. This operation mode is suitable for long-term multi-patient (lower risk of sudden death than the previous class) cardiac arrhythmia event surveillance.
3. **Level 3:** *textual emergency message*. In this mode, only a short textual emergency message will be sent to the physician when a cardiac arrhythmia event is detected. According to the gravity of the symptom the physician can decide to intervene immediately or later. This mode may be operated on any access medium (wire or wireless).
4. **Level 4:** *diagnosis report email*. This is the lowest-level operation mode. The local server will periodically use the e-mail interface to send a report (much like the Holter report) to the remote server. The interval is defined by the physician. This mode is suitable for monitoring a large number of patients.

It has to be noted that the physician can remotely reconfigure the operation mode to adapt it to the evolution of the patient's status.

## 2. Technological Overview

In terms of software development, the platform contains four main configurable modules. These modules are configurable and geared at making appropriate use of system resources, to meet users' requirements.

***ECG acquisition module***: The WES can capture 4-lead ECG signals sampled at 500Hz in real time. The sample frequency and the lead numbers are programmable to meet users' requirements. Raw digital ECG input signals are filtered by a band pass (0.05Hz, 125Hz) and a notch (50Hz). Furthermore, in order to satisfy real-time multi-processes operation, an adaptable embedded real-time microkernel is integrated into the WES.

***ECG diagnosis module***: Another key feature of this platform is a real-time effective ECG detection and diagnosis algorithm. This algorithm can automatically diagnose (in real time) tachycardia ventricular (TV), brachycardia ventricular (BV) and fibrillation ventricular (FV), as well as and other anomalies. Moreover, the algorithm is developed with easy VLSI implementation in mind.

***Embedded real-time communication module***: The platform provides an embedded real-time TCP/IP stack to supply network functions for the WES. This minimal TCP/IP stack contains essential real-time communication elements that support the following protocols: TCP, UDP/IP, ICMP and PPP. It also provides remote surveillance functions for system management of the SNMP standard and PING services.

***Telemedicine communication module***: Reliable and effective remote network communication is the main foundation of telemedicine. The telemedicine communication module provides a high-layer adaptive communication protocol to overcome network access medium bandwidth fluctuation. Moreover, a compression algorithm is implemented to reduce network traffic. Because of the different priority levels between ECG and image data, a competition algorithm is designed to ensure real-time transmission of ECG signals. The telemedicine communication module ensures data reliability, network security and peer-to-peer quality service.

## 3. Conclusion and Ongoing Work

Currently, the platform dedicated to the real-time remote continuous cardiac arrhythmia detection is being evaluated on about 10 patients at the C.H.U. of the Gabriel Montpied hospital in Clermont-Ferrand (France). Detection algorithms have also been evaluated by using the MIT-BIH database [14]. Concerning VT and ESV, the detection rate is about 96%. It is to be noted that, the quality of the ECG signal on our platform is better than for HP telemetry systems.

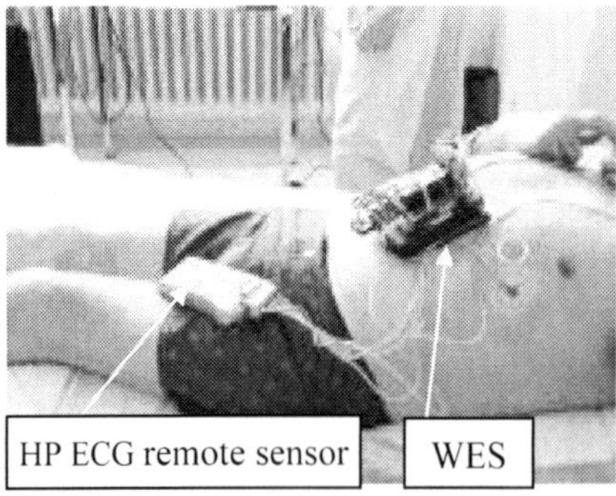


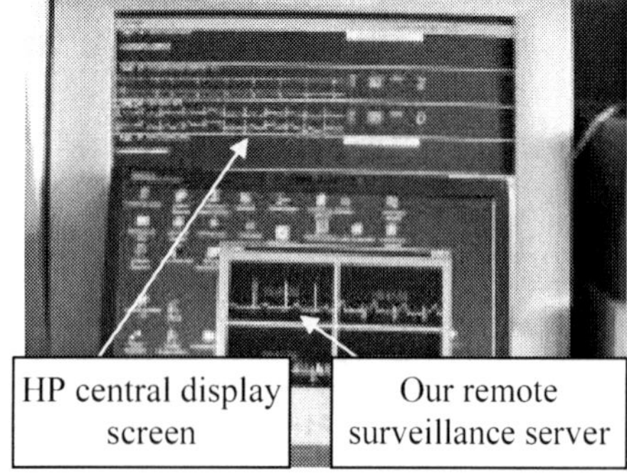


**Fig. 3.** Test and evaluation at the Gabriel Montpied hospital in Clermont-Ferrand

Our platform allows continuous remote cardiac arrhythmia monitoring and permits the patient to lead a normal life, indoors and outdoors, thus being an efficient system for diagnosing cardiac arrhythmias.

The results of the tests and evaluations are satisfactory. We believe that our platform enables a new clinical approach to more accurately evaluate a large number of high-risk patients. Furthermore, it may be used by cardiologists to remotely monitor and evaluate the efficiency of drugs or to discuss difficult cardiac pathology cases with other colleagues.

We are currently working on the implementation of an Intelligent Wireless ECG Sensor (IWES) by integrating the cardiac arrhythmia detection algorithm on a chip (ICAC). The ICAC is currently under evaluation and testing on an FPGA. Thus, the new platform contains both IWES and a remote server, and it will be more reliable and user-friendly. With the IWES, when the patient leaves home and wireless communication is impossible, the sensor will automatically disconnect from the remote server. Thus, when cardiac rhythm disturbances are detected, ECG signals will be recorded locally on a flash card. Therefore, only emergency short messages will be sent to the remote WAP server through a mobile phone (SMS). The emergency message may be defined by the cardiologist according to the physical state of the patient. In fact, IWES will periodically attempt to connect to the remote server and if the connection is established, a cardiac rhythm disturbance report along with all the recorded events may be sent.

**Acknowledgements.** We would like to thank the MENRT, the ANVAR and the Conseil Regional d'Auvergne for their support in this project.

## References

[1] P. Palau, K.M. Hou et J. Ponsonnaille, «TelmedTCP: Protocole TCP/IP temps réel dédié à la télémédecine», revue Informatique et santé, Télémédecine et e-santé, 2002 vol 13, pp 53-60, Springer-Verlag France.

[2] D. Perrot, M. Dabonneville, K.M. Hou et J. Ponsonnaille, "Plate-forme de validation dédiée à la télémédecine – Application à la détection d'arythmie dans les signaux ECG", revue Informatique et santé, Télémédecine et e-santé, 2002 vol 13, pp 149-156, Springer-Verlag France.

[3] C. de Vaulx et K.M. Hou, "DREAM: un micro noyau réparti, temps réel orienté pour la tolérance aux fautes", revue Informatique et santé, Télémédecine et e-santé, 2002 vol 13, pp. 63-69, Springer-Verlag France.

[4] Zhou H., Palau P., De Vaulx C., Li J.J., Guo C., Quilliot A. and Hou K.M., A Configurable Micro Network Kernel dedicated to real-time distributed embedded network sensor: Telemedicine application. 2002 6th international conference on signal processing proceedings, August 26-30, 2002, Beijing China, pp. 1748-1752.

[5] Jenkins J.M. and Caswell S.A., Detection Algorithms in Implantable Cardioverter Defibrillator. Proceeding of the IEEE. March 1996; pp. 428-445.

[6] Bailey J.J., Berson A.S., Garson A., Horan L.G., Macfarlane P.W., Mortara D.W. and Zywietz C., Recommendations for standardization and Specifications in automated electrocardiography: Bandwidth and digital signal processing. Special report Circulation, February 1990; 81 (2): pp. 730-739.

[7] Berbari E.J., Scherlag B.J. and Lazzara R., A computerized Technique to Record New Components of the Electrocardiogram. Proceeding of the IEEE. May 1977; pp. 799-802.

[8] Collins S.M. and Arzbaecher R.C., An Efficient Algorithm for Waveform Analysis Using the Correlation Coefficient. Computers and biomedical research 14, 1981, pp. 381-389

[9] Koyrakh L.A., Gillberg J.M. and Wood N.M., Wavelet Transform Based Algorithms for EGM Morphology Discrimination for Implantable ICDs. Computers in Cardiology, 1999, No 26, pp. 343-346.

[10] Swerdlow CD et Al. Discrimination of Ventricular Tachycardia from Supraventricular Tachycardia by a Download Wavelet-Transform Morphology Algorithm: A Paradigm for Development of Implantable Cardioverter Defibrillator Detection Algorithm. Journal of CARDIOVASCULAR Electrophysiology, Vol 13, No 5, May 2002.

[11] *http://www.novacor.com*

[12] Gineste L. Plate-forme de suivi à distance d'arythmie cardiaques. Rapport de DEA CSTI, Université Blaise Pascal Clermont-Ferrand II, 2002.
[13] Texas-Instruments. MSP430x13x, MSP430x14x MIXED SIGNAL MICROCONTROLLER. July 2000, pp. 1-67.
[14] *http://www.physionet.com*
[15] *http://www.who.int* (Who: World Health group)
[16] K.A. Ellenbogan, Cardiac Pacing, Chapter 1, pp. 1-10, Blackwell Scientific Publications, 1992.
[17] "Sudden death and how to prevent it" A commentary from Internet Medical Education, Inc.
[18] "The Electrocardiogram (ECG)", Richard N. Fogoros, M.D. *http://heartdisease.about.com*
[19] "Holter Monitors and Event Recorders" Richard N. Fogoros, M.D. *http://heartdisease.about.com*
[20] C. Partridge, "The End of Simple Traffic Models", (Editor's Note), IEEE Network, Vol. 7, No. 5, September 1993, page3-3.
[21] *http://www.intel.com/support/proshare/8150.htm#5*

# Cardiological Telemonitoring in Rehabilitation and Sports Medicine

Alfonsas VAINORAS[1], Vaidotas MAROZAS[2], Stasys KORSAKAS[1], Liudas GARGASAS[1], Laimonas SIUPSINSKAS[1], Vytenis MISKINIS[1]
[1]*Institute of Cardiology, Kaunas University of Medicine, Sukileliu av. 17, 50167 Kaunas, Lithuania*
[2]*Biomedicine Engineering Institute, Kaunas University of Technology, Studentu str. 51424 Kaunas, Lithuania*
*e-mail: alfavain@kmu.lt*

**Abstract.** The paper presents the development results of teleconsultative cardiology systems and their application in rehabilitation and sport medicine. The first teleconsultative cardiology (TELECARD) system was developed for outpatient departments in the city of Kaunas, using Internet links. It was based on the CompCardioSignal terminal. One branch of the TELECARD system with a mobile CompCardioSignal terminal was used for functional state evaluation of Lithuanian sportsmen during the 2000 Sydney Olympic Games. The examined results have shown that every sportsman responded differently to acclimatization and the TELECARD system provided support to physicians and coaches for making optimal decisions regarding the sportsmen's adaptation and other situations. The final telemetry system was used for rower monitoring. It was based on the new CompCardioSignal terminal with three EASI ECG leads and synchronously recorded motion signals for evaluation of human reaction to physical load. The developed telemonitoring systems were a useful tool for evaluation of human reaction to physical load in rehabilitation and sports activities.

## Introduction

The basis for telecommunications in cardiology is formed by electrocardiographic and ultrasound clinical data transmission and acquisition. At the present time, the systems for electrocardiographic data transmission are widely used in clinical practice, epidemiological studies and research on common consultations, database collection and interchange. Advanced telecommunications, the Internet, robotics, and other automation/computer technologies have significantly changed the nature of healthcare [1-2].

In order to improve better training performance by individualization of activities, a technology is needed that could monitor and provide feedback on mechanical as well as on physiological parameters. Physiological parameters are needed for functional state evaluation of sportsmen for optimizing their performance during the training process [3].

New technologies in sports and clinical medicine typically allow us to collect detailed information on the human body processes under investigation. Achieving deeper insight into these processes requires collecting larger amounts of data. In order to evaluate this data, special analysis methods are required. Integration of data usually is performed on the basis of mathematical methods, however in real life, different data pieces are connected to each physiological mechanism. Activation of one organ evokes changes in others. Integration of such changes in diagnostic systems must account not only for the functionality of separate organs systems, but also the links between such systems.

Literature analysis suggests that most commercial monitoring systems in sports currently use indoor training simulators (ergometers) [4]. They provide minimal information in the time and frequency domain and can display information regarding speed and distance. Usually only one physiological parameter, i.e. the heart rate is measured. Investigation with an indoor ergometer is therefore not suitable for real training conditions and it cannot accurately reflect conditions in watersports such as boat drag races and the effect of the rower's mass on the motion of the boat. There are commercial solutions that can be used in this scenario [5]; however, the amount of information they provide is not sufficient for the coach. Additionally, most of them are not intended to provide information to in real time, because they just log the data in memory during training. Even worse, the provided information is mostly averaged, hence trends cannot be discerned. The shortfalls of current technology – the high cost of commercial sports data logging systems, combined with the lack of acquisition of physiological parameters and the lack of wireless devices leave room for improvement.

In order to reduce the initial amount of data being transmitted, the EASI lead ECG system [6] has been chosen for rower monitoring. It has some advantages compared to a standard 12-lead system: it uses only 5 electrodes (the 12-lead ECG uses 10), and these 5 electrodes are more rapidly and easily located than the 6 chest electrodes of standard ECG. It also seems that this system is less sensitive to noise and artifacts than conventional 12-lead ECG. Using synchronous ECG and body movement recording, it is possible to calculate physical load and power and compare them with organism reactions. The selected EASI ECG system allows to evaluate not only the heart rate, but also ischemic changes, disturbances of heart conduction and other disorders [7].

Physicians or physiotherapists can use an online mode for monitoring cardiovascular diseases or other disorders in the rehabilitation phase to evaluate the applied physical exercise or any other physical load. They can monitor heart function, rhythm disturbances as well as physical load. In sports activities, the coach can use the online mode during training, and, according to the obtained online data, he can correct the sportsman's actions. This is especially needed in water sports, such as rowing and paddling, when the distance between the sportsman and the coach is significant. The offline mode can be used for detailed data analysis, to evaluate strategic features of the influence on the investigated person. Cardiological telemonitoring systems are a useful means of evaluation of human organism reactions to load in rehabilitation and sports activities.

## 1. Background of Teleconsultative Cardiology Systems

There are a lot of situations where we need to evaluate organism reactions to physical load. In sports physiology, military medicine, as well as in kinesiology or physiotherapy or even in clinical medicine during functional diagnostics, the exact evaluation of organism reactions helps manage the restoration of functional abilities and improves diagnostics as well as the monitored person's functional state. It has to be noted, that abnormal functional interactions can be amplified through the involvement of a regulatory system. When the performance of a working system is failing, the regulatory system is activated. If the working system is still capable to produce an adequate response to the regulatory input, its functional failure is not apparent. However, with the progressing pathological process or other limiting factors (overtraining), the activation level of the peripheral systems lags behind the activation level of the regulatory system. Finally, even maximal activation of the regulatory system cannot further augment the performance of the working system, and the latter's functional failure becomes evident. Hitherto, there has been no readily-accessible method to evaluate these functional interactions of the peripheral and regulatory systems in health and disease, even though such integrative information would be very important in assessing the progression of a pathological process or in evaluating changes in the functional status of a healthy individual.

According to physiological changes in human organisms during load, the main system responsible for organism functionality is a working muscle, for energy supply – the cardiovascular system, for oxygen supply – lungs and for coordinating all these systems – the regulatory system (which covers the central nervous system, the peripheral nervous system, humoral regulation etc.) All the mentioned systems are joined through functional, synergetic links, allowing the organism to work as one integral unit. The proposed model lets us to account for that and reflect main functional links. Such a structure of evaluation of the human organism is novel in sports and medical practice.

In our model, the main processes recorded to evaluate the organism's functions during load are muscle function (evaluated by the exerted power), changes in blood pressure (by the arterial blood pressure) and heart function (by ECG parameters). Other parameters could also be added, for example – breathing and biochemical parameters, if they can be recorded online, etc.

Under load conditions – for instance during typical bicycle ergometry, when the Bruce protocol for load is used – a computerized system measures about 10,000 initial parameters. Every process is measured in detail, and maximal decomposition of the scenario is achieved. Through physiological analysis, a group of complex parameters with special physiological meaning is created. This group consists of only about 100 parameters. Some of them are used to build an integral evaluation – one parameter, which describes the main changes in the organism. In this way, the composition of parameters is finished and a pyramid of analyzed parameters is formed.

In the group of complex parameters there are some which reflect links between the regulatory system and acting peripheral systems. When the organism needs to make some changes, for example during load, during adaptation to different heights, or to different time areas, difficulties can appear in the weakest system, which has the most problems in fulfilling this adaptation. Changes in the parameters reflecting that link show in which way the organism can be helped to adapt.

The model allows us to solve the problem of joining of decomposition and composition methods as one diagnostic tool for the evaluation of human organism functionality, taking into account that the human organism under load conditions acts as a complex system with synergetic links between its elements.

### *1.1 The Integrative Model*

When skeletal muscles are contracting during exercise, several bioactive substances accumulate and cause the dilatation of the vessels in the periphery (P) in skeletal muscles (Figure 1). To meet the growing oxygen demand, the regulatory system is further activated. This augments the functional capacity of the heart, the supplying system (S) and the respiratory system, i.e. lungs (L). At least four systems are activated during this exercise: (1) the vessels in the working skeletal muscles; (2) the heart, responsible for maintaining adequate blood supply; (3) the lungs, responsible for maintaining adequate oxygen supply and (4) the regulatory system. These four elements make up a working complex of adaptive systems, the model of which can be represented as a kind of pyramid. Its apex represents the regulatory system, which affects all three remaining parts – the blood vessels, the heart and the lungs.

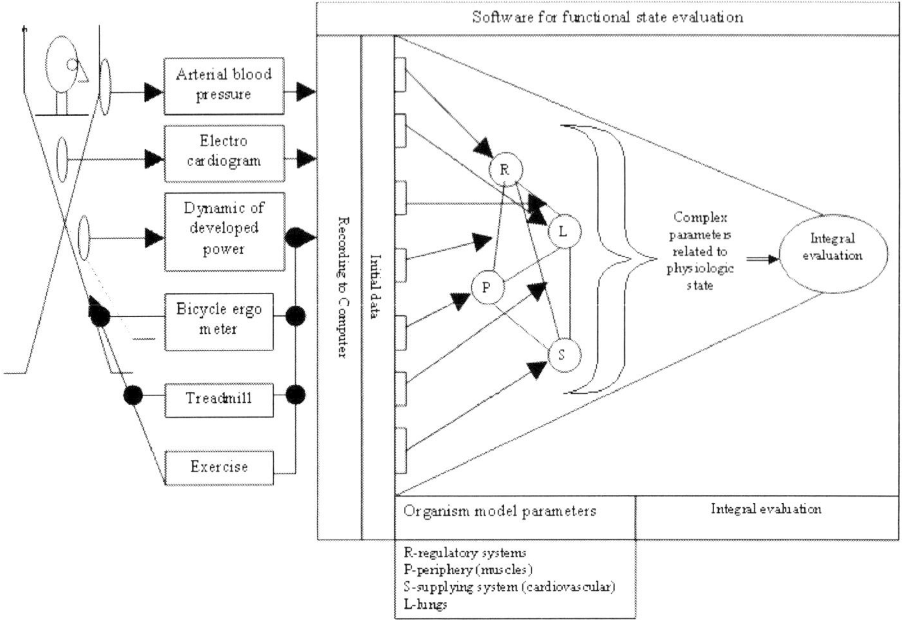


**Fig. 1.** Integrative model for evaluation of changes of the organism's functional state under load conditions

The pyramid could be reduced to a triangle by joining the lung function (the L element in Figure 1) with the S element (the supplying system). Integral evaluation (Sv), which embraces changes of the triangle (R, P and S elements) has been studied [8]. For integral description, the power exerted and the arterial blood pressure (ABP) have been used, along with twelve synchronous ECG leads, recorded continuously into computer memory during rest, load and recovery [9].

The developed integrative model is the basis of functional state evaluation in the telemonitoring system.

## 2. Teleconsultative Cardiology System Using the Internet

The Teleconsultative Cardiology System (TELECARD) is a project aiming at improving the quality of the process of patient care [10]. The main purpose of the system is to provide teleassistance in urgent cases in acute cardiac incidents as well as consultation for diagnostics and treatment in common cases. The clients (users) of system include paramedics; outpatient departments; hospitals; clinics; sports, fitness and rehabilitation centers, and GP in primary healthcare.

To achieve the main aim of the TELECARD project, some intermediate goals have been identified:

- the definition and development of an architecture allowing access to remote consultative centers and databases through the Internet,
- the design and implementation of a clinical application (the TELACARD system prototype) which allows a GP to send ECG and clinical data from his office or from home to a consultative center for teleconsultation,
- the unification of clinical data used for teleconsultations.

### *2.1 System Architecture*

The TELECARD system architecture is presented in Figure 2.

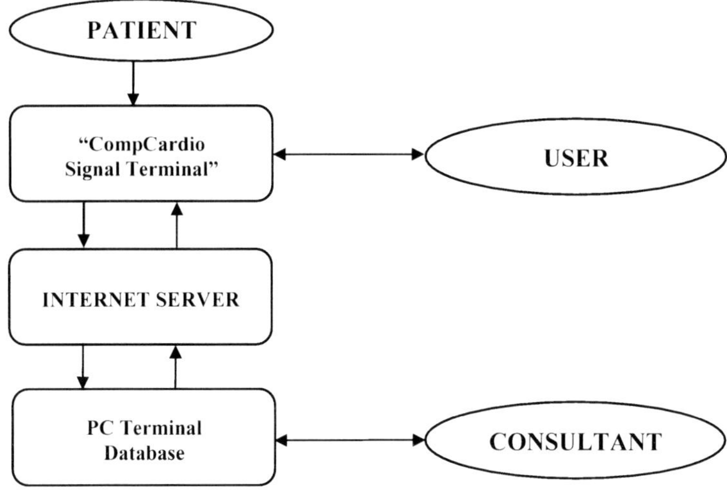


**Fig. 2.** TELECARD system architecture

When designing the system architecture three different parts were considered: the client (remote) part, the Internet server and the consultant (host) part. The client part was based on a computerized ECG analysis terminal called CompCardioSignal [10]. The CompCardioSignal terminal consists of a 12-lead ECG recorder, a personal computer (PC) and two program packages for ECG analysis at rest and during functional tests. It also provides tools for communication, i.e. a modem or mobile phone with special software [11]. Special software for data transmission has been developed, which allows to formulate queries and replies between clients and consultants. Queries and replies were sent as e-mails with attached ECG data files. Software requirements are limited to an operating system supporting Internet network protocols.

The Internet server consists of a computer and the appropriate software. It handles queries coming from the clients and consultants. The consultant part consists of a computer with a database, and software. This part of the system handles functions related to ECG data analysis, visual representation, data management, data storage, access control, concurrency control and recovery.

### *2.2 System Data*

The TELECARD medical record consists of clinical data and ECG obtained at rest or during functional tests. A standard form was elaborated for clinical data. It includes personal data (name, sex, personal code, birth date), demographic data (place of data transmission, institution), date of clinical incident, objective data (blood pressure, heart rate, temperature), subjective data (stress, anxiety, emotional discomfort, weakness, chest pain, non-specific chest pain, dizziness, vertigo, dyspnea), anamnesis (date and localization of myocardial infarction, unstable angina pectoris, dangerous rhythm disturbances, congestive heart failure, cerebral vascular accident, cardiosclerosis, diabetes mellitus, tumors and others), procedures and treatment before the incident (defibrillation, cardiostimulation, coronary bypass, coronary angioplasty, coronary stenting, aspirin, heparin, anticoagulants, β-blockers, ACE inhibitors, nitrates, Ca antagonists, cardiac glycosides, antiarrhythmics, diuretics and others).

### *2.3 A teleconsultative Cardiology System for the City of Kaunas*

The structure of a teleconsultative cardiology system for the city of Kaunas has been developed [12]. The system consists of hardware and special software. Its two main parts are terminals for consultants and users. The structure of the system is presented in Figure 3. The first version of the Kaunas TELECARD system consisted of three consultant centers and seven user points. Six users used stationary CompCardioSignal terminals and one used a mobile ECG terminal. The mobile terminal consisted of an ECG recorder, a portable computer and a mobile phone. Usually, the mobile terminal was used in rehabilitation and sports medicine. It proved particularly useful for sportsmens' functional state evaluation during acclimatization in training camps and competition venues. Both consultants and users can connect to the teleconsultative cardiology system without problems, but they must use specialized hardware and software. The hardware consists of a 12-lead ECG recorder and a computer. The main functions of the software are to prepare an e-mail for consultants and users, to attach ECG data and statements, to display ECGs on a screen, to print e-mails and ECG diagrams, to analyze ECG parameters, to transmit ECG and additional data to databases and to evaluate the functional state.

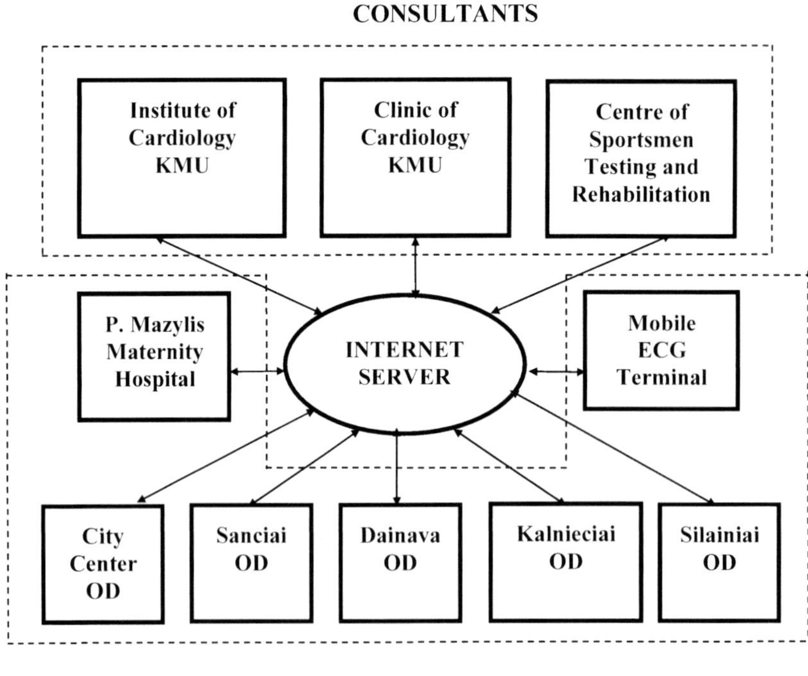


**Fig. 3.** The structure of the TELECARD system of the city of Kaunas (KMU – Kaunas Medical University; OD – outpatient department)

### 2.4 TELECARD System Testing

The TELECARD system was tested in real-life conditions. The mobile ECG terminal was used for evaluation of the functional state of Lithuanian sportsmen who participated in the Sydney 2000 Olympic Games [13]. 28 sportsmen were examined and 141 Ruffje exercise tests were performed. Measurements were taken every second day in the morning before first training and in the evening after training during the acclimatization period. Data was analyzed with a mobile computerized ECG terminal (CompCardioSignal). The integrated functional state evaluation of sportsmen was subsequently presented. If the sports physician had some doubts about computer ECG analysis results, data was transmitted (in a compressed form) to Kaunas. At the consulting center, data was analyzed and compared to past data from the database. Consultants identified changes and sent back recommendations to the terminal terminal. The examined results showed that every sportsman expereienced different changes of organism functions during acclimatization and TELECARD gave support to sports physicians and coaches to make optimal solutions under various conditions.

## 3. New Wireless Telemetry System for Rower Monitoring

A new wireless telemetry system for rower monitoring has been developed. The schema of the proposed and implemented system, with all components for real-time monitoring of mechanical and physiological parameters reflecting the status of the rower and the canoe is presented in Figure 4.

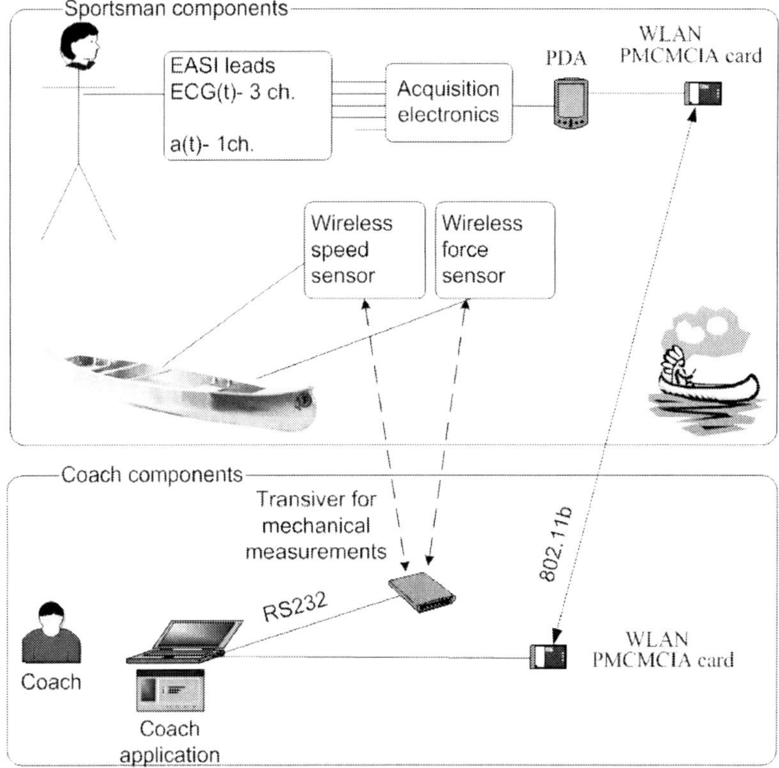


**Fig. 4.** The functional scheme of the telemetry system for real-time monitoring of rowers

The telemetry system consists of sportsman and coach components. The sportsman component includes acquisition devices for of physiological and mechanical parameters and a personal digital assistant (PDA) with a WLAN PMCMCIA card. The coach component consists of a WLAN PMCMCIA card, a transceiver for mechanical measurements and a portable computer.

### *3.1 Acquisition of Physiological Parameters*

The functional state of the rower was evaluated using an integrative model [3]. However, that model is based on standard 12-lead ECG. This configuration of leads is not convenient for the rower and, in addition, it generates excessive amounts of artifacts when the rower is in motion. Thus we decided to use an ECG lead configuration named EASI [14]. The 3 EASI ECG leads (5 electrodes) of this configuration are less sensitive to noise. The required 12 leads for sportsman functional state evaluation are recalculated from EASI by a transformation matrix [6].

Physiological signal acquisition hardware includes three amplifiers for three EASI ECG leads, a low-pass filter, a high-pass filter and a microcontroller with ADC. One additional channel is set for acquisition of motion signals. An Analog Devices Inc. accelerometer was used as a motion signal sensor [15]. The acquired signals were transmitted to a personal digital assistant (PDA) via a serial interface (RS 232). The recorded motion signal was used to estimate mean power, frequency of paddling (strokes per minute) and correlation to boat motion parameters.

### *3.2 Wireless Communication*

The acquired mechanical parameters were sent online directly to the coach's computer. Radiometrix Ltd. BiM2-433-160-3V modules were used for sustaining the bidirectional link. Physiological parameters were sent using different communication links. A large amount of physiological data was generated, and for its transmission, a broader channel was required. GPRS modems were tested, but the results were unsatisfactory due to the unreliable links. Better results were achieved by using wireless LAN (WLAN) (802. 11b) communication. This kind of wireless link satisfies portability requirements as it is already integrated in modern PDA and laptop computers. The declared communication ranges are 300-500 meters in an open area. The UDP protocol was used to reduce data transmission overhead and to meet real-time requirements.

### *3.3 Telemetry System Software*

The developed software included firmware for sensors, software for PDAs as well as software for the laptop (coach's computer). All digital signal processing - digital filtering, transformation of EASI leads to the 12-lead system and evaluation of the functional state is concentrated in the laptop computer of the coach. The C++ and C# languages were used for laptop and PDA software development.

### *3.4 Telemetry System Testing*

The ECG and motion recorder have been tested on 30 healthy persons. The obtained results have shown that the quality of EASI ECG and motion signals was good enough and could be used for further, detailed analysis. Attempts have been made to perform ECG analysis by using earlier software [16] and to calculate power averaged from the motion signal. A resultant example of ECG analysis and averaged power is presented in Figure 5. Testing revealed some methodological shortcomings in motion evaluation: the method requires that the single-direction motion sensor must be aligned very precisely to the movement vector's direction. Low-weight sensors are sensitive to high-frequency vibrations and noise, thus exacerbating potential errors. Additionally, the motion often has a spin component, which also introduces errors. These shortcomings will be eliminated in the future through improvements of the movement evaluation method.

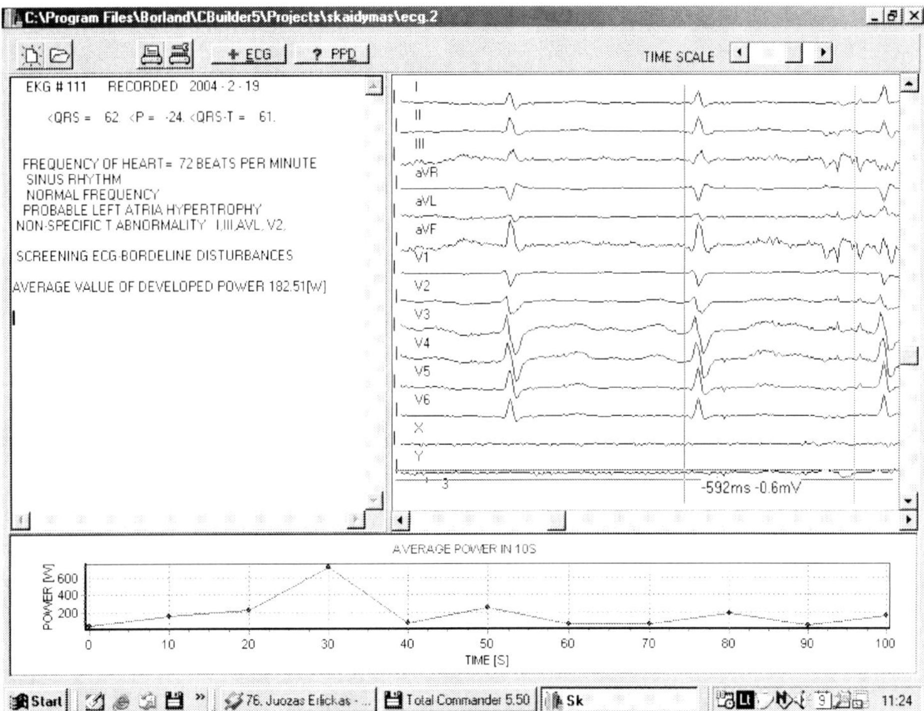


**Fig. 5.** Screenshot of reconstructed ECG with statements and a motion signal with averaged power

## 4. Conclusion

The described teleconsultative cardiology systems have been tested in real-life conditions. Test results have shown that cardiological telemonitoring systems are a useful tool for the evaluation of human organism reaction to load in rehabilitation and sports activities.

## Reference


[1] Bertrand Ch.A., Benda R.L., Mercando A.D., Faddeo M.M., Bailey K.E., Effectiveness of the Fax Electrocardiogram. *The American Journal of Cardiology*. 1994, **74**, pp. 294-295.

[2] Moertl D., Halter O., Dombrowsk T., Porenta G., Reengineering a Cardiology Information System for Intranet Use and Web Technology, *Computers in Cardiology*, 1997, **24**, pp. 275-278.

[3] Vainoras A. Functional model of human organism reaction to load – evaluation of sportsman training effect, *Education Physical Training Sport*, 2002, **3**, pp. 88-93.

[4] Ergometer "Rowperfect". Internet site address: *http://www.rowperfect.com/index.htm*.

[5] NK rowing computers. Internet site address: *http://www.nkhome.com/rp/rpindex.html*.

[6] Dirk Q., Feild D.Q., Feldman Ch.L., and Horaček B.M., Improved EASI Coefficients: Their Derivation, Values, and Performance, *Journal of Electrocardiology*, 2002, **35** Suppl., pp. 23-33.
[7] Rautaharju P.M., Zhou S.H., Hancock E.W., Horaček B.M., Feild D.Q., Lindauer J.M., Wagner G.S., Pahlm O. and Feldman Ch.L. Comparability of 12-Lead Derived from EASI Leads with Standard 12-Lead ECGs in the Classification of Acute Myocardial Ischemia and Old Myocardial Infarction, *Journal of Electrocardiology*, 2002, **35** Suppl., pp. 35-39.
[8] Vainoras A., Gargasas L., Ruseckas R., Miskinis V., Jurkoniene R., Schwela H., Bauer U.J. Computerized exercise electrocardiogram analysis system "Kaunas-Load". "Electrocardiology'97" Bratislava, Slovak R., Ed.Bacharova L., Macfarlane P., World Scientific, 1997, pp 253-256.
[9] Schwela H., Vainoras A., Gargasas L., Bauer U., Ruseckas R., Miskinis V., Evaluation of systolic blood pressure response during veloergometry performed by computer analysis system "Kaunas-Load". *Lith. J. of Cardiology*, 1997, **4(1)** pp 34-39.
[10] Korsakas S., Gargasas L., Vainoras A., Bluzas J., Miskinis V. Teleconsultative cardiology system: Application Development Using the Internet, *Med. Biol. Eng. Comput.*, 1999, **37**, suppl. 1, pp. 119-120.
[11] Gargasas L., Korsakas S., Vainoras A. and Miskinis V., Teleconsultative cardiology system using conventional and cellular telephones, *Med. Biol. Eng. Comput.*, 1999, **37,** suppl. 2, pp. 1408-1409.
[12] Korsakas S., Vainoras A., Gargasas L., Ruseckas R. Cardiological teleconsultative system of Kaunas city, Biomedical Engineering, Proceedings of International Conference, Ed. Lukosevicius A., Kaunas Technologija, 1999, pp. 84-87.
[13] Korsakas S., Vainoras A., Gargasas L., Poderys L., and Jurkonis V. Telecardiology system: methods and results of sportsmen functional state evaluation. IFMBE Proceedings, Medicon 2001, 12-15 June, Pula, Ed.Magjarevic R., Tonkovic S., University of Zagreb, 2001, pp. 94-95.
[14] Horacek B.M., Warren J.W., Field D.Q., Feldman C.L. Statistical and deterministic approaches to design transformations of electrocardiographic leads, *J. Electrocard.* 2002, **35**, pp. 41-52.
[15] Bussmann J.B, Hartgerink I, van der Woude L.H, Stam H.J. Measuring physical strain during ambulation with accelerometry', *Med Sci Sports Exerc.*, 2000, **32(8),** pp.1462-1471.
[16] Korsakas S., Gargasas L., Vainoras A., Torrau I., Jurkoniene R. The ECG Analysis System SAA ECG Kaunas-02, Ischemic Heart Disease, Ed. J. Bluzas, Vilnius: Mokslas, 1987, pp. 116-120.

# Development of Methods for Monitoring of Electrocardiograms, Impedance Cardiograms and Seismocardiograms

Liudas GARGASAS[1], Arturas JANUSAUSKAS[2], Arunas LUKOSEVICIUS[2], Alfonsas VAINORAS[1], Rimtautas RUSECKAS[1], Stasys KORSAKAS[1] and Vytenis MISKINIS[1]

[1] *Institute of Cardiology, Kaunas University of Medicine, Sukileliu avenue 17, 50167 Kaunas, Lithuania*

[2] *Biomedicine Engineering Institute, Kaunas University of Technology, Studentu street, 54, 51424 Kaunas, Lithuania*

**Abstract.** Cardiovascular diseases remain the main cause of morbidity and mortality in Lithuania, and early detection of those diseases is one of opportunities to reduce this problem. Usage of information technologies including clinical decision support systems, telemedicine networks and computer analysis of cardiac signals, can serve this purpose. Therefore, the presented paper deals with development of a system for the analysis of 12-lead electrocardiograms (ECG), impedance cardiograms (ICG) and seismocardiograms (SCG) in the aim to use it in a wider cardiologic teleconsultative system. Such a complex set of signals makes it possible to monitor the electric (ECG), hemodynamic (ICG) and mechanical (SCG) properties of cardiac activity. The hardware for synchronous recording of 12-lead ECG, ICG and SCG as well as the software containing programs for signal input, recognition, measurement, analysis and data transmission has been developed.

## Introduction

Ischemic heart disease (IHD) and other cardiovascular diseases remain a major cause of morbidity, disability and mortality among adults in economically developed countries, as well as in Lithuania. Contrary to many countries, however, both Lithuania and Eastern Europe in general have seen recent increases in cardiovascular mortality. The IHD is a myocardial dysfunction due to insufficient oxygen supply in the myocardium, and it is well established that early diagnosis of IHD and proper elimination of the cause of ischemia can improve both the quality of life and life expectancy, and reduce expenses on healthcare services. Therefore, early detection of IHD is a very important, albeit difficult, aim in cardiology [1]. One of ways of solving this problem could be the development and introduction into clinical routine of information technologies such as clinical decision support systems and computerized systems for cardiac signal analysis. Lithuanian cardiologists have great experience in developing diagnostic and therapeutic IHD methods, much of it concentrated at the Kaunas Institute of Cardiology. Several versions of ECG computer analysis systems for assessment of ECG parameters during rest, physical load and other functional tests have already been created and introduced into practice at more than 30 medical institutions of Lithuania [2-6]. This approach has also allowed us to accumulate useful databases [7,8]. Methods of biophysical mathematical modeling were thus introduced for ECG analysis, increasing the clinical value of ECG methods [9,10]. Additionally, methods of ECG mapping and analysis of impedance cardiograms (ICG) and seismocardiograms (SCG) have been investigated [4,6,11], and expert system for early detection of IHD designed [1,12]. The "Kaunas" ECG computer analysis system software has been tested according to EU standards for ECG [13], and comparatively good results were received. However, new information and computing technologies enable us to use even more efficient methods for analysis of cardiac signals and clinical decision support, and this paper describes a new program for recognition of the basic points of ECG and ICG signals, and improvements in other programs of cardiac signals analysis as well.

## 1. Methods of Computerized Analysis of Electrocardiograms, Impedance Cardiograms and Seismocardiograms

### *1.1 Structure of System Hardware and Software*

The structure of the developed computer analysis system is presented in Figure 1.

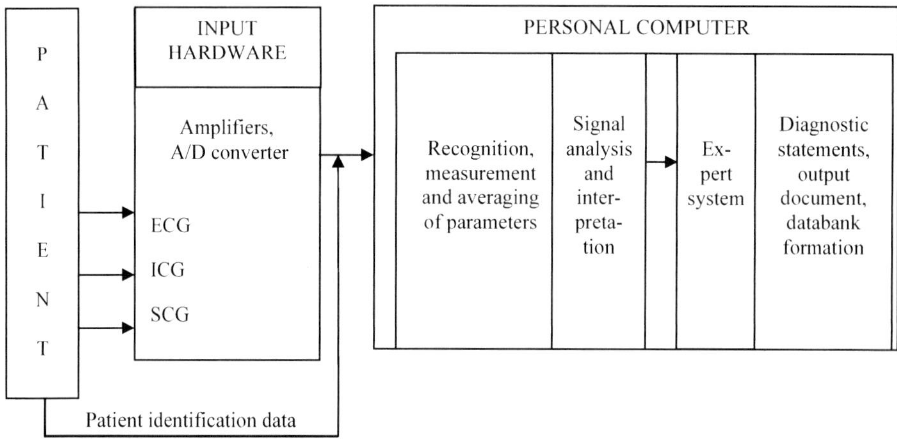


**Fig. 1.** The architecture of the ECG, ICG and SCG analysis system

The hardware consists of a device for recording conventional 12-lead ECG, tetrapolar ICG and SCG. SCG was recorded by a low-frequency piezoelectric accelerometer with a linear response of 0.5-600 Hz, a sensitivity of 0.9 V/g (g = 9,8 m/s$^2$, a weight of 0.8 kg and a sampling rate of 500 samples/second. Synchronous recording of complex of signals creates possibilities for evaluating the electric (ECG), blood circulation (ICG) and mechanical (SCG) properties of the heart; moreover, it enables us to recognize more precisely the waves and characteristic points in each signal, and to derive additional diagnostic information from the relations of time and frequency domain parameters between separate signals. The software contains programs for signals input, recognition, measurement, analysis, data compression and transmission. The results of signal analysis are transmitted to the external database of an expert system designed for diagnosis of ischemic heart disease.

### *1.2 Recognition of Basic Points on ECG and ICG*

Signal processing has been implemented using Matlab software, integrated into standalone applications. A four-stage algorithm has been developed for ECG and ICG signal analysis:

- detection of R peaks in the ECG signal;
- detection of QRS onset and offset points,
- ICG basic time point detection,
- calculation of time and amplitude parameters.

In all stages the, 4th-order Butterworth IIR bi-directional filters were used for removing movement, power line induction and other subject- and equipment-related noise.

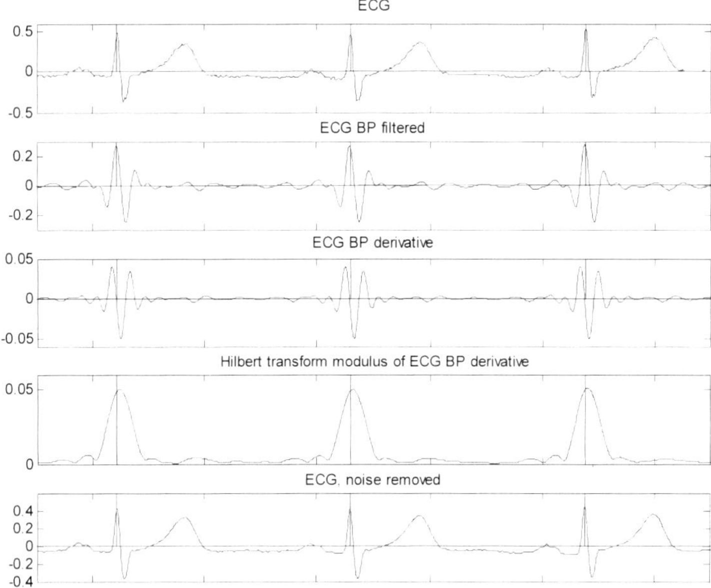


**Fig. 2.** Illustration of the R wave detection algorithm

The ECG R peak detection algorithm is based on the Hilbert transform as described by Benitez D. and co-workers in 2001 [14]. First, the ECG signal is band-pass filtered, between 8 and 20Hz, thus enhancing highest QRS energy frequency components and significantly enhancing the signal to noise ratio (Fig. 2). Subsequently, a derivative of the signal is calculated. The position of the most prominent ECG R peak can then be defined as a zero crossing point of this derivative. In the case of noisy signals, the use of this criterion is rather complicated and therefore the modulus of the Hilbert transform derivative is calculated in order to enhance the time regions of QRS waves. During the next stage, the positions of peaks in the result signal are detected, using the adaptive threshold technique [14]. In this way, however, the detected peaks usually fall within a few milliseconds of the actual R peak position. Real R peak positions are detected by finding the maxima of filtered original ECG signals (between 1 – 45Hz) in the time regions bordering preliminarily-defined R peak positions (Fig. 2). A search interval of ±30ms has been used.

This method has shown very good performance both in terms of immunity to noise and its precision. A similar method can also be implemented for near-real-time QRS detection.

Detection of QRS onset and offset points has been implemented by an algorithm based on the above described method. The first stage of this method is the calculation of Hilbert transform modulus $h(n)$ of the ECG band-pass filtered between 8 and 20Hz (Fig. 3). A derivative of the result signal is then calculated in order to detect changing slope points in signal fronts, which are assumed to correspond to Q and S wave positions in the QRS complex. In order to simplify detection for different QRS shapes, the modulus of the derivative signal is calculated (Fig. 3). Onset $N_{QRSON}$ and offset $N_{QRSOFF}$ points of QRS complexes are defined as the most prominent signal maxima positions in the time region around each R wave:

$$N_{QRSon}(m) = coord\left[\max\left\{h_1\left(N_R(m)-\Delta\right)\right\}\right], \tag{1}$$

$$N_{QRSoff}\left(m\right) = coord\left[\max\left\{h_1\left(N_R\left(m\right)+\Delta\right)\right\}\right], \tag{2}$$

where

$$h_1(n) = \left|H\left[\frac{d}{dn}(h(n))\right]\right|, \tag{3}$$

and $N_R(m)$ denotes m-th R peak position in the signal ($H[]$ – Hilbert transform; coord – position of maximum; $\Delta$ – the search interval, narrower than the offset of the adjacent R peak, but wider than half of the possible QRS complex). This method has shown good performance results and acceptable accuracy both for high-quality and noisy ECG signals.

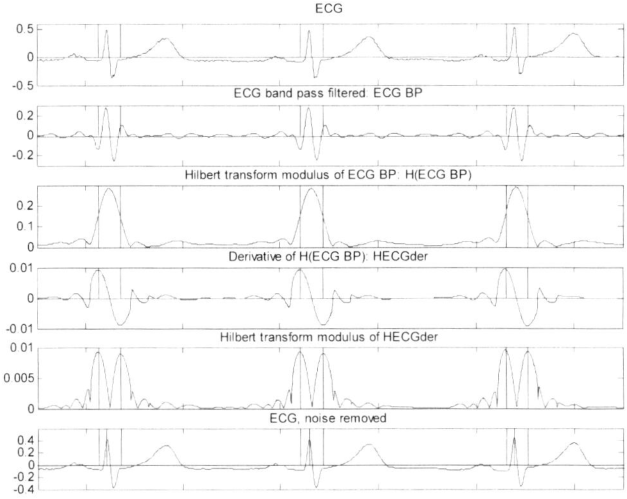


**Fig. 3.** Illustration of the QRS onset and offset detection algorithm

ICG basic point detection involved finding the positions of ICG onset, ICG wave derivative maxima, ICG wave maxima and the points of ICG wave descending slope changes (minima of the ICG derivative). Detection of ICG characteristic points is a very complicated task because of the low signal to noise ratio. The detected QRS basic points are therefore used as reference points for synchronously-recorded ICG characteristic point detection. The ICG wave itself was also filtered between 0.7 and 20Hz in order to remove baseline trends and high-frequency noise. These cut-off frequencies were chosen as a compromise between signal to noise ratio enhancement and preserving the main ICG signal features. The ICG onset point for each ICG wave was detected as negative minimum of the ICG derivative signal in time intervals corresponding to R peaks – QRS offset in synchronously-recorded ECG signals (Fig. 4). The maxima of the ICG derivative were defined as derivative maxima points between ICG wave onset and second zero crossing points in the derivative signal. Peaks of ICG waves were defined as initial zero crossing points in the ICG derivative signal following ICG derivative maxima. Points of ICG waves slope changes were detected as the tive minima in low-pass-filtered (4 Hz) ICG derivative signals between ICG wave maxima and the onset of successive ICG waves (Fig. 4). Detection of these characteristic points is usually most problematic, because of the high number of negative peaks in ICG derivative signal corresponding to small noise-induced waves superimposed on the ICG slopes. Low-pass filtering sometimes reduces the accuracy of this basic point detection in high-quality ICG signals, but significantly improves the performance in noisy cases (Fig. 5).

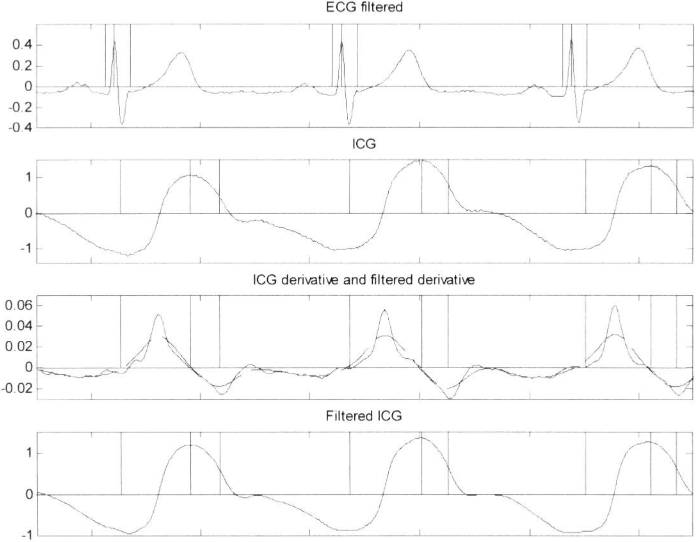


**Fig. 4.** Illustration of ICG basic points detection algorithm. High-quality ICG signal case

The overall performance of the described ICG basic points detection method was acceptable both in high-quality and noisy cases. Nevertheless, in a number of ICG signals recorded during the stress test, this method was unreliable.

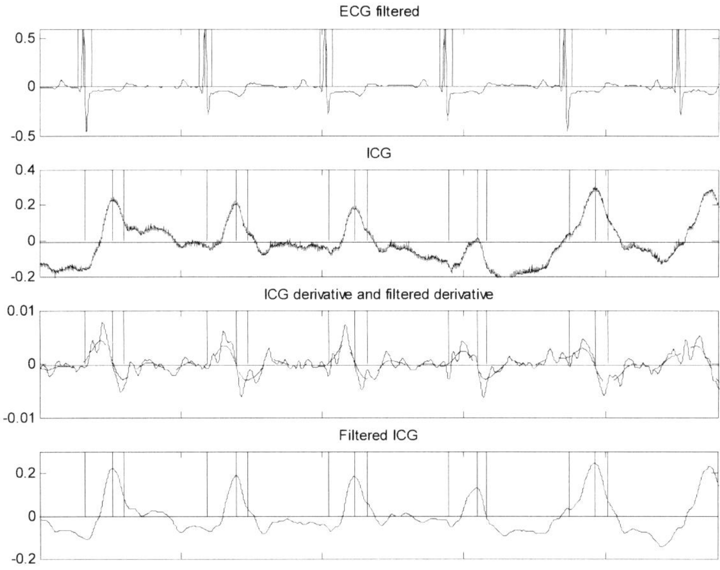


**Fig. 5.** Illustration of the ICG basic points detection algorithm. Noisy ICG signal case

The following parameters were calculated using the detected points (Fig. 6): $t_1$ – pre-ejection period; $t_2$ – duration of early systole; $t_3$ – duration of late systole; $t_4$ – duration of diastole; SA – systole amplitude; DA – diastole amplitude; dZ/dt max – velocity of impedance change.

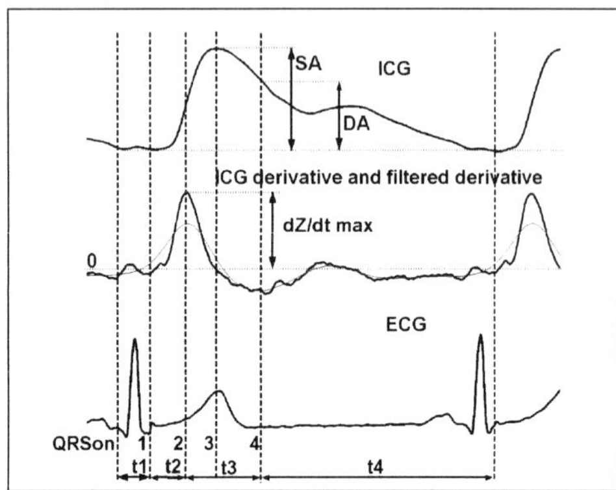


**Fig. 6.** Definition of ICG wave physiological parameters

### *1.3 The Accuracy of Program Performance*

Testing of the program for detection of basic points on ECG (R wave position, onset and offset of QRS complex) and ICG (ICG onset, position of ICG derivative maximum, positions of ICG wave maxima, point of ICG wave descending slope change, minima of ICG derivatives) signals has been performed on 60 ECG and ICG records of 20 healthy volunteers and 40 patients with cardiovascular and pulmonary pathologies. For this purpose, an expert analyzed the program windows (Fig. 2-5), detected the basic points and fixed the degree of differences in time units between manually- and automatically-detected localizations of points. In cases, when these differences exceeded the appropriate threshold (10ms), an error was logged. The number of errors when detecting various basic points varied substantially. There were several errors in the detection of R wave positions and positions of ICG derivative maxima, but the other five points of QRS and ICG were detected with a mean accuracy of 91-96%. Such a comparatively high accuracy of determination of ECG and ICG basic points allows us to draw positive conclusions regarding the effectiveness of the means that were used for noise filtering, as well as for detection of basic points on ECG and ICG.

### *1.4 Interpretation of ECG and ICG Parameters and Making Diagnostic Statements*

A program for interpretation of parameter changes in ECG was developed some time ago [2,3], and it enables us to receive routine ECG diagnostic statements about cardiac rhythm and conduction disorders, heart hypertrophy and ischemic ECG changes. Additionally, some ECG parameters which could serve as markers of IHD have been investigated and implemented into the program of ECG analysis, and one of those parameters is the ventricular gradient [15,16]. The ventricular gradient is the electric vector of the heart, characterized by magnitude, azimuth and elevation, and it could be determined either for the frontal plane or for a three-dimensional space. The ventricular gradient magnitude and its coefficient of beat-to-beat variation are computed from the orthogonal VCG Frank leads system. Since our system is based on recording of standard 12-lead ECG, the Dower matrix for reconstructing the Frank VCG from 12-lead ECG has been used [17]. The QRS complex, the ST segment and T wave integrals are used for computing the ventricular gradient magnitude for each heart beat. The mean and standard deviation of the ventricular gradient magnitude (SD), as well as the coefficient of the ventricular gradient magnitude beat-to-beat variation (SD/mean x 100) have been calculated. The Receiver Operating Characteristic Curves of the ventricular gradient magnitude and coefficient of beat-to-beat variation are presented in Figure 7. The coefficient of variation of the magnitude of the ventricular gradient for patients with IHD was significantly higher than for healthy control subjects. A variation coefficient value equal to 8.8 permits with a sensitivity of 70% and a specificity of 95% indicate IHD (Figure 8). On the other hand, the absolute value of the ventricular gradient magnitude is less important, although a mean value of the magnitude is observably higher for healthy persons than for patients with IHD ( 98 uVs vs. 79 uVs ).

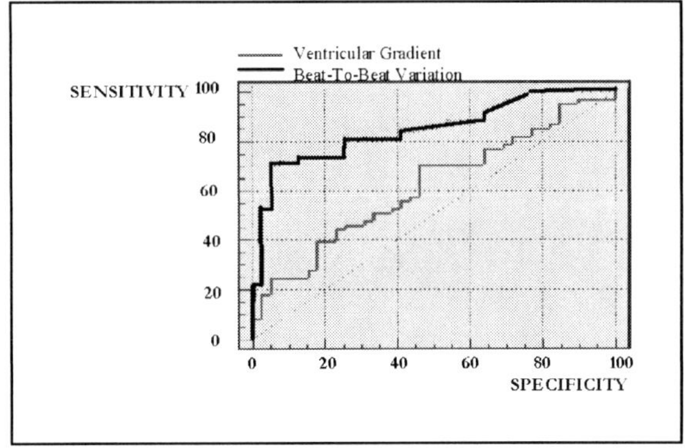


**Fig. 7.** ROC curves of ventricular gradient and its beat-to-beat variation

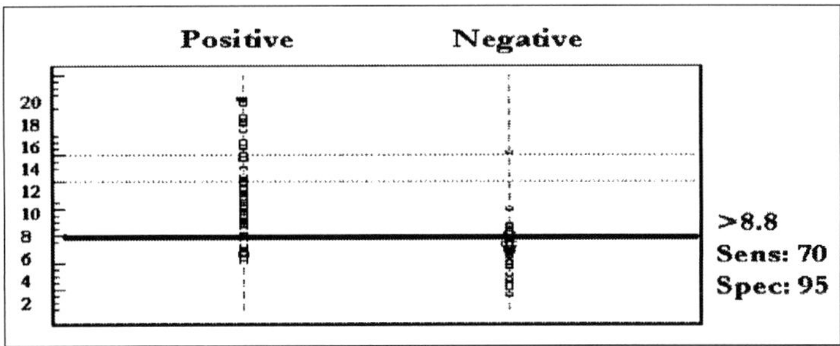


**Fig. 8.** Distribution of ventricular gradient variation values in groups of healthy persons and patients with ischemic heart disease

The impedance cardiogram was introduced over 30 years ago as a non-invasive, harmless and cost-effective method of measuring systolic time intervals, cardiac output and other parameters of the cardiovascular system [18-24]. In spite of the fact that commercially-available ICG analysis systems exist [18], new developments of the ICG method reveal its positive features [19-24]: ICG as a cardiac performance method has been compared with radionuclide ventriculography and heart catheterisation methods [20,24], and with the indirect Fick's method of measuring cardiac output [23]. New methods of ICG recording and analysis have been proposed [21,22]. Besides, the ICG method could be used not only for investigation of the systolic function, but for detection of diastolic dysfunctions of the heart as well [20].

The presented ICG analysis program allows us to receive 13 parameters that reflect such features of the cardiovascular system as global blood flow, left ventricular performance, pumping efficiency, stroke volume, cardiac output, index of contractility, systemic vascular resistance, left ventricular ejection time, pre-ejection period, diastolic – systolic index, cardiac index, stroke index, cardiac output reserve, systolic and diastolic pressure in pulmonary arteries and common resistance in the pulmonary arteries. Finally, according to the degree of deviation from normal values of those parameters and by adding some ECG and blood pressure measurements, conclusions about the type of circulation (hyperkinetic, normokinetic, hypokinetic), degree of circulation insufficiency (slight, moderate, significant) and degree of pulmonary hypertension ($I^0$, $II^0$, $III^0$, $IV^0$) can be formulated.

### *1.5 Methods and Results of Seismocardiogram (SCG) Analysis*

Seismocardiography is a noninvasive method for recording cardiac vibratory activity as a measure of cardiac contractile performance [25]. SCG devices detect and provide recordings of low-frequency cardiac vibrations on the chest wall during ventricular contractions and during both early and late ventricular filling [25,26]. Several clinical trials have proven the SCG as an informative and useful test for diagnosing IHD [26,27,28]. According to the methodology proposed by D.M. Salerno and co-workers [25], the following waves and points are recognized on SCG (Fig. 9): in the systole – mitral valve closure (MC), isovolumic movement (IM), aortic valve opening (AO), onset of rapid ejection in the left ventricular outflow tract (RE) and aortic valve closure (AC); in the diastole – mitral valve opening (MO), early rapid filling (RF) and atrial systole (AS).

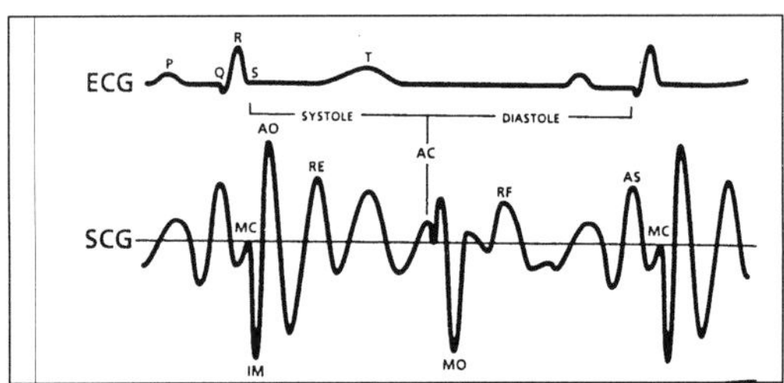


**Fig. 9.** Characteristic points on a seismocardiogram

During pilot tests of the developed system, the diagnostic efficacy of SCG has been assessed. The signals were obtained in a supine patient position, during rest and immediately after bicycle load. In resting and post-exercise SCG, two criteria – systolic and diastolic – were estimated [28]: systolic criteria – $[(AO\text{-}IM)/(IM\text{-}MC)_{Load} < (AO\text{-}IM)/(IM\text{-}MC)_{Rest}]$; diastolic criteria – $[(RF)_{Load} > (1.2RF)_{Rest}]$, where AO-IM and IM-MC are distances between points of SCG and RF is the amplitude of this wave (Figure 9). 73 healthy persons and 46 patients with confirmed moderate IHD were investigated. The sensitivity of SCG systolic parameters was 59%, with a specificity of 89%; for diastolic parameters the sensitivity was 77%, with a specificity of 90%. Summarized values for both parameters were 87% and 89% accordingly. The sensitivity of ECG parameters (depression of ST interval more than 0.1 mV in any ECG lead) was 48%, and the specificity – 89%. It can be concluded, that the sensitivity of the SCG method for detection of IHD is significantly higher than that of the ECG method. Further investigations into the proposed methods and developed systems are required before introducing them into clinical practice.

## 2. Implementation of the System for Computer Analysis of Cardiac Signals in a Cardiologic Teleconsultative System

A cardiologic teleconsultative system with distributed intelligence has been designed [29], and it structure is presented in Figure 10. The developed system is based on flexible methods of telemonitoring, and the hardware and software of this system use modern electronics and telecommunications mechanisms, such as Bluetooth modules for data transmission, a knowledge base formed by data mining and other methods in the aim

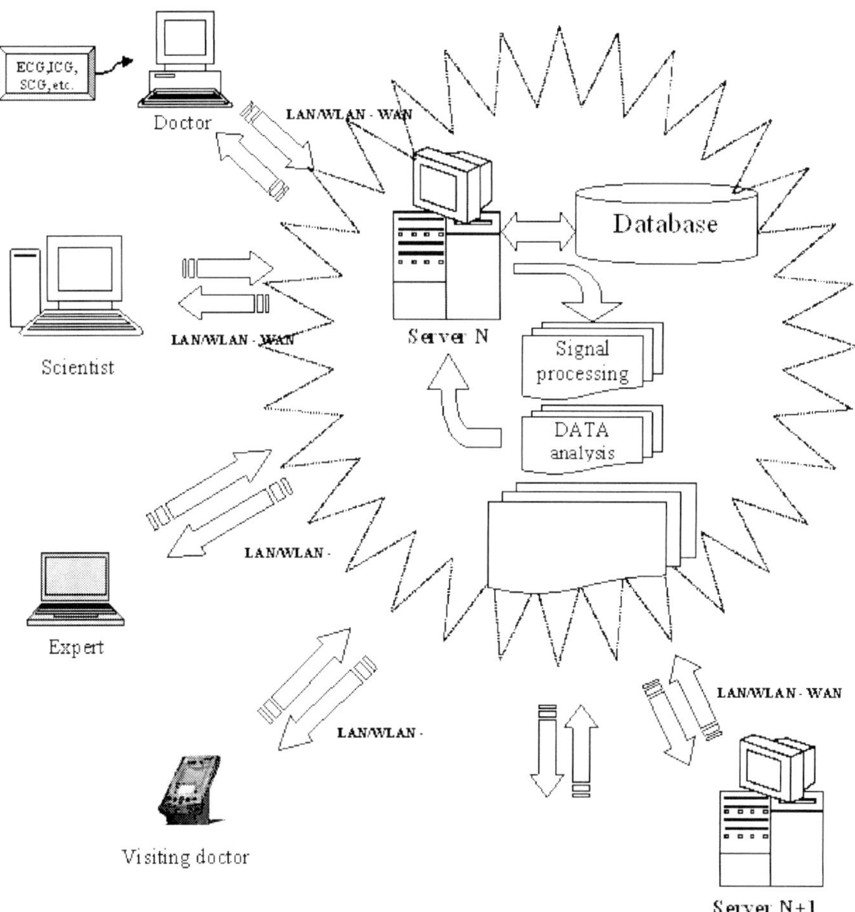


**Fig. 10.** Structure of the cardiac teleconsultative system with distributed intelligence

to search for informative parameters. This system permits us to perform teleconsultations by means of intellectual terminals, which are provided by laptops or pocket PCs, including hardware and software for monitoring of cardiac signals. It can be supposed that the developed methods of cardiac signal analysis as well as the cardiologic teleconsultative system will serve as valuable assistants for Lithuanian cardiologists and will play their role in decreasing the morbidity caused by cardiovascular diseases.

## References


[1] Gargasas L, Ruseckas R, Torrau I, Miskinis V, Jurkoniene R, Cizas M, Kirmonas A. An expert system for early recognition of ischemic heart disease. *Medical & Biological Engineering & Computing* 1996; 34, Suppl. I, Part I: 401-402.

[2] Korsakas S, Kirmonas A, Gargasas L, Miškinis V. Testing of ECG computer analysis system. Building Bridges in Electrocardiology: Procceedings [of] the XXIInd International Congress on Electrocardiology, Nijmegen, The Netherlands, 25 - 29 June 1995 / Eds.: A. Van Oosterom, T.F. Oostendorp, G.J.H. Uijen/, Nijmegen : University Press, 1995, p. 210-21

[3] Korsakas S, Vainoras A, Gargasas L, Ruseckas R, Miškinis V, Jurkonienė R. The computerized analysis of cardiac signals. Proceedings of First Austrian Symposium on Noinvasive Magnetic and Electrical Source Imaging within the Human Heart and Brain, Graz, Austria, September 25-28. *Biomedizinische Technik* 1997; 42, Erg. 1: 114-117.

[4] Gargasas L, Vainoras A, Jaruševičius G. Diagnostic Efficacy of Seismocardiography for the Diagnosis of Coronary Artery Disease During Veloergometric Test. Electrocardiology'97: Proceedings of the XXIV International Congress on Electrocardiology; Bratislava, Slovak Republic, 24-28 June 1997 / Ed. Ljuba Bacharova, Peter W Macfarlane/, World Scientific, 1998, p. 320- 323.

[5] Gargasas L, Vainoras A, Jurkoniene R, Korsakas S. Computer Analysis of Pediatric ECG: Problems, Methods, Results. *Medical & Biological Engineering & Computing* 1999; 37, Suppl. 1: 734-735.

[6] Korsakas S, Gargasas L, Kriščiūnas A, Andziulis A. Evaluation of Functional State in Disabled Patients with Cardiopulmonary Diseases: Computer Analysis of Cardiosignals. Electrocardiology'98: Proceedings of the XXV International Congress on Electrocardiology, Budapest, Hungary, 3 - 6 June, 1998 / Ed. I. Preda/ , World Scientific, 1999, pp. 412-415.

[7] Korsakas S, Gargasas L, Vainoras A, Bluzas J, Miškinis V. Teleconsultative Cardiology System: Application Development Using the Internet. *Medical & Biological Engineering & Computing* 1999; 37, Suppl.1: 119-120.

[8] Gargasas L, Korsakas S, Vainoras A, Miškinis V. Teleconsultative Cardiology System Using Conventional and Cellular Phones. *Medical & Biological Engineering & Computing* 1999;37, Suppl.2, Part II:1408-1409.

[9] Gargasas L, Gelmanas G, Jurkonis V. Biophysical Analysis of Electrocardiogram (ECG) for Assessment the Luminal Narrowing of Coronary Arteries. *Medical & Biological Engineering & Computing* 1999; 37, Suppl.1, Part II: 1212-1213.

[10] Bluzas IN, Bastys AI, Gargasas LI, Tamosiunaite MR, Kaminskiene SS, Matiukas AP, Urbonaviciene GA, Jurkonis VK, Vaisnys IM. Computer Analysis of Cardiological Signals for Diagnosis of Ischemic Heart Disease. *Kardiologiia* ( in Russian) 2004; 44(2); 8-10.

[11] Gargasas, L. ECG Mapping, Impedance Cardiography and Seismocardiography for Diagnostication of Coronary Artery Disease. Proceedings of First Austrian Symposium on Noinvasive Magnetic and Electrical Source Imaging within the Human Heart and Brain, Graz, Austria, September 25-28. *Biomedizinische Technik* 1997; 42, Erg. 1: 111-113.

[12] Gargasas L, Ruseckas R, Jurkoniene R. An Expert System for Diagnosis of Coronary Heart Disease (CHD) with Analysis of Multicardiosignals. *Medical & Biological Engineering & Computing* 1999; 37, Suppl.1, Part I: 734-735.

[13] Commission of the European Communities, Medical and Public Health Research. Common Standards for Quantitative Electrocardiography – CSE, 9th Progress Report, Leader Jos L. Willems, 1989.

[14] Benitez D, Gaidecki PA, Zaidi A, Fitzpatrick AP. The Use of the Hilbert Transform in ECG Signal Analysis. *Computers in Cardiology* 2001; 31: 399-406.

[15] Gargasas L, Vainoras A, Kaminskiene S, Urbonaviciene G, Ruseckas R, Miskinis V. Dependence of the Ventricular Gradient Beat-to-Beat Variability upon Severity of Ischemic Heart Disease Syndromes. *International Journal of Bioelectromagnetism* 2003; 5(1): 263-264.

[16] Gargasas L, Ruseckas R, Miškinis V. The ventricular gradient and heart rate variability for detection of ischemic heart disease. Electrocardiology 2000: Proceedings of the XXVII International Congress on Electrocardiology, Milan, June 27 - July 1, 2000 / Ed. Luigi de Ambrogi/. Milan, 2001. p. 241-244.

[17] Edenbrandt L, Pahlm O. Vectorcardiogram Syntesized From a 12-lead ECG: Superiority of the Inverse Dower Matrix. *Journal of Electrocardiology* 1988;21:361-367.

[18] Impedance Cardiography (ICG) Technology Parameters, CardioDynamics, Internet site address: *http://www.cardiodynamics.com/cdprod41.html*

[19] Kerkkamp HJJ and Heethaar R.M. Thoracic electrical bioimpedance assessement of left ventricular diastolic function. Proceedings of the IX International Conference on Electrical Bio-impedance, Heidelberg – Germany, 1995, p. 129-132.

[20] De Vries PMJM, Woltjer HH, Van Der Meer BJM, Vonk Noordegraaf A and Bogaard HJ. Impedance cardiography gives a complete picture of cardiac performance. Proceedings of the IX International Conference on Electrical Bio-impedance, Heidelberg – Germany, 1995, p. 189-191.

[21] Woltjer HH, Bogaard HJ and De Vries PMJM. The technique of impedance cardiography. *European Heart Journal*, 1997; 18: 1396-1403.

[22] Kauppinen PK, Hytinen J, Koobi T, Kaukinen S, Malmivuo J. Impedance Cardiography. *International Journal of Bioelectromagnetism* 2000;3, *www.ee.tut.fi/rgi/ijbem*.

[23] Pianosi P, and Garros D. Comparison of Impedance Cardiography With Indirect Fick ($CO_2$) Method of Measuring Cardiac Output in Healthy Children During Exercise. *The American Journal of Cardiology* 1996; 77: 745-749.

[24] Drazner MH, Thomson B, Rosenberg PB, Kaiser PA, Boehrer JD, Baldvin BJ. Comparison of Impedance Cardiography With Invasive Hemodynamic Measurements in Patients With Heart Failure Secondary to Ischemic or Nonischemic Cardiomyopathy. The *American Journal of Cardiology* 2002; 89: 993-995.

[25] Salerno DM, Zanetti J. Seismocardiography: A New Technique for Recording Cardiac Vibrations. Concept, Method and Initial Observations. *Journal of Cardiovascular Technology* 1990; 9:111-118.

[26] Crow RS, Hannan P, Jacobs D, Hedquist L, Salerno DM. Relationship between Seismocardiogram and Echocardiogram for Events in the Cardiac Cycle. *The American Journal of Noninvasive Cardiology* 1994; 8: 39-46.

[27] Wilson RA, Bamrah VS, Linsay J, Schwaiger M, Morgganroth J. Diagnostic Accuracy of Seismocardiography Compared with Electrocardiography for the Anatomie and Physiologic Diagnosis of Coronary Artery Disease During Exercise Testing. *The American Journal of Cardiology* 1993;71: 536-545.

[28] Salerno DM, Zannetti JM, Poliac LC, Crow SC, Hannan PJ, Wang K, Goldenberg IF, Van Tassel RA. Exercise Seismocardiography for Detection of Coronary Artery Disease. American Journal of Noninvasive Cardiology 1992;6:321-330.

[29] Vainoras A, Korsakas S, Gargasas L, Ruseckas R, Miskinis V, Juodenas G, Lukosevicius A, Janusauskas A, Marozas V, Poderys J. Monitoring system with distributed intelligence for cardiology and kinesiology. Biomedical Engineering: Proceedings of International Conference, Kaunas University of Technology, 23-24 October 2003; pp. 28-31.

# 3. Electronic Healthcare Record and Decision Support

*Transformation of Health Care with Information Technologies*
*M. Duplaga et al. (Eds.)*
*IOS Press, 2004*



# Relationships between Healthcare and Research Records[1]

Helmut DUWE
*Institute of Aerospace Medicine, German Aerospace Center (DLR), Linder Höhe, 51170 Köln*
*e-mail: helmut.duwe@dlr.de*

**Abstract.** The ultimate end-point of healthcare and health-related life sciences, more or less as regulatory idea, is the prevention and cure of diseases, considering the fate of individual patients as well as the challenge of providing sufficient care for all. However, all undertakings stand under the "proviso of rightness of action". The movement of evidence-based medicine has triggered a renaissance of systematic self-assurance of best practise.

The systematic utilization of healthcare records and research study recordings in an inter-linked manner provides a better enabling environment to improve evidence. Good e-health must contribute to accumulate inter-generation clinical experience. Qualified research should ensure methodological strictness via gold standards like controlled, randomised and masked trials.

Building information systems for e-health as well as for e-science bears as a special focus the mutual cross-fertilization of these application domains. Analysing a variety of building blocks shows that both areas can benefit from generic solution pattern, keeping in mind that each domain has distinguished knowledge realms. Generic patterns as well as distinguished special features are illustrated by analysing state of the art solutions plus some experimental approaches, as there are: the generic part of the HL7 V3 RIM, the RCRIM work, laboratory information handling, vital sign standardization efforts, like ECG information models.

Finally, the precision of the usage of the ubiquitous term "metadata" is taken as example of an open issue.

## Introduction

It is obvious that novel approaches of healthcare are inspired by basic and applied research. Evidence-based medicine (EBM) is a movement which aims to ensure the usage of care approaches motivated by a scientifically well-founded knowledge base. Whether or not EBM has been introduced in a too rigid manner shall not be addressed in this document. However, the impetus of EBM to assure the quality of care by recurring on scientific proof is taken as master problem to be dealt with. It is stated here that the fundamental link between healthcare records and research study records will surely gain momentum as powerful, long-term measure to increase evidence of e-health actions.

A central issue is the question to what extent can the time shortage ("time-to-practise"), evident in scientific undertakings and practical healthcare settings, be lessened. On the one hand, whimsical treatment methods may actually cause more harm than good. On the other hand, promising new interventions being tested too extensively may arrive too late for many people: the patient may die before the treatment is sufficiently evidence-based.

[1] The views and conclusions contained in this paper are those of the author and should not be interpreted as representing the official policies of any organization.

Basic science-theoretical connections between research and medical practise have to be explicated to understand the necessity of feedback loops between practise and theory, between research knowledge generation and healthcare action. One connection has to deal with the principle of scientific methodology to restrict the causal factors under investigation. A physiology lab type of research study reduces the complexity of life and isolates the subject of investigation to a certain extent from its normal surroundings to control the interaction of causal factors. When research is conducted as a field study, a more complex interaction of all system factors has to be taken into account.

Finding clear causal relations in a practical care setting is more like conducting a field study than a lab study. Nevertheless, the effects of medical treatments have to be assured in the "non-lab" situation of daily life. From the science-theoretical standpoint the relationship between the methodology of clear-cut lab research and research-oriented daily practise in medicine is similar to the complementary methodologies of the kinds of science that deal with "lab-like experiments" and those which use other approaches. Historical science, for example, is a research discipline which cannot do prospective experiments and investigate the causes by testing a fallible hypothesis. Yet, such types of science can conduct retrospective studies to understand causes-and-effect structures. The individual history of individual patients and patient collectives can be investigated alike. What's more, with "predictive" settings of a hypothesis even a "quasi-prospective" design can be envisioned, but, research team have then to wait until the time of the onset of the predicted event occurs.[2] Inter-individual variations and multi-factorial determination pattern can tremendously increase the complexity of the analysis.

The healthcare record has a dimension which comes quite close to the methodology of advanced historical science (e.g. using – for example – hermeneutical techniques). This issue has been discussed also under the heading of "narrative objectivation" of human thinking. Kay and Purves [see Kay, 1996] have – a while ago – introduced a so-called «narratological framework» for medical records. For Alan Rector these considerations place the literature-like logbook writing of healthcare professionals somewhere between arts and science[3]. New technologies, such as the XML Schema, have shown up, holding the promise to better bridge the gap between the richness of clinical narration and the need to enable computers to operate with powerful computational capacities on such "sign-based output" of professional thinking as "medical writing". After all, years after Hay et al. have promised a narratological framework for health informatics the "puristic" XML community now operates with terminological distinctions like "narrativ-centric" XML documents in contrast to "data-centric" XML-applications.

## 1. A Relationship Example: Water and Electrolyte Homeostasis

Investigating the role of the skin as sodium storage, researchers are confronted with vague up to detailed descriptions of the structure and dynamics of sodium in the human body. It has been known for more that 20 years that the majority of sodium present in the human body is in a dissolved form. The degree and fine-tuned kinetics of interchange of the so-called "non-dissolved", osmotic inactive form of sodium has been less well investigated. Besides bones, the skin[4] has lately (re-)gained interest as an important repository of "less soluble" sodium [5].

[2] This can take a while, e.g. when the outbreak of a "silent" infection takes years.

[3] Besides Kay et al. and Rector see also Kluge, Grémy, van Ginneken in this special issue of Methods of Information in Medicine on the narrative aspects of the medical record.

[4] Truninger and Richards have stated the role of the connective tissue for sodium storage already in 1985 [6], bone as storage has been mentioned as early as the fifties [5].

Ongoing studies now attempt to improve the knowledge about this kinetics. A practically-oriented researcher is certainly interested in assessing the clinical impact of these investigations. The pathophysiology and healthcare problem space regarding sodium interchange is centred around the health state of patients – for example – with cardiac insufficiency, with diabetes mellitus, with pheochromozytoms, with severe burns, etc.

From a physiology viewpoint, the situation of a diabetes mellitus becoming uncontrolled has been described by Truniger and Richards with regard to water and electrolyte homeostasis. Here, the patient may experience a hypernatremia and a parallel depletion of sodium reserves. Therefore, infusion of free water is suggested, as opposed to the withdrawal of sodium. In the case of severe cardiac insufficiency, the same authors describe that these patients may get a hyponatremia, while at the same time having surplus sodium reserves. They therefore propose, as therapeutic measure, fluid retention and not sodium intake.

The question is now if an improved knowledge on the kinetics of filling and depletion of sodium storages may improve the evidence of the effectiveness of such treatment advises, or at least give hints for causal plausibility. Despite the fact that recent excellent review articles are available regarding the treatment of water and electrolyte disorders, of diabetes mellitus, cardiac insufficiency, etc.[5], the role of sodium storage mechanism in physiology, pathophysiology, preventive medicine and acute healthcare still awaits a sufficient endeavour to gain the needed insight.

To gain progress here the combined usage of research study and healthcare records may provide evidence how the kinetics of sodium behaves in relationship to more or less soluble forms of body sodium. It is not within the scope of this paper to report further insight into these questions. The example shall just illustrate a practical need for alignment between e-science and e-health.

## 2. Building Blocks of the EHCR and the ERSR

To generalize the alignment of the Electronic Healthcare Record (EHCR) with the Electronic Research Study Record (ERSR) the following outline description shall deliver a "bird's view".

A general difficulty when talking about healthcare records is the underlying understanding and mental concept of the discussion participants. German industry stated for example in an official statement that the national industry is able to build an electronic healthcare record system within 6 month, others speak about the electronic healthcare record as the central issue of health informatics for the next two decades. This is not necessarily contradictory, but, the story which it tells is that a clear indication of the scope and dimension of the "electronic healthcare record" project should be given when using the term. The same holds also true for the electronic research record.

To provide a kind of "sketchy" roadmap the following extract of a matrix shall indicate which conceptual approaches should be considered when building electronic healthcare (Table 1) as well as research study record systems (Table 2). Even the underlying matrix of the depicted extract is not complete at all and driven by practical needs of real implementation projects in Germany. Other projects may set up a similar matrix with generic components and national specialties.

---

[5] Some authors point to the importance of hyperosmolarity, yet implicitly seem to neglect the role of hypernatremia at all for diabetes mellitus, others describe decreased salt elimination capabilities of patients with cardiac insufficiency via the kidney and the occurrence of low sodium levels as late effect of the disease without a complete picture of the end-to-end dynamics, yet others generally give warnings to use free water infusions, but do not mention the role of sodium storage [4].

**Table 1.** Structure matrix of a Frame Data Model for the Continuous Evolutionary Development of a Integrated Electronic **Healthcare Record**

| **Kind of Data** / **Medical Subdomain** | **Patient Basic Data** | **Image Data** | **Lab Data** | **Vital Sign Data** |
|---|---|---|---|---|
| **Ambulatory Settings** | Basic Data Sets: HL7, DICOM, national standards like BDT (D)[6] ,... | DICOM, self-made products | Lab data, e.g. HL7, LOINC, national standards like LDT (D) | Measurement device data, e.g. CEN Vital Sign Representation, SCP-ECG, GDT (D), ... |
| **General Stationary Clinical Settings** | Basic Data Sets: HL7, DICOM; CEN EHR, not BDT for example | DICOM, IHE | HL7, LOINC, interfacing eventually to LDT (D) | Integrated approaches are wishful, VITAL, SCP-ECG, HL7 ECG, ... |
| **Radiological Settings** | Basic Data Sets: HL7, DICOM | DICOM as classical application domain with image handling | Lab data as complementary to images | Vital sign data as complemen-tary to images, e.g. ECG-triggered NMR imaging |
| **Laboratory Medical Settings** | Basic data of lab orders and reports | Special techniques: e.g. fluorescence microscopy | Main responsibility area of lab physician | Vital sign complementing lab results, e.g. ECG + Troponin test for myocard diagnosis |
| **...** | | | | |

The comments in the matrix cells can just indicate the degree of complexity when the design of Electronic Healthcare Record systems is being undertaken with a scalability scope from small office computer systems up to national platforms. The same holds true for large scale distributed systems for reseach. Table 2 lists a selected set of issues to be considered when designing larger applications for health research.

[6] See explanation of some abbreviations later in the text.

**Table 2.** Structure matrix of a Frame Data Model for the Continuous Evolutionary Development of an Integrated Electronic **Research Study Record**

| **Kind of Data**<br><br>**Research Subdomains** | **Test Subject Basic Data** | **Image Data** | **Lab Data** | **Vital Sign Data** |
|---|---|---|---|---|
| **Clinical Trials** | Good Clinical Practise guidelines, HL7, RCRIM, Janus, … | DICOM is relevant | HL7, LOINC, LDT(D) | CEN Vital Sign standards, SCP-ECG, FDA ECG approach, HL7 ECG, … |
| **Fundamental and applied physiology** | Revised GCP, HL7, RCRIM approaches needed, wishful: integrated approach | DICOM, … Standardized technology lacking behind, XML and DICOM (Philips), IHE | National standards like LDT (D) have to be analysed and integrated (existing lab infrastructure) | Cardiology research uses an extended set of instruments (basic ones like blood pressure and ECG devices, experimental ones: impedance cardiography up to ballistocardiographics) |
| **Health related life sciences** | Growing importance of cell and molecular biology within health related research | High demand on 4-D modelling of original images | Advance devices like Fluorescence Correlation Spectroscopy | Is it reasonable to talk about the "vital sign" of cells (e.g. patch clamps techniques)? |
| **Laboratory Investigative Settings** | Basic data of lab orders and reports, similarities with healthcare | Special techniques: e.g. fluorescence microscopy, high demand on evalution | Advanced techniques: e.g. for protein separation, equal to university hospital infrastructure | Complex protocols, e.g. tilt table instrumentation |
| **…** | | | | |

Leaving the "bird eye" perspective, the content of each framework matrix cell has to be considered, elaborated, and driven up to functioning implementation level. As a concrete breakdown of the core elements of an ERSR, a logical view of the designed components of the DLR Electronic Study Record Manager (openESRM) is presented in Figure 1. For each component a UML- and XML Schema-oriented information model is elaborated as baseline version. The full-flagged components shall grow in iterative, incremental extensions and refinements up to a "component suite". The whole application layer is designed in such a way that it can be connected to an open Telematics Platform, the latter being component-based middleware itself.

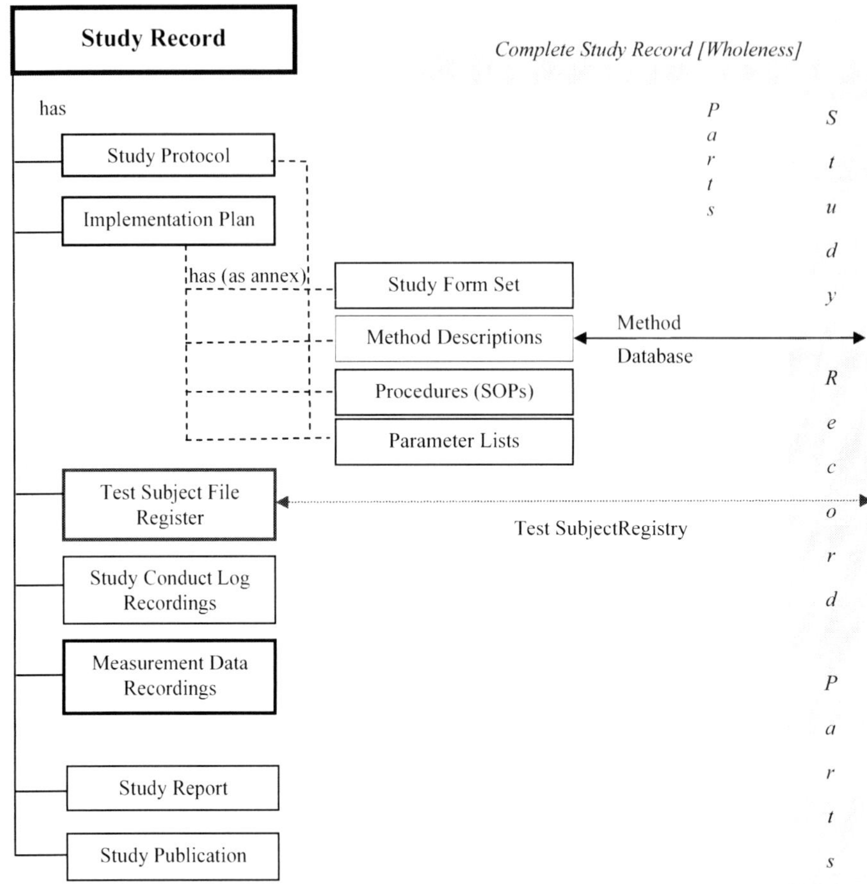


**Fig. 1.** A Component Overview (extract) of the open ESRM (logical view)

## 3. EHCR-ERSM-Relationship in Different Areas of Interest

Four kinds of activities shall be considered as worth of further investigations: (A) defining generic components usable for EHCR as well as ERSR, (B) identification of common components, (C) areas of specialization, and (D) inter-working structures between EHCR and ERSM.

A master example of **generic component** specification can be the top level layer of the HL7 V3 Information Model, namely the four core concepts and classes; respectively: Entity, Role, Participation, and Act.

Generally speaking, this top level of the RIM has no domain vocabulary in it. The four terms (entity, role, participation and act) are useful for numerous domains. The domain vocabulary does appear in the RIM on the next lower level, e.g. "Observation" as a specialization of "Act" carries a special medical connotation (despite the fact that the "observation" as such may take place in many areas). A complement of "observation" in research could be an "investigation" or a special research connotation of "observation" (as in "observational studies").

An obviously convincing example of a **common component**, used by healthcare as well as research, is a laboratory system. It is very common that a research team sends samples to external laboratories to perform a lab analysis. Such lab units can be settled outside or inside larger healthcare facilities, independent of acute care settings as part of larger research establishments. In case of the latter setup there is generally a house-internal subsystem border. All these settings require the regulations of interfaces between IT systems. This holds true even for the reverse case, e.g. when an acute healthcare entity requests the lab analysis of probes in a severe, complex scenario and sends it to the lab of a research institution.

The **specification of the differences** between EHCR and a ERSR is the major bulk of work when developing two different product line, on top of the same middleware. Some specialties are indicated in section 5. A systematic description of relevant, detected, and envisioned differences should be left to a dedicated publication.

The investigation of **inter-relationships** between the use of EHCRs and ERSRs has to consider the following utilization profiles: (i) re-purposing research data gained with research tools for healthcare, (ii) re-purposing healthcare data gained with healthcare tools for research, but also (iii) directly generating research data with healthcare tools, and (iv) healthcare data with research tools. All four profiles involve issues of cross-utilization, either retrospective or prospective.

## 4. Building Blocks and Components

Only a very limited set of building blocks and components can be described here in detail. To illustrate the relationship between EHCR and ERSR the following components have been chosen for an illustrative detail presentation: (a) the Research Study Protocol, (b) Lab Data Handling, and (c) Vital Sign Management.

The **study protocol** in a scientific study is a document which has to state precisely and clearly the scientific intent of the study. It is a typical document which can be classified as a more "narrative" full text component than a data-centric component. But, with the power of advanced techniques like XML, former long, free text can be transformed to "structured full text". As a start up configuration for a structured information decomposition, the RCRIM Model of a Study Protocol is given in Fig. 2.

One of the central issues when discussing the transfer between EHCR and ERSR technologies is the exchange of components with advanced planning functionalities, based – for example – on a concept of nested tasks.

A very important standard for building **lab data handling** systems for healthcare as well as for research is LOINC (Logical Observation and Identifier Names and Codes), a good example of a medical terminology system. The main difference between the LOINC usage profile of healthcare in contrast to the ones of research is surely that research generates more new concepts by itself. Before an observation method is used in daily healthcare settings, a certain time of testing will be needed. Before terms are "born", phenomena may appear as diffuse problems in healthcare. For example, before the HIV was detected by researchers, some clinicians observed some strange cases of deaths, naming conventions of HIV research and AIDS healthcare followed soon. After these initial phases, clinicians or researchers coin terms, more or less systematically: Sudden Infant Death as example of a healthcare related term is, analytically seen, a quite imprecise term (still alive, decades after creation, due to the complex of the underlying phenomenon, actually being more an ICD[7] problem, than a LOINC problem).

[7] International Classification of Disease

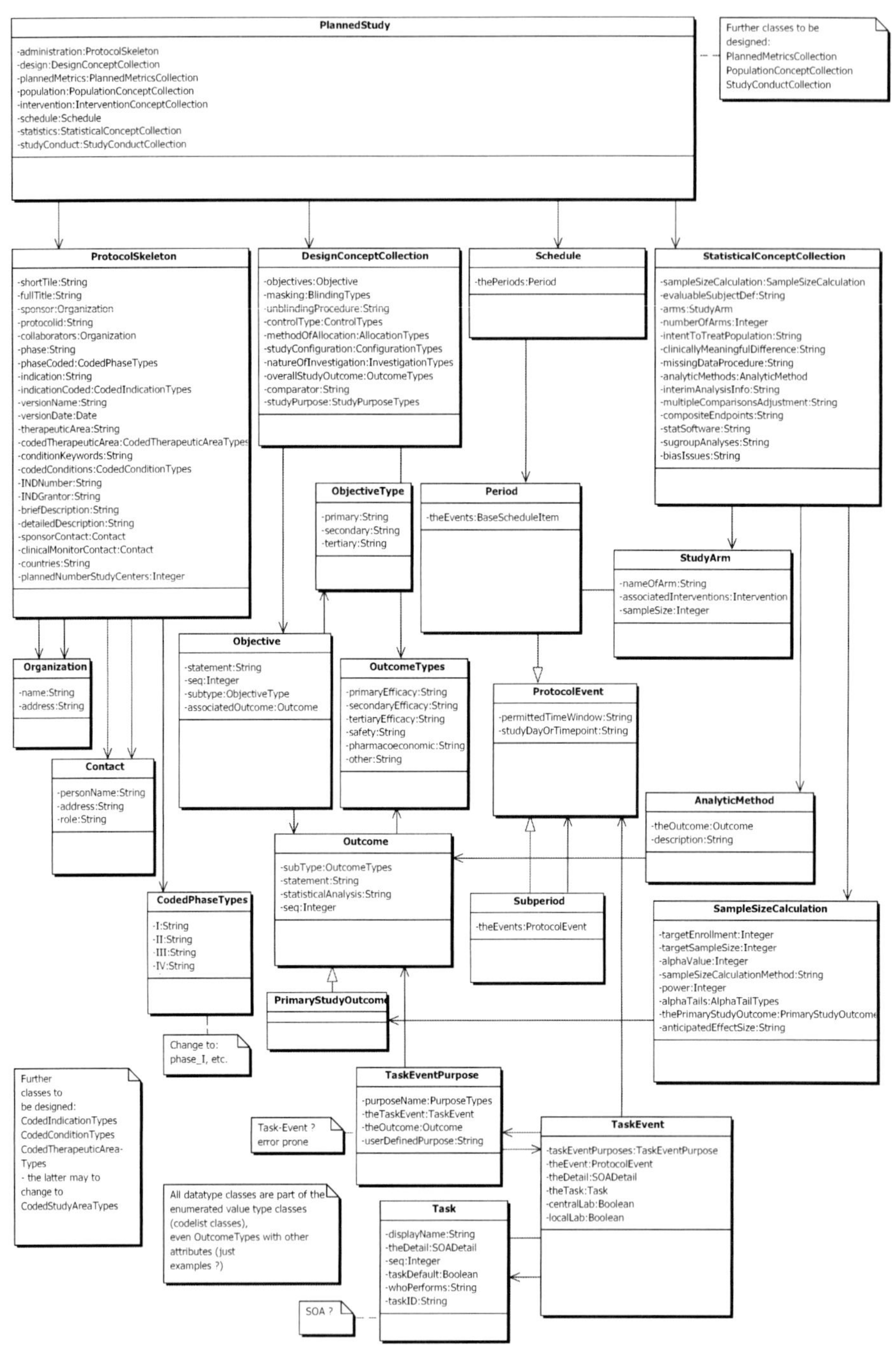


**Fig. 2.** The RCRIM Model of a Study Protocol [8]

[8] partially modelled according to available RCRIM material, see [9]

Due to the need for precision, terms systems like LOINC become cumber stone, e.g. there are – for example – 29 variations of sodium-related observational methods, and hence names. Some names change, as it was the case of adiuretin, later named antidiuretic hormone, then arginine vasopressin (argipressin). Therefore, a higher set of current research concepts may not have been inserted in LOINC and research may be a major deliverer of new terms. Furthermore, these considerations have influence on implementation issues like the different ease to set up coded lists for healthcare and research.

Another issue of lab data handling is the still prevailing co-existence of international and national standards. For example, in Germany the "Labordatenträger-Satz" (LDT, lab data carrier set) still plays a vital role independently from HL7. The German Association of Ambulantory Physicians (KBV) had standardized (beginning in the late eighties) the data exchange between physician office computer systems. The set of KBV standards had been defined and maintained for a long time, independently from the U.S.-driven HL7 standards[9] The KBV has defined – besides the LDT – a "Basisdatenträger-Satz" (BDT, Basic Data Carrier Set), an "Allgemeiner Datenträger-Satz" (ADT, General Data Carrier Set), a "Gerätedatenträger-Satz (GDT, Device Data Carrier Set) and more.

Due to the fact that a re-definition of the term set will take time, the German SCIPHOX project has chosen an interim solution by handling the KBV data sets via XML namespace techniques. This does not solve the semantic unification problems, but it is at least a step towards a higher level of interoperability.

The generation of **vital sign data** and image data in healthcare as well in research very often result in huge amounts of data (e.g. in some clinics and research institute this can grow up to terabyte levels). An important topic to be reflected in this area is the work done by CEN TC251 under the title "Vital Sign Information Representation". The issue is too complex to be considered here en passant. Nevertheless, the following remarks may introduce some useful thoughts for practical implementations. It would be ideal to be able to trigger common implementations in the Frame of Common European initiatives.

Furthermore, dealing with the vital sign issue has to be limited to some aspects of ECG data handling. The usage of ECGs can be seen with regard to conceptual data modelling and actual data handling of e-health and e-science as a quite uniform and well established process. A simple example of a necessary distinction of differences is given by discussing issues of handling so-called personal and demographic data of a patient. These data have, for example, been incorporated in the SCP ECG[10] header, which is well-suited for healthcare, but can create some problems for researchers. ECG devices with a fixed SCP ECG header would be too rigid. In order to preserve blind—trial conditions, the name field of the SCP ECG header must be left empty during the conduct of an investigational ECG measurement. Instead, the subject code and study participation data have to be handled somehow. The patient name segment in the SCP ECG header could be used for inserting the Test Subject Code. However, in the end, the personal and complete demographic data of a test subject should be inserted in the overall data header of the ECG measurement, when it comes to data archiving after de-blinding. Either the SCP ECG header has to be handled in a flexible way or a fixed header has to be used with some specially tailored workarounds.

Another interesting approach to improve the interoperability of ECG data was elaborated in the context of clinical trial submissions to FDA (U.S. Federal Drug and Food Administration). The FDA reviewers of drug approvals wanted to check the quality of the undertaken measures by requesting the submission of pieces of the original ECG measurement data. After a first standardisation round, an XML approach of device-

---

[9] This had been different in the German hospital scene. The Hospital Information System (HIS) developers have soon adapted HL7 standards, including the HL7 lab standards.

[10] Standard Communication Protocol ECG, a CEN standard

independent ECG data was drafted. It turned out, that the semantics of the developed XML DTD[11] was actually representing a "plotter semantics". Therefore, more effort was undertaken to specify an ECG measurement activity as a special form of observation. The HL7 Class "Observation" was extended by a subclass group which enables to define "series of observations", regions of interest and more. The value attribute of such an "Observation" class should not only contain single values, but should be able to manage time series.

## 5. The bIT4Health Initiative of the German Government

The German Federal Ministry of Health and Social Affairs (Bundesministerium für Gesundheit und Soziale Sicherung; BMGS) has initiated an ambitious project to implement a crypto-processor-based health card no later than 2006. In a short time window every German citizen should obtain a second generation health card. 72 million cards have to be issued; a first cost estimation for the introduction came up with figures of about 1 billion Euro. Additionally, special arrangements have to be made for children and persons not mentally able to handle such a device. The "bIT for Health" project shall deliver a framework architecture enabling the German software industry to build up a national telematics platform for health. The health smart card is seen as key infrastructure element to modernize the German health system.

The Telematics Platform shall be designed in a way that further applications can be added in an incremental fashion. A nation-wide distributed system architecture, which enables the virtual arrangement of electronic health records across organizational borders, could be the next logical step in this endeavor. A consortium led by IBM Germany[12] (on behalf of the BMGS) has started to specify a detailed, feasible architecture for the health card. Work is already underway and currently comprises primarily the analysis of the requirements and a business process model of the services linked to the health card. This business process model is seen as highly necessary to be able to focus the preparation of a data model and data flow descriptions.

The interest of the author is now focused here on following the initiative of the BMGS and trying to identify in the coming years the prospect of inter-connecting healthcare and research via electronic record systems in a more systematic way.

## 6. Open Issues

Some central issues related to interchanging the concepts used for the development of EHCRs and ERSRs need further clarification of the underlying concepts. One of these issues is a more elaborated use of the term "**metadata**". Some authors equate metadata with header data or reference data, others distinguish between header data and metadata, while a central group of authors work with an understanding that metadata being constituted via IT-technological decisions. The last group distinguishes metadata from data by pointing to the manner of implementation. Metadata are interwoven in code, for example as class, attribute, method names in object-oriented programming, as table and column names in relational database technology, as element and element attribute names in XML, etc.. In this way, a clear distinction can be made between metadata as named system containers and data as content. Technologies like the Java reflection methods can handle metadata in a powerful way. The interchange between different techniques is possible, e.g. generating XML tags from the RDBMS table with the name "Table" (actually a meta-table).

---

[11] Document Type Definition

[12] The other partners are FhG, SAP, InterComponentWare and Orga.

Distinctions between metadata and data not based on technical implementation decisions are in danger on relying too much on the subjective, arbitrary will of the person making the distinction. It happens very often that one person -classifies data as data and another as metadata, introducing unwanted subjectivity. In the "research" application field distinctions like "science data" and "house keeping data" are common, but they depend on the scientific question, on when and how the border between the two is shifted. Furthermore, it can be questioned whether house keeping data is metadata or simply another kind of data[13]. The subject matter here has to deal with topical subjects like data dictionaries, repositories, etc., eventually a distinction between "explicit" and "implicit" metadata is helpful. The term field of "metadata" contains and extends to such concepts as meta-language, meta-class, meta-objects, meta-model, meta-meta-model (Meta-Object-Facility), meta-signs, meta-relationships, meta-schema, etc. As it is very often when trying to elaborate semantic precision, the players have to accept that a term is used as homonym.

To establish a clear non-technological distinction of the relationship between metadata and data in a discipline, a foundational ontology[14] may disengage from too subjective constructs and pave the way for an inter-subjective consensus on the matter.

**Acknowledgement.** The author thanks Andrea Nitsche for critical-constructive proofreading.

## References

[1] Duwe H., Schwartmann D., Bartels E.: The Relevance of System Modeling and Semantic Analysis for the Development of E-Health Applications, International Conference on E-Health in Common Europe, Kraków, 2003

[2] Duwe H.: Managing Information Model via Planned Evolutionary Pathways, in press

[3] Kay S., Purves I.: Medical Records and Other Stories. A Narratological Framework, Methods of Information in Medicine, Volume 35, 2/1996, p. 72 – 87

[4] Verbalis J.G.: Disorders of body water homeostasis, Best Practice and Research Clinical Endocrinology and Metabolism, Vol. 17, No. 4, 2003, pp. 471-503

[5] Titze J. et al: Osmotically inactive skin Na+ storage in rats, Am J Physiol Renal Physiol, 285, 2003, pp. F1108-F1117

[6] Truniger B., Richards R.: Wasser- und Elektrolythaushalt. Diagnostik und Therapie, Stuttgart, 1985

[7] Heer M. et al: High dietary sodium chloride consumption may not induce body fluid retention in humans, Am J Physiol Renal Physiol, 278, 2000, pp. F585-F595

[8] Logical Observation Identifier Names and Codes (LOINC). User Guide, edited by McDonald et al, *http://www.regenstrief.org/loinc*

[9] Regulated Clinical Research Information Model, *http://www.hl7.org/Special/committees/rcrim/rcrim.htm*

---

[13] Setting "data" and "content" as synonym, as it is done in DLR-Medical Telematics Platform development, is a pragmatic decision, well suited, but not solving the problem to establish a conceptual foundation, clarifying possible derived constructs as "meta-content", a term naming the union set of metadata and data, "metadata" as distinct from "content-data", etc.

[14] For the meaning of the term „foundational ontology" see the works of the Institute of Formal Ontology and Medical Information Science (Leipzig). After all, this requested kind of foundation will surely require to clarify the role of "meta-data" as special "signs" within the semiotic triangle (C.S. Peirce), the meta-language approaches of Bertrand Russell, the speech act theory of Austin and Searle, and more.

*Transformation of Health Care with Information Technologies*
*M. Duplaga et al. (Eds.)*
*IOS Press, 2004*

# Integrating Electronic Guidelines into the Diagnostic Cycle

Ole Martin WINNEM
*SINTEF ICT*
*S.P. Andersensvei 15b, 7465 Trondheim, Norway*

**Abstract.** Clinical guidelines have been used for diagnostic and treatment purposes, and lately much of this information has become available in electronic formats. In Norway a medical electronic handbook has been developed [1] to give support for the physician, deciding upon diagnoses and treatment. This electronic handbook is now widely used, but not in a systematic fashion – due to lack of user-friendliness. The lack of integration with EPR systems and, more importantly, the lack of integration with the working process, are additional obstacles.

In order to improve the usability of the electronic handbook, we have developed a prototype where the commercially-available handbook is tightly integrated with the EPR system and where the EPR system is based on a problem-based approach. The prototype is focused on providing support to the diagnostic process, treatment planning, documentation and pointers to extended knowledge support. The integration of knowledge support and the EPR system was based on a semantic model representation in the middleware and an XML-based representation of the knowledge content within a SQL database. In addition to clinical guidelines, the ICPC-2[2] codes and their inclusion and exclusion criteria are used to support the diagnostic task

## Introduction

Improving the care and treatment within 1st-level care (general practitioners) is a major concern. An important contribution to the field is a set of clinical guidelines, used to support the clinician in the diagnostic and treatment process. Clinical guidelines have, until now, been based of textual descriptions of diagnostic procedures and treatment. Development has been driven by medical experts with focus on content, using well-known concepts for presentation, and the systems have been used separately from diagnostic or documentation tools. In our proposed framework, we have focused on creating a solution where a semantic network explains the relations between textual knowledge and the user context. We have chosen to use the Creek [3] semantic network because of expression strength and due to the fact that it enables the representation and retrieval of cases. Case retrieval is not further discussed within this article, since it will only be used for creating patient plans.

The most important tool for GPs is an EPR system. The purpose of the system is to make the GP able to remember events of importance. Since our overall objective is to support continuity of care, we base the indexing of patient information on a problem-based approach where almost all patient-related information provided by GPs is related to defined episodes of care. The problem-oriented patient record [4] was first introduced by Lawrence L. Weed in the late 1960s. He suggested to index patient information based on problems in order to improve the structure of the medical record and make it easier to use. So far, the approach has not been followed up in commercial EPR systems, but we have reasons to believe that this will be seen as a necessity in the future. With today's EPR systems it is nearly impossible to keep track of the history of a complex problem, but still the problem-based EPR has not been successful. We believe this is due to lack of user-friendly solutions available. With our approach, we want to demonstrate that it is possible to make the problem-oriented EPR time-effective compared to today's chronological-based EPR.

This paper is structured into four sections. The first section presents the knowledge base and identifies its limitations, the second section discusses how problem-based EPR is able to improve the quality of GP work. The third section describes the GP working style and the fourth section suggests a design for a helpful problem-based EPR system. The last section presents concluding remarks and further work.

## 1. Norwegian Electronic Physician Handbook (NEL)

NEL is an electronic handbook that was developed by GPs with support from hospital experts in order to allow for better diagnostic decisions and treatment. The early initiative was taken in relation with a NTNU/SINTEF project in the early 90s and a company (NHI) was later established to exploit the developed product. At that time, more than 90% of GPs in Norway were using EPR systems [5] to document diagnostic and treatment information as fairly skilled computer users. The handbook had been based on a hierarchy of HTML pages, but it has later been transferred into an XML-based database structure.

The handbook has evolved into a generic support system for both GPs and hospital experts searching for knowledge within areas outside their expertise. This extended use has made the handbook a tool for all health providers in Norway.

The handbook tries to follow a natural diagnostic process where the physician can input the most important symptoms and retrieve information about how to go about making diagnoses, known pitfalls, differential diagnoses, examinations, treatment and references to documentation. The approach constitutes a great improvement in the area of knowledge support to GPs by providing best practice information, updated four times a year and even more frequently, if critical changes to diagnostic standards are introduced.

The content of the handbook varies from information about children psychiatry and working medicine to cardiac diseases and orthopedic treatment. It is divided into chapters describing different medical sub-domains, all of which fall into five focus areas:

- symptoms and signs,
- conditions and diseases,
- examinations,
- patient information,
- illustrations.

Each area is, of course, further structured: while selecting one of the possible symptoms and signs, the information is presented in a structured way, starting with general definitions, occurrence, diagnostic thinking, diagnostic pitfalls and ICPC and ICD-10 classifications. The next chapters describe differential diagnoses, related diseases, clinical examination, treatment and advice, patient information, illustration and, at the end, sources of knowledge.

The handbook has a predefined structure that is easy to navigate, but this structure has been developed in order to make it easier for human experts to find information. The structure is not coded in a way that makes it easy for the computer to find relevant information, except for searching special phrases. Information is coded, using XML, but XML is also used to identify the type of font for the information and not for structuring the content. The figure below shows that XML markers do not tell anything about what kind of information is shown below.

```
<document>
    <title>Kronisk obstruktiv lungesykdom (KOLS)</title>
    <content>
    <section>
       <heading>Kjerneopplysninger</heading>
       <section>
            <heading>Definisjon</heading>
            <ul>
                <li>Samlebetegnelse for lungesykdommer med
                luftstrømshindring som ikke er fullt reversibel</li>
                <li>Luftstrømshindringen er vanligis både progressiv og
                assosiert med unormal inflammatorisk reaksjon i
                lungene</li>
                <li>Definisjonen inneholder ikke betegnelsene kronisk
                bronkitt eller emfysem, og den utelukker astma</li>
            </ul>
       </section>
    </section>
    </content>
</document>
```

**Fig. 1.** Typical coding of information within NEL (the information is written in Norwegian)

By developing a more advanced metamodel describing the structure of the content, the handbook can be integrated with other programs and be used in other, more advanced ways than just for providing information to the user through a Web interface. In the section of system design we are suggesting a solution where a semantic network is used to identify relevant information.

## 2. Problem Based EPR – a Holistic View of Patient Information

With today's chronological approach to indexing record information, GPs face significant challenge when attempting to identify all information that is relevant for current consultations. Some systems provide limited search tools in order to support the solution, but this will never give a complete view of related information. With today's working style of Norwegian GPs, where they document several problems in one note[6] and relate this to only one diagnosis, it becomes impossible to identify relevant information. In order to structure the information in an adequate way, new documentation practices must be introduced. The problem with introducing new practices is that the new practice must reduce the work that the GPs have to do. This is again related to identifying the tasks required in order to perform an activity. If the number of tasks increases, this will boost the cognitive load of the GP and focus will drift away from their core mission.

The main argument for problem-based EPR has so far been that the user should receive a holistic view of the patient's situation. This is a very important argument, but the demand for problem-based EPR becomes even more important when close, cross-level collaboration is introduced. Sharing information about a specific problem across various levels of care creates the need for problem-based indexing. Such indexing will provide an opportunity to share relevant information about the patient without having to invest effort in deciding what is relevant and what is not.

To be able to create a holistic view of the patient for all relevant caregivers, the system should provide all relevant information about a given problem, including all documentation from each episode of care, as well as shared plans. This is especially important when related to chronic patients, where a shared understanding of the patient's situation for both caregivers and the patient is required [7]. The information on the patient must be viewable with different granularities, based on the role of the caregiver.

## 3. GP Working Process and System Task Model

Several task models related to the GPs examination of patients have been developed and elaborated, but the successful models have so far had little impact on EPR systems. Early systems, based on DOS, required a good task model and a clear understanding of the working process, but when Windows-based systems were introduced in the early 90s, this focus and knowledge seamed to dissipate. EPR systems have since then focused on keeping all options open for each user. This lack of understanding on the part of providers has led to a very diverse working style among Norwegian GPs, switching between modules and with minor focus on the patient problem.

It is therefore important to redesign the system in order to fit it to a generic working process and identify a task model proper to problem-based EPR. In this approach we have chosen to use the generic working process as shown in Figure 3. The initial part of our approach involves investigating the reason for encounter; hence information related to this reason plays an important role. By identifying the reason for encounter, the GP is able to prepare herself even before the patient is invited into the office in order to delve more thoroughly into the reason for encounter (subjective and objective). When applied to chronic patients (eg. suffering from diabetes), this solution gives the GP the opportunity to prepare for annual physicals, etc.

The SOAP model illustrates the main tasks of the GP, but it is not compatible with the way GPs works today. One of the main problems related to today's working process is the documentation of several problems within one note [8]. In order to overcome this obstacle, we have created a simple task structure that covers the most common user tasks and makes it easy to change between selected problems. The first step in a normal process related to a patient visit is the reason for encounter registration. This is normally done by an assistant and is less time-critical (may even be performed within another system). In our prototype we have focused on creating relations to the structured information captured within objective (laboratory requisition), assessment (diagnosis) and plan (medication) tasks. In our approach, we have focused on how we are able to connect the assessment and plan and support these steps through providing an integrated solution of the knowledge base (NEL).

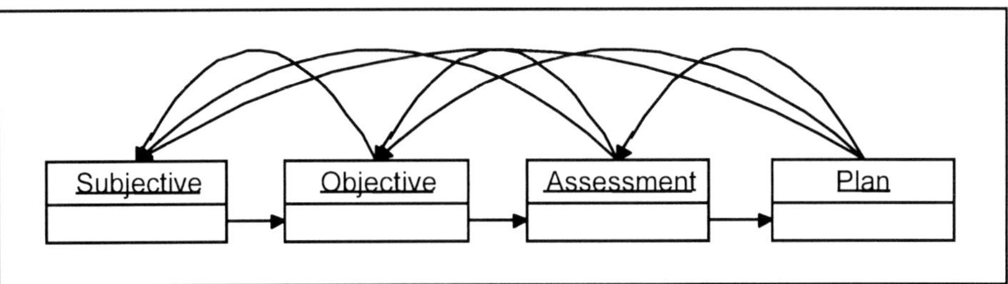


**Fig. 2.** The SOAP model is a well-known solution for the medical diagnostic process

## 4. System Design

Understanding the working process is critical when introducing problem-based EPR because it requires indexing on more than one parameter. In our approach we have created a system with minimal navigation. By this we understand that the user, when dealing with a patient, is always circling around one overview picture where all important information is present and where changing problems is supported with an open tree model that simplifies navigation. Since we are focusing on the increasingly important problem of chronic care [9], we have also chosen to introduce new information in this central view. Through this view, the GP is always informed about the long-term treatment objective and the treatment plan for the selected problem. The system is designed to support collaboration with other caregivers through the planning module. In this module all caregivers are able to share information about the patient regarding treatment goals and activities.

### *4.1 Three Modules Covering the user Needs*

The system has been developed with three modules. The administrative module covers tasks related to setting up the system and patient administration. This unit is developed in order to create a framework for the patient module and make the user able to configure the system. The patient module is the main module and the one discussed in detail within this article. It exemplifies some of the principles that must be discussed when introducing problem-based indexing within the EPR. The planning module provides support for taking care of chronic patients (it is not discussed within this article). The rest of the system design is focused on the patient module.

### *4.2 Semantic Model for Retrieving Information from the Knowledge Base*

The described system has a limited number of tasks related to the SOAP process. This gives a limited knowledge model identifying relevant information from the knowledge source to the GP. The semantic model describes the user tasks and their relation to the working process. Dependent on process steps, tasks and input information, pointers to relevant sources are created. The system then displays the referenced information. In figure 3, a part of the semantic structure is shown. The structure shows how the knowledge model links information about the tasks performed and the knowledge source. Dependent on which component[1] the selected ICPC code contains, different relations have to be introduced into the knowledge base (e.g. signs and symptoms are described differently than conditions and diseases).

[1] The ICPC is structured into 7 components where component 1 relates to symptoms and complaints, components 2-6 are process codes and component 7 involves disease codes.

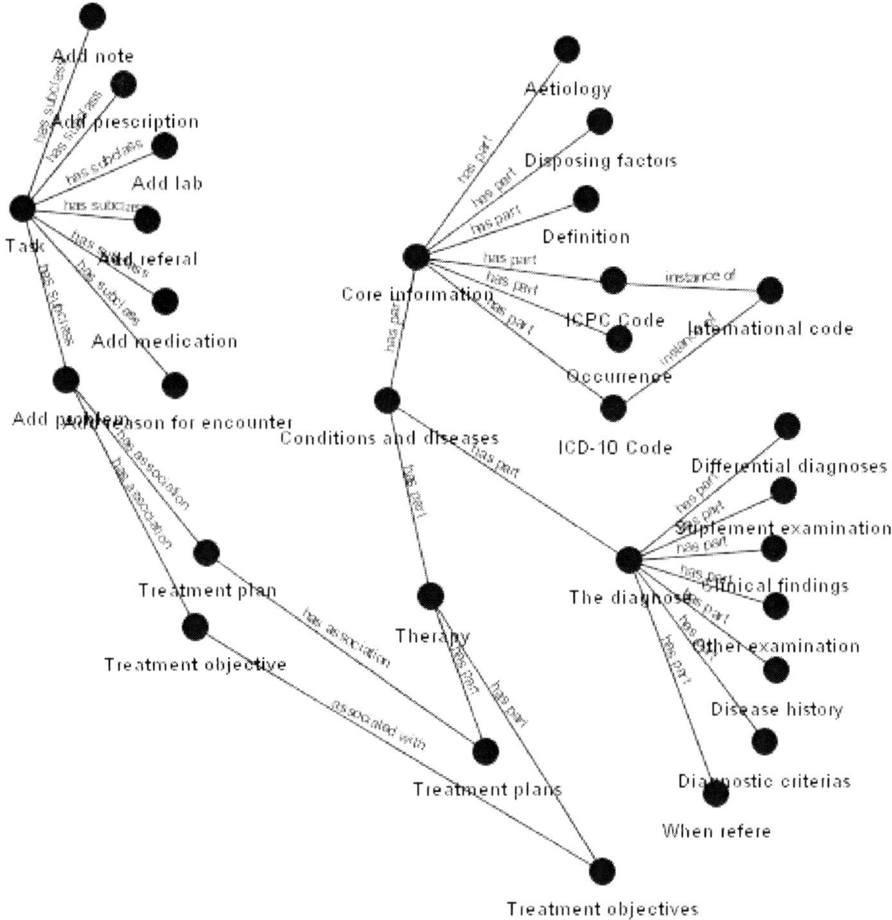


**Fig. 3.** Part of the semantic network connecting the partly-structured information from NEL to information elements in the user interface[2].

## 4.3 The Patient Examination Task Model

In the task model shown in Figure 4, all tasks are tied up to the examination activity. The idea is to have one view that all tasks can be performed from. We call this a zero-navigation approach since the user is not switching between views or modules when working with a patient. The figure only identifies the major tasks related to patient examination, but we have focused on the tasks that normally occupy the GP during consultation. When introducing problem-based EPR one of the most important tasks is the creation of problems and switching between problems. Since this is a task that imposes additional load on the GP, it is a challenge to integrate it into the natural process and not make the GP spend extra time. The system is designed in order to always return to the main activity when a task is performed and we are using a modal dialog approach. The referral task is the most

[2] The model has been created with the Creek browser (*www.idi.ntnu.no/~frodeso/*).

advanced task with several dialog options available, but we have solved this issue by making it easy to select the type of referral within the dialog.

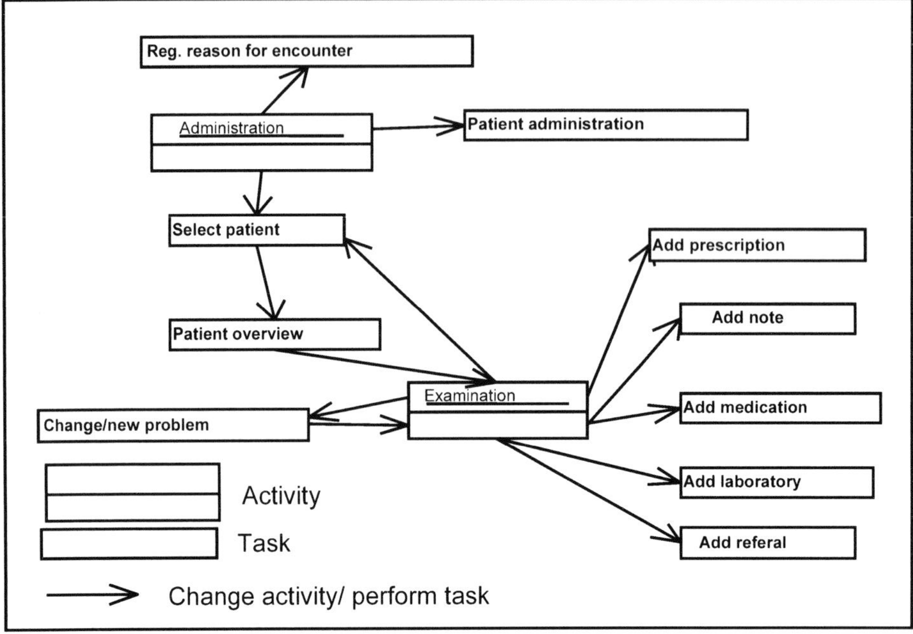


**Fig. 4.** A zero-navigation alternative for a problem-based EPR solution

The registration of the reason for encounter is the first step in a sequence of tasks that are performed in relation to a patient visit. This is a task that is not time-critical and that is often performed by administrative workers. By making the patient selection task easy (choosing the next item on the list of patients) the GP is led into a patient overview task where the reason for encounter is presented along with a list of related documents within the EPR. If the reason for encounter is not related to earlier problems, then the most recent documents are presented. The registration of the reason for encounter does not support structured records of several reasons, but this is an improvement that might be added in the future. When the GP has performed the patient overview study, the patient is invited into the GP's office to undergo further examination. At the point the patient is presented, the problems related to the reason for encounter are selected by the system and the GP can focus on acquiring more information about the visit. In this process, all tasks performed by the GP are related to the selected problem.

### *4.4 Naming and Clustering of Problems*

When designing a problem-based EPR, one of the problems involves creating a naming strategy for problems. We have evaluated three possible solutions. One solution is to keep the initial name of the problem. An example of this is when a problem is created based on symptoms and signs as "SHORTNESS OF BREATH" (ICPC: R02). The diagnosis might, over time or following further investigation, end up with COPD (ICPC: R95). The initial problem name may be kept or it may evolve over time (second solution). A third solution is to have the problem name only as an open text field. Each solution has its advantages as well as drawbacks. It can be argued that the third option keeps the GP updated about ongoing diagnoses, but from a research point of view, where the initial reason for encounter is used for preparing statistics about what initial complaints end up with a specific diagnosis, it may be more natural to maintain the initial diagnosis. Others will argue that the problem should not be directly connected to a diagnosis. An important argument related to the last naming convention is the issue of problem clustering. We know many cases of parallel diseases, including they relate to each other. In our solution, we have chosen to implement a system where each case is related to the last given diagnosis for the evolving problem. Furthermore, we have created a solution where two levels of problems can be described simultaneously. With our two-level design, we cover the issue of problem clustering. This is kept as an open solution where the GP can attach several diagnoses to one main diagnosis. Since this is realized in a tree structure, the total overview remains intuitive. Figure 5 shows an example a of tree structure where one diagnosis is stored as a subdiagnosis of other, higher-level diagnosis.

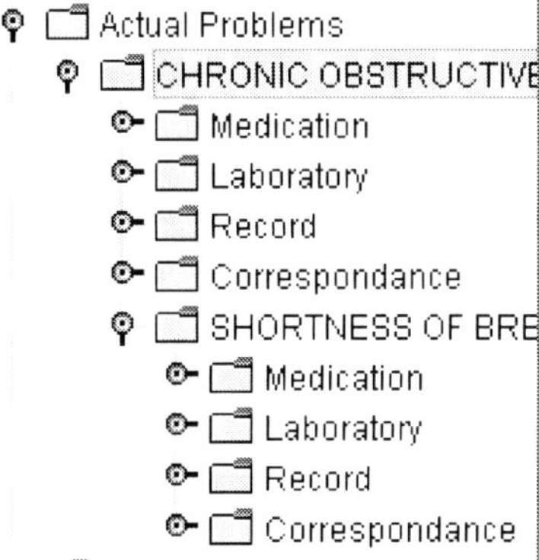


**Fig. 5.** The tree model in the user interface

### *4.5 Knowledge Support Related to New Problems*

The use of knowledge support has been focused on the interaction related to creation of new problems. We have integrated support from both ICPC II and NEL. They are both reached through knowledge middleware using the Creek semantic network. When an ICPC code is chosen, the middleware identifies what kind of relevant information should be displayed to the user. This is needed, because the NEL knowledge base is not well structured as described earlier. Dependent on whether the ICPC number identifies a symptom or a diagnosis and dependent on which type of diagnosis/symptom is identified, the middleware helps find the relevant information for diagnostic reasoning, treatment objectives etc. In Figure 6, COPD is chosen and the system presents inclusion/exclusion criteria along with treatment objectives and treatment plans. If the information presented is insufficient, then all the available information about the problem can be reached through a Web browser.

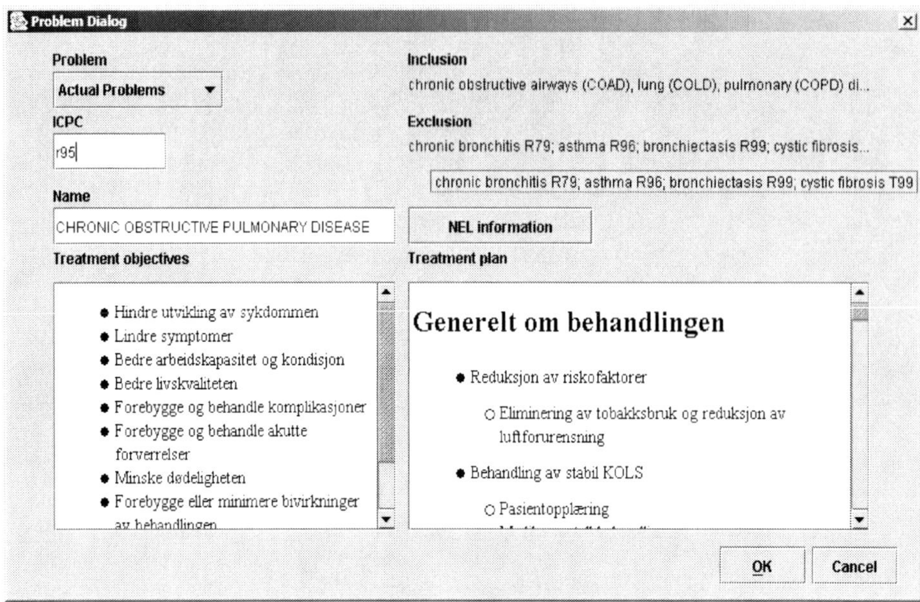


**Fig. 6.** The Problem Dialog is used to input new problems. Within the dialog, the GP is able to obtain all relevant information for the chosen diagnosis[3]

## 5. Conclusions and Further Work

Electronic medical records have had major success with improving the administrative work, such as billing, prescription etc.; however diagnostic-related activities have not used the potential advantage that modern software methods provide. The EPR systems have so far been used as a kind of a typewriter, with documentation based on free text. Developing new methods provides great potential for the improvement of diagnostic and treatment work.

Within this article, we have presented a framework for integrating knowledge support within a problem-based EPR. We have focused on problems related to how a partly-structured knowledge base can be used to support a diagnostic process and which challenges related to the design of a problem-based EPR that must be overcome before this approach can be successful. The most important challenge when developing a problem-based EPR is deciding on how to relate clustered problems to each other. We have used what we think is the most promising approach, with one main problem to which all others relate in a two-layer model. Still, this approach must be further investigated and validated in order to make conclusions.

When it comes to using a electronic knowledge base originally built to support GPs in a separate solution, we have fond that it is possible to create close integration, but this depends on building up context middleware, able to identify where to find the relevant information, given the user needs. Another approach that should be investigated is to create a metamodel and transform the markup of the knowledge base to structured content, understandable for the EPR software.

In order to create a holistic view of a patient, documentation of plans is needed. The development of a planning system integrated with the problem-based solution is important. Our approach demands some changes in working style of the GP, but we see this as needed

[3] Some of the text elements within the figure are written in Norwegian.

to improve the quality of care. The changes in working habits have to be further evaluated and monitored in order to identify whether they are a viable solution.

**Acknowledgement.** Tom Christensen and Anders Grimsmo, NTNU, Faculty of Medicine.

## References

[1] Johannesen, T.L., I., *Norsk elektronisk legehåndbok*. 2004, NHI.

[2] WONCA, I.C.C., *International Classification of Primary Care ICPC-2*. 2 ed: Oxford Medical Publications.

[3] Aamodt, A.P., E, *Case-Based Reasoning: Foundational Issues, Methodological Variations and System Approaches*. AICom - Artificial Intelligence Communications. Vol. 7:1. 1994: IOS Press. 39-59.

[4] Weed, L.L., *Medical records that guide and teach*. The New England Journal of Medicine, 1968. 278(12).

[5] Grimsmo, A., EPJ in General Practice. 1994.

[6] Bayegan, E., Knowledge Representation for Relevance Ranking of Patient-Record Contents in Primary-Care Situations, in IDI. 2002, NTNU: Trondheim. p. 203.

[7] Hernandez C., C.A.E.J., Alonso J., Puig-Junoy J., Farrero E., Vilagut G., Collvinent B., Rodriguez-Roisin R. and Roca J., *Home hospitalisation of exacerbated chronic obstructive pulmonary disease patients*. European Respiratory Journal, 2003. 21(1): p. 68-73.

[8] Bayegan, E.N., Ø.; Grimsmo, A. Ontologies for knowledge representation in a computer-based patient record. in 14th International Conference on tools with Artificial Intelligence. 2002.

[9] WHO, *Innovative care for chronic conditions*. 2002, World Health Organization: Geneva. p. 61.

# Presentation of Medical Guidelines on a Computer

David BUCHTELA[1,2], Zdeněk ANGER[1,3], Jan PELESKA[1,3], Arnost VESELY[1,2], Jana ZVAROVA[1,2]
[1]*European Center for Medical Informatics, Statistics and Epidemiology – Cardio*
[2]*Institute of Computer Science ASCR, Prague, Czech Republic*
[3] *2nd Dept. of Medicine, General Faculty Hospital, Prague, Czech Republic*
*e-mail: buchtela@euromise.cz*

**Abstract.** Free-text forms of medical guidelines that are used in medical care are often cumbersome and difficult to memorize. Therefore a system that is able to present guidelines in a user-friendly manner has been designed. Guidelines are at first formalized by means of the popular GLIF3 model. Subsequently, the GLIF3 model is coded in XML. The system uses patient data and an XML-coded GLIF3 model graph evaluating the conditions of decision steps. If some conditions cannot be evaluated, (due to the unavailability of required data items), the system stops and highlights a branch from the root of the decision tree to the final step. Then, the user can input missing data into the system so that the system can continue to provide visualization. Thus, the presentation of guidelines is data-driven, making its use easier. The visualization system and the Electronic Health Record can be integrated in a system that can, during examination of a patient, suggest subsequent medical actions according to medical guidelines. Such a system has been designed and is now under development.

## Introduction

Many medical guidelines have been elaborated to improve the quality of medical care and to achieve standardization of treatment. Typically, the first version of medical guidelines is worked out by a group of medical experts in a free-text form. For computer implementation and processing, it is necessary to explicitly structure the guidelines. Numerous modelling techniques have been suggested for this purpose. The most important and, nowadays, most popular one seems to be the GLIF (Guideline Interchange Format) model. The GLIF model is a result of collaboration among Columbia University, Harvard University, McGill University and Stanford University. Version 2.0 of GLIF (GLIF2) was published in 1998 [1].

The main goal of GLIF was to enable sharing of guidelines among institutions and across computer applications. GLIF specifies an object-oriented model for guideline representation and syntax for guideline utilization in software systems as well as for their transport. GLIF guidelines are mostly given as a flowchart representing a temporally-ordered sequence of steps. Different types of steps in the flowchart represent clinical actions and decisions [1]. To enhance the usability of GLIF, a new version (GLIF3) has been developed. GLIF3 builds upon the framework set by GLIF2, but augments it by introducing several new constructs and extending GLIF2 constructs to allow a more formal definition of decision criteria and patient data [2]. In the following parts of the paper, by GLIF we mean the GLIF3 model [3].

## 1. Guideline Representation Model

The GLIF model provides a process-orientated view on guidelines. It is also object-orientated. The model consists of a set of classes for guideline entities, attributes of these classes and data types for attribute values. Instances of classes (objects) have only attributes and no methods.

Particular guidelines encoded in GLIF are instances of a general guideline model. They can be represented in the form of an orientated graph. The nodes of the graph are guideline steps and edges representing continuation from one step to another. Guideline steps include the following: *action step*, *decision step*, *branch and synchronization steps* and a *patient state step*.

*Action steps* specify clinical actions that are to be performed. This can be an application of some therapy, carrying out some examination or measurement, etc. Action steps may also contain sub-guidelines, which provide greater detail for actions. (Fig. 1)

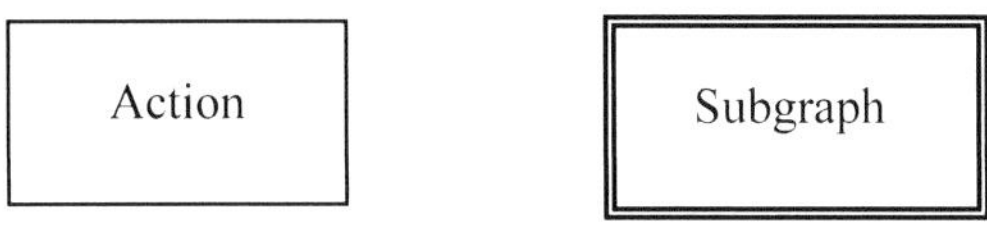


**Fig. 1.** Action steps

*Decision steps* are used for conditional branching. There are two kinds of decision steps: *case step* and *choice step*. *Case step* is used, when branching is determined by evaluation of predefined logical criteria based on data items. *Choice step* is used when the decision cannot be precisely specified in guidelines themselves and the decision should be made by the user (Fig. 2).

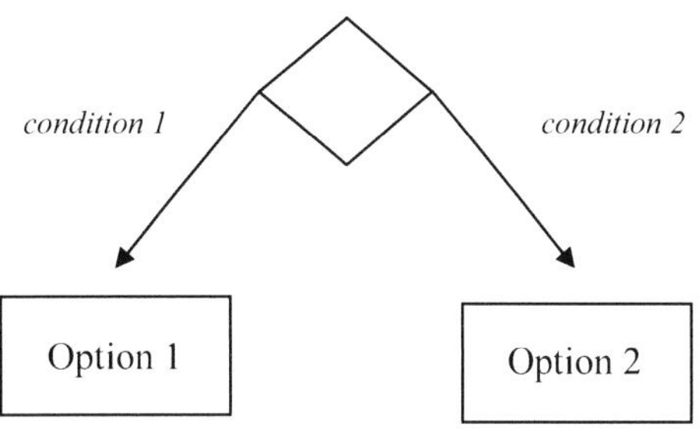


**Fig. 2.** Decision step

The decision step specifies strict-in, strict-out, rule-in and rule-out conditional criteria for each decision option. The strict-in attribute is used to specify a decision condition that could be computed automatically. If a strict-in attribute is evaluated as true, then control flows to the guideline step that is specified by that decision option's destination. The strict-out attribute is analogous to an absolute contraindication. If a strict-out attribute is evaluated as true, then that decision option's destination is forbidden. The rule-in criterion ranks a choice as the best among several options. For example, when there are competing diagnoses for a disease, a pathognomonic condition would be a rule-in for the disease. A rule-out takes precedence over rule-in when ranking options. If an option contains both a rule-in criterion and a rule-out criterion, and both are evaluated as true, then that option should be the last choice. The ranking of rule-ins and rule-outs is left to the user who may use his or her clinical judgment or may develop custom ranking schemes.

*Branch and synchronization steps* enable concurrence in the model. Guideline steps that follow branch steps can be performed concurrently. Branches with roots in branch steps eventually converge in a synchronization step. In this step, all branches are synchronized. This means that actions following the synchronization step cannot be performed unless all actions following the branch step and preceding the synchronization step are finished. (Fig. 3).

**Fig. 3.** Branch and synchronization step

The *Patient state step* characterizes a patient's clinical state (Fig. 4).

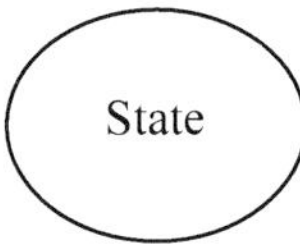


**Fig. 4.** State step

## 2. XML Implementation of GLIF 3.5

The guideline model can be equivalently expressed in the XML (*eXtensible Markup Language*) form. The syntax for guideline description language is a part of the guideline model specification. In the language form, encoded guidelines consist of a sequence of guideline steps. Some attributes of a guideline step contain subsequent guideline steps. This enables sequential representation of a graph structure in the guideline language.

### *2.1 Syntax of GLIF-XML*

**<GLIF>**
**<Step>** = start of step
    **<name>** = name of step – identification (ID)
    **<type>** = type of step: *action*
        *case*
        *state*
        *subgraph*
    **<note>** = short description of step
    **<text>** = text in a graphical symbol of step
    **<tag>** = shared actions
        **<T>**

```
                <ttype>        =     get     = input parameter get
                                     put     = output parameter set
                                     open    = open of subgraph or HTML file
                                     run     = service application run
                <tparam>       =     list of parameters
           </T>
           <T>
           ...  other shared actions
           </T>
  <x>           = x-coordinate of graphical symbol
  <y>           = y-coordinate of graphical symbol
  <w>           = width of graphical symbol
  <h>           = height of graphical symbol
  <focus>       = highlighting of step:      0 = no
                                             1 = yes
  <status>      = status of step:      1 = start step of a graph
                                       2 = end step of a graph
                                       0 = other steps
  <next>        = next step(s)
           <F>  = one of option attributes
                <nname>        = identification of option
                <nstep>        = name of destination (target step)
                <ncaption>     = caption of option
                <nnote>        = description of option
                <nline>        = coordinates of line to target step
                <nstrictin>    = strict-in criterion
                <nstrictout>   = strict-out criterion
                <nrulein>      = rule-in criterion
                <nruleout>     = rule-out criterion
           </F>
           <F>
           ...  = other options
           </F>
  </next>
</Step>         = end of step
<Step>
...             = other steps
</Step>
</GLIF>
```

## 3. Presentation of Medical Guidelines

Computerized GLIF guideline models provide the possibility of presenting them to a user in an easily-readable manner. The first simple version of the GLIF browser was developed and tested on the GLIF model of WHO/ISH Hypertension Guidelines 1999 (Fig. 5) and unstable angina pectoris guidelines.

In the meantime, a general browser has been developed in order to visualize any computerized GLIF model. The functionality of the browser is verified using models of 2003 ESH/ESC Hypertension Guidelines (Czech version) (Fig. 6).

The new system is of a client-server architecture. The GLIF online server stores GLIF models with different medical guidelines. Assuming that during examination of a patient the physician is working with an electronic health record (EHR) – if he requires decision support, he may choose one of the available guidelines provided by the GLIF server and start the GLIF client. The main part of the GLIF client is the browser that goes through the GLIF model graph evaluating the conditions of each decision step.

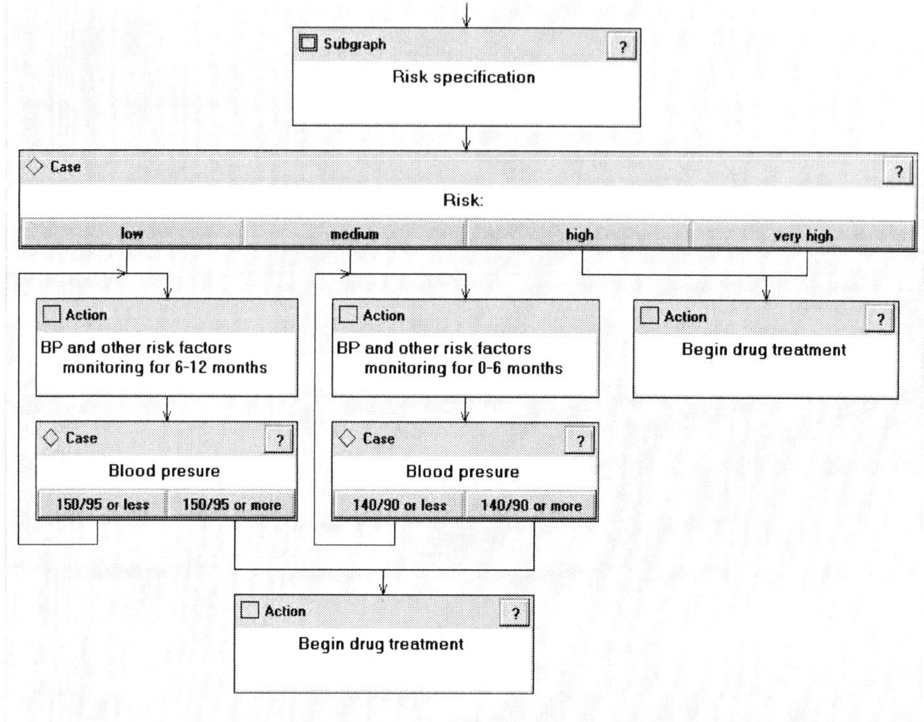


**Fig. 5.** GLIF model of 1999 WHO/ISH Hypertension Guidelines

The computer system uses patients' data and goes through the GLIF 3.5 model graph evaluating conditions of decision steps. If some condition cannot be evaluated, because the required data items are not available, the system stops and highlights the branch from the root to the current step. Thus it can serve as a reminder of the missing data necessary for a correct decision. Then, the user can input the missing data manually (or simulate data) in the system to continue visualization.

## 4. Conclusion

The GLIF browser is designed as a general tool that can present any formalized medical guidelines in a user-friendly manner. It could be used for education of students and as a decision support system in medical practice.

The GLIF model of formalized 2003 ESH/ESC Hypertension Guidelines offers to physicians an automated reminder system and a check of their decision algorithm in comparison with that of hypertension guidelines. In future, it will be able to obtain values of GLIF model parameters directly from the electronic health record.

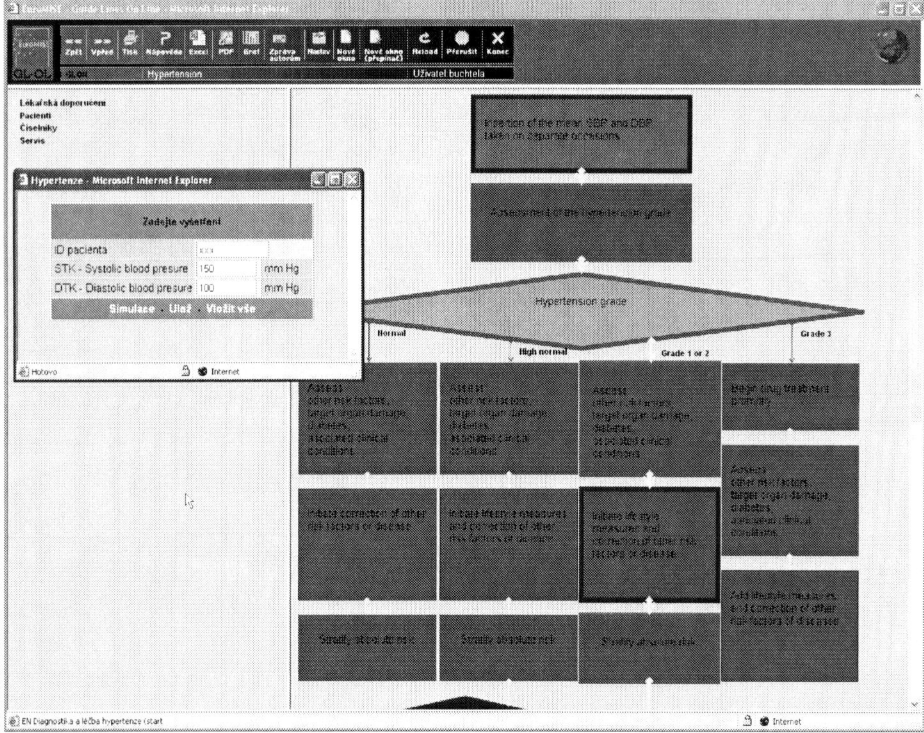


Fig. 6. GLIF model of 2003 ESH/ESC Hypertension Guidelines (Czech version)

The system, based on the proposed method, can work with arbitrary guidelines. Only at first the guidelines must be transformed into a GLIF graph model. Transformation of free-text guidelines into the GLIF model or a similarly structured and precisely defined formal model should be accomplished anyway, because only in this way guidelines can be expressed as unambiguous and non-contradictory.

When certain guidelines are changed, it is not necessary to correct the set of rules used for checking input data. Making corresponding changes in the guideline model is sufficient.

**Acknowledgement.** The research was supported with the LN00B107 project of the Ministry of Education CR.

## References

[1] Ohno-Machado L., Gennari J.H., Murphy S.,N., Jain N.,L., Tu S.,W., Oliver D., et al.: The Guideline Interchange Format: A model for representing guidelines, Journal of the American Medical Informatics Association 1998, 5(4), pp. 357-372.

[2] Peleg M., Boxwala A.A., et al.: GLIF3: The Evolution of Guideline Representation Format, In: *http://smi-web.stanford.edu/projects/intermed-web/guidelines*, 2000.

[3] Patel V.L., Branch T., Wang D., Peleg M., Boxwala A.: Analysis of the Process of Encoding Guidelines: A Comparison of GLIF2 and GLIF3, Methods Inf. Med., 2002, no.2, pp. 105-113.

# Caseview: Building the Reference Set

Pierre P. LÉVY
*Hôpital Tenon (Assistance Publique Hôpitaux de Paris),*
*INSERM U444, Unité de Biostatistique et Informatique Médicale, 4, rue de la Chine,*
*75970, Paris Cedex 20*
*e-mail: pierre.levy@tnn.ap-hop-paris.fr*

**Abstract.** There is a worldwide consensus for using the diagnosis related groups (DRG) when considering hospital activity. This tool leads to the production of tables of numbers (case mix), the interpretation of which is difficult. Therefore, methods aimed at facilitating this interpretation are needed.

One of such methods is the case view, i.e. a graphical representation of the case mix. It reduces, in a way, each DRG to a "pixel", the set of the DRGs being an image (the case view). The reference set should be organized according to three criteria: medical/surgical, nosological and economic. This method can be used to answer theoretical questions or to visualize activity at the level of a hospital or at the level of a department.

The purpose of this paper is to present important principles inherent in this graphic representation, both at the level of the method and at the level of the user.

## Introduction

There is a worldwide consensus for using the Diagnosis Related Groups (DRG) when considering hospital activity [1]. This approach leads to the production of tables of numbers (case mix), the interpretation of which is difficult (Figure 1).

**Table 1.** Part of a list of French DRGs

| DRG | NAME | Nb |
|---|---|---|
| 689 | Autres techniques d'irradiation externe, en séances | 5000 |
| 681 | Chimiothérapie pour tumeur, en séances | 4210 |
| 680 | Épuration extra-rénale, en séances | 2950 |
| 688 | Techniques complexes d'irradiation externe, en séances | 1697 |
| 876 | Nouveau-nés de 2500 g et plus, avec autre problème significatif | 675 |
| 540 | Accouchements par voie basse sans complication | 642 |
| 823 | @Motifs de recours de la CMD n°23 : ambulatoire, sans acte opératoire | 531 |
| 587 | Chimiothérapie pour autre tumeur, sans CMA | 484 |
| 685 | Préparations à une irradiation externe avec une dosimétrie | 468 |
| 686 | Autres préparations à une irradiation externe | 444 |
| 675 | Autres facteurs influant sur l'état de santé | 343 |
| 777 | Dilatations et curetages au cours de la grossesse, en ambulatoire | 307 |
| 684 | Autres séances sans acte opératoire | 272 |
| 830 | Endoscopies sous anesthésie, en ambulatoire | 266 |
| 127 | Œdème pulmonaire et détresse respiratoire | 264 |
| 182 | Cathétérismes cardiaques ou coronarographies pour une pathologie autre | 252 |
| 539 | Accouchements par voie basse avec complications | 234 |
| 874 | Nouveau-nés de 2500 g et plus, sans problème significatif | 209 |
| 549 | Affections de l'ante partum, avec ou sans intervention chirurgicale, sans | 201 |
| 690 | Transfusion, en séances | 200 |

The issue is to translate these tables of numbers into an image, to make them easier to use (Figure 1).

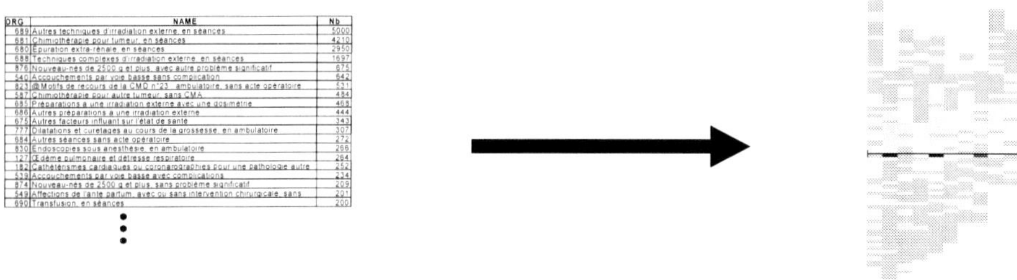

| DRG | NAME | Nb |
|---|---|---|
| 689 | Autres techniques d'irradiation externe, en séances | 5000 |
| 681 | Chimiothérapie pour tumeur, en séances | 4210 |
| 680 | Épuration extra-rénale, en séances | 2950 |
| 688 | Techniques complexes d'irradiation externe, en séances | 1697 |
| 876 | Nouveau-nés de 2500 g et plus, avec autre problème significatif | 675 |
| 540 | Accouchements par voie basse sans complication | 642 |
| 823 | @Motifs de recours de la CMD n°23 , ambulatoire, sans acte opératoire | 521 |
| 587 | Chimiothérapie pour autre tumeur, sans CMA | 484 |
| 685 | Préparations à une irradiation externe avec une dosimétrie | 468 |
| 686 | Autres préparations à une irradiation externe | 444 |
| 675 | Autres facteurs influant sur l'état de santé | 343 |
| 777 | Dilatations et curetages au cours de la grossesse, en ambulatoire | 307 |
| 684 | Autres séances sans acte opératoire | 272 |
| 830 | Endoscopies sous anesthésie, en ambulatoire | 266 |
| 127 | Œdème pulmonaire et détresse respiratoire | 264 |
| 182 | Cathétérismes cardiaques ou coronarographies pour une pathologie autre | 252 |
| 539 | Accouchements par voie basse avec complications | 234 |
| 874 | Nouveau-nés de 2500 g et plus, sans problème significatif | 209 |
| 549 | Affections de l'ante partum, avec ou sans intervention chirurgicale, sans | 201 |
| 690 | Transfusion, en séances | 200 |

**Fig. 1.** Issue

In this approach, the definition of the reference set of the image appears to be crucial. The reference set is a framework, which allows data analysis. It has to be built from three points of view:

- from the point of view of the DRG classification;
- from the point of view of the user: it is the building of a structure in the mind of the user. This step is obligatory if one wants the user to be able to understand the image. The mechanism of interpretation of the image will be outlined in the final part of the paper;
- from the point of view of the reader of this paper, as a future user of the method: many results will be presented to familiarize the reader with the method.

## 1. Method

The main idea is to reduce a DRG to a "pixel", the set of all DRGs being an image called a case view (Figure 2).

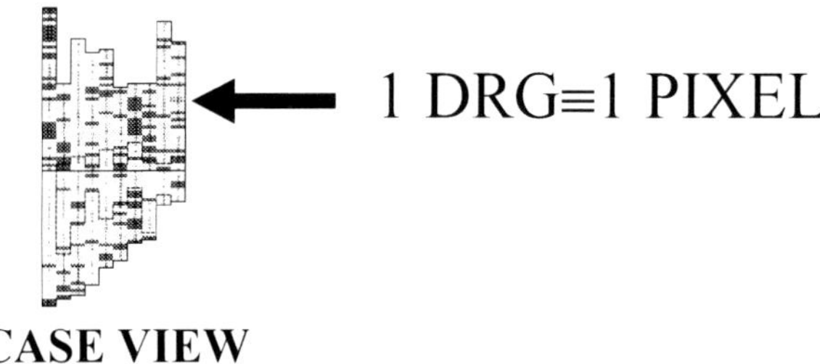


**Fig. 2.** Main idea

The method consists of two steps: building the reference set and visualizing the data.

### *1.1 Building the Reference Set*

This step involves the ordering of the "DRG pixels". Three main criteria are necessary [2] (Figure 3) to define the reference set. The first one is the surgical/medical dichotomy. The second one is the nosological criterion, i.e. the clustering of DRGs belonging to the same system or presenting a common characteristic. The third one is the "cost" criterion or, more exactly, the notion of "intensity of resource utilization" common to every classification in the world.

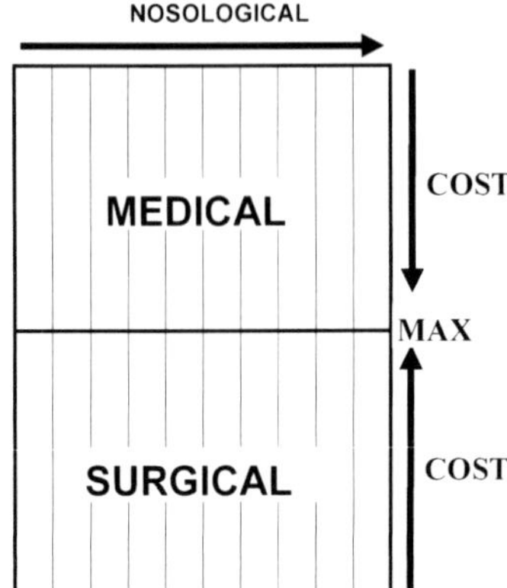


**Fig. 3.** The three main criteria enabling the construction of a reference set

Examples

In the French reference set [3] (Figure 4), the medical DRGs are in the upper part of the image and the surgical DRGs are in the lower part of the image (surgical/medical dichotomy). Each column contains a major category of diagnoses or a set of major categories of diagnoses (nosological criterion). Inside each column, the DRGs are sorted according to their cost: the heaviest DRGs, medical as well as surgical, are localized at the center of the reference set, close to the horizontal line.

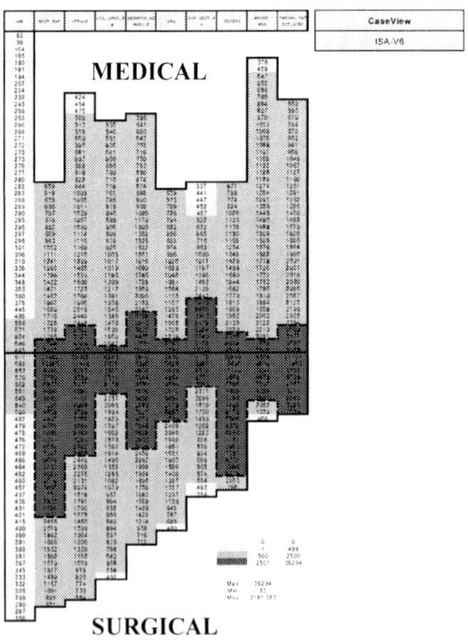


**Fig. 4.** The French reference set

The Hungarian reference set [4] (Figure 5) has been built in a way analogous to the French reference set.

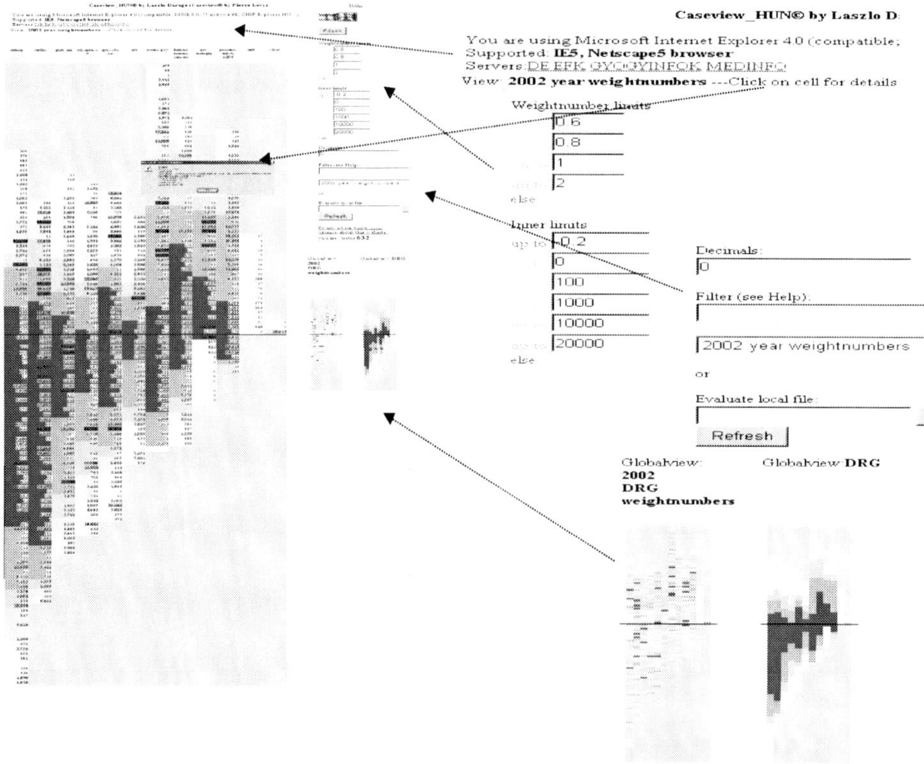


**Fig. 5.** The Hungarian reference set *(http://www.gyogyinfok.hu/darago/caseview/caseview.php)*

## 1.2 Visualizing the Data

This step corresponds to dispatching of the data associated with each DRG into the corresponding cell ("pixel") of the DRGs in the reference set. Then, to be able to display the image, the user has to define a colour scale.

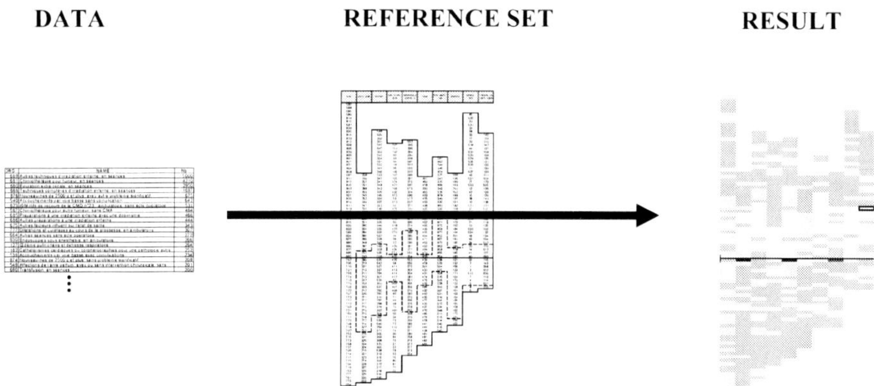


**Fig. 6.** Visualizing the data using the reference set

## 2. Results: Building the Reference Set for the Reader

The results show the case mix of a department, the case mix of a hospital, the variation of the French scale of cost between years 2003 and 2002, resource utilization of the French scale of cost and the case mix of a set of departments.

### *2.1 Case Mix of a Department*

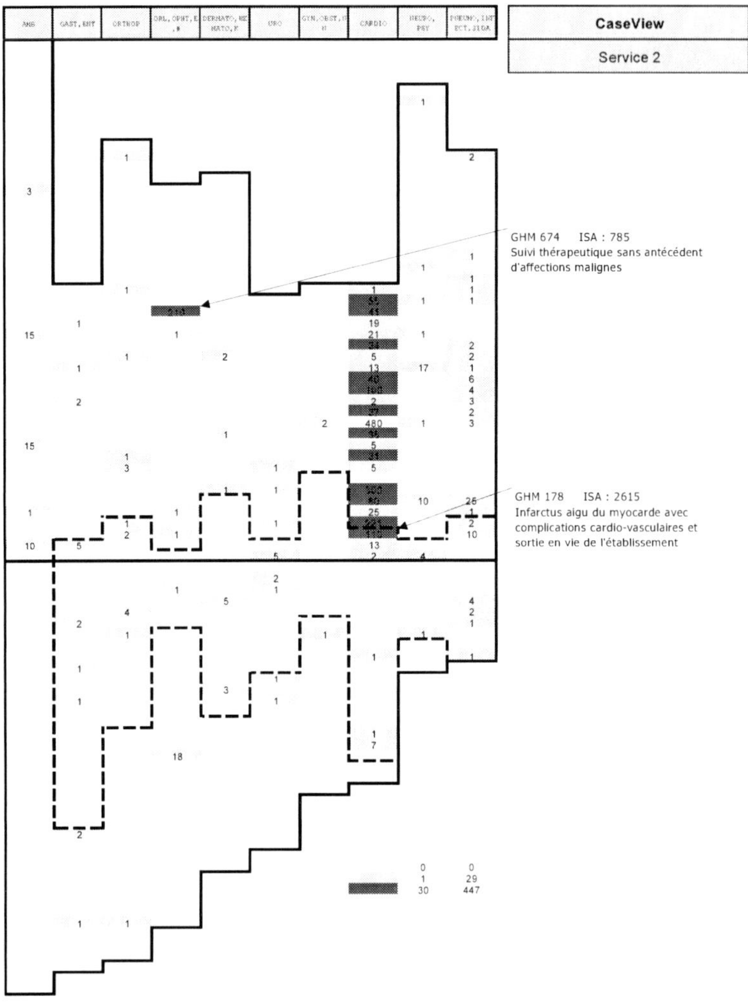


**Fig. 7.** Case mix of a cardiology department

It is clear that the activity of this department (Figure 7) is specific: its main body is located inside one column of the case view. Moreover, it is a medical department, with activity mainly in the upper part of the image. Finally, it is a cardiology department (the title of the column which contains most of the activity).

## 2.2 Case Mix of a Hospital

The activity of a sample hospital (Figure 8) is diversified. The hospital in question has little emergency activity (leftmost column in the reference set) and it has no heavy cardiac surgery.

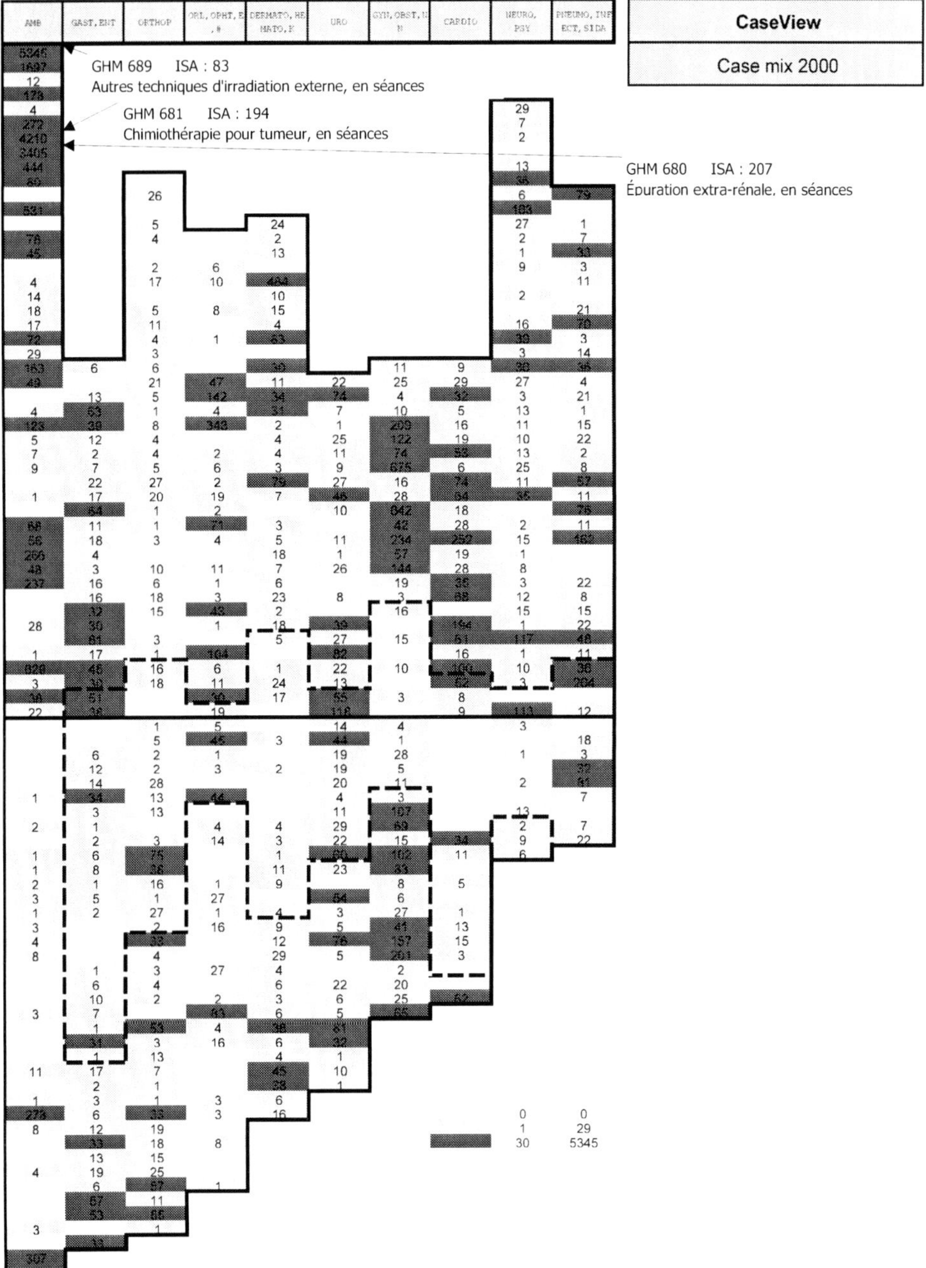


**Fig. 8.** Case mix of a hospital

## 2.3 Cost Scale (2003 – 2002)

This is an important result (Figure 9) which shows that the French cost scale between years 2002 and 2003 has increased the weight of heavy medical DRGs and decreased the weight of all other DRGs.

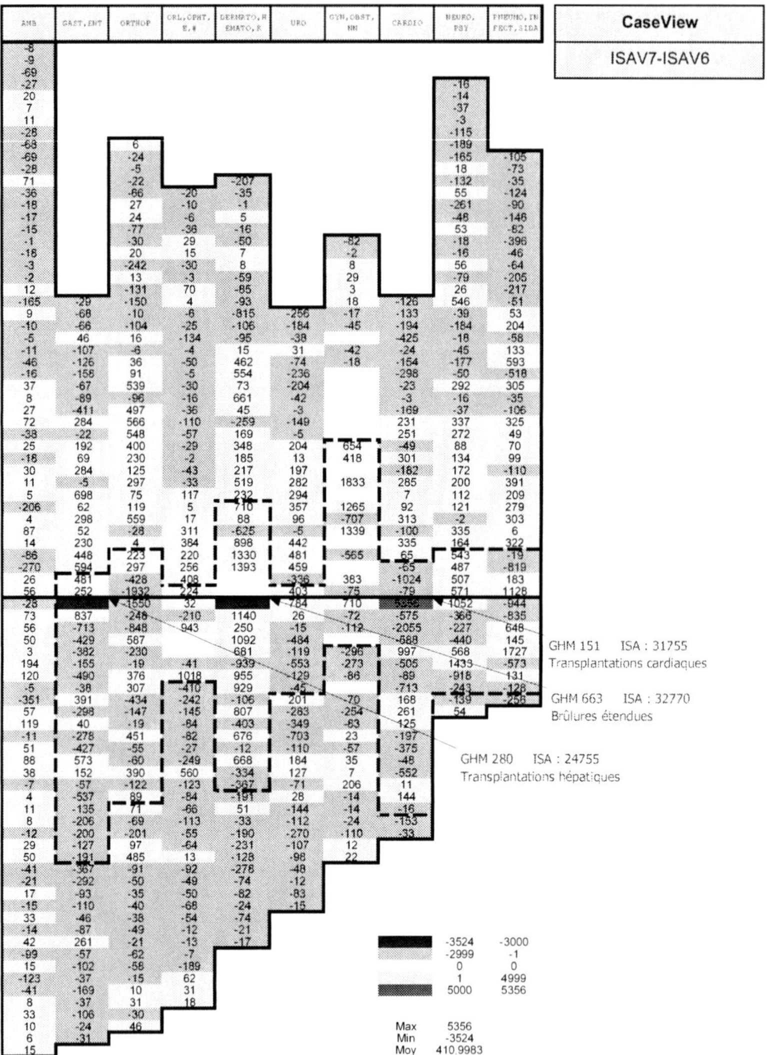


**Fig. 9.** Cost scale (2003 – 2002): positive values are in yellow or red, while negative values are in blue

## 2.4 The French Scale of Cost: Resources Utilization

Figure 10 shows all the resources utilization, from which the 2003 French cost scale has been constructed. Average costs are displayed using the same colour scale. The case views are displayed in a descending order left to right and from top to down. The highest costs are associated with nurses (IDE) and the lowest – with radiotherapy.

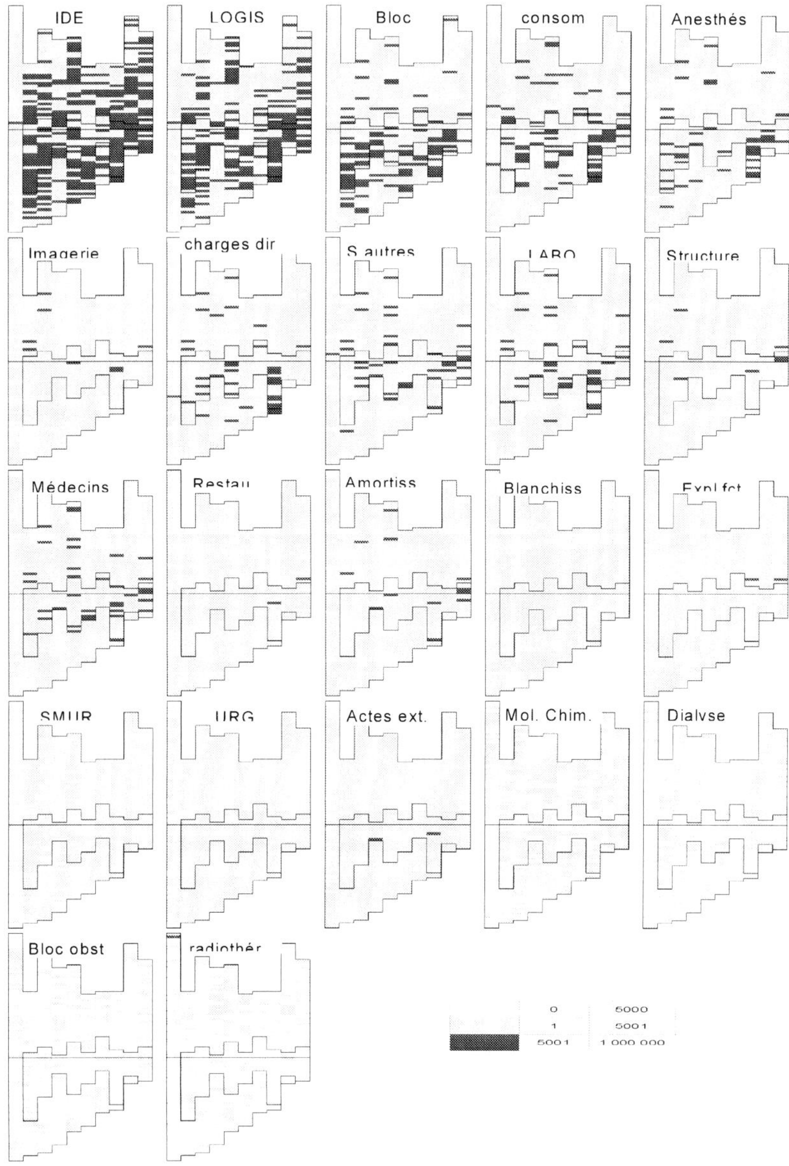


**Fig. 10.** Resources utilization in the French cost scale

## 2.5 Case Mix of a Set of Departments

Figure 11 shows the case mix of the departments of the hospital from Figure 8. The medical departments are reflected in the three upper rows and the surgical departments – in the two lower rows. One immediately sees that, on the one hand, the activity of the surgical departments is more specific than the activity of the medical departments, and on the other hand, most of the surgical departments conduct both medical and surgical activities, contrary to purely medical departments.

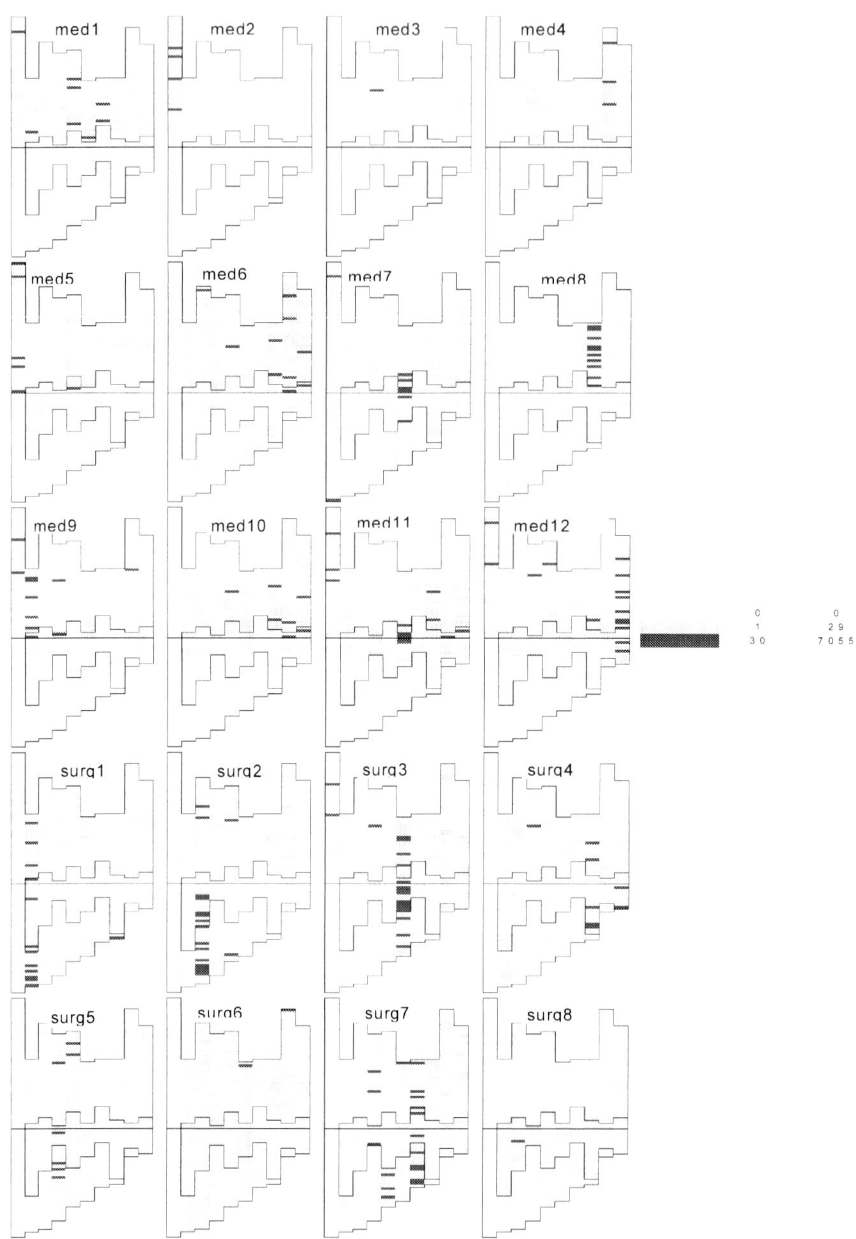


**Fig. 11.** Case mix of a set of departments

## 3. Building the Reference Set from a Cognitive Point of View

The interpretation of the user results from matching new images with the reference set present inside his brain. Thus, the existence of this reference set (from the user's perspective) is crucial for this interpretation to be possible. And the best way to build this reference set is to use the method as often as possible, within various contexts.

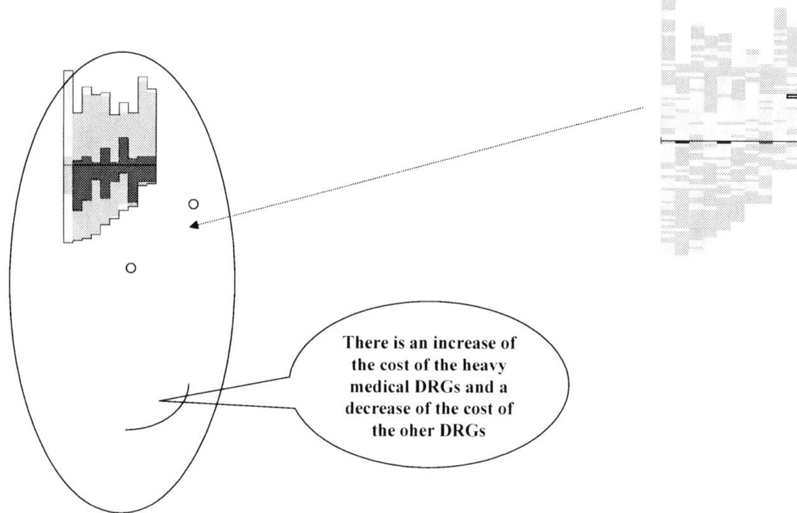


**Fig. 12.** Matching a new image to the reference set, to generate an interpretation

## 4. Conclusion

When building the reference set, from the point of view of the method, we can provide assistance for defining the reference set, while, from the point of view of the user, the use of this tool ought to enable and amplify his interpretative capabilities regarding the case mix number table.

## References


[1] R.B. Fetter & al. Case Mix definition by diagnosis Related groups. Med care 1980; 18 (suppl): 1-53.

[2] P.P. Lévy the case view, a generic method of visualization of the case mix. International Journal of medical Informatics. To be published.

[3] P.P. Lévy, le case view, une méthode de visualisation du case mix, Journal d'Economie médicale, mars 2002, vol 20, n°2 , pp.118-127

[4] L. Darago, P.P. Lévy, Caseview_HUN un outil internet pour appréhender les DRG hongrois. Journal d'Economie médicale, 2003, vol 21, n°7-8

# Caseview_HUN: Easy DRG Overview

László DARAGÓ
*University of Debrecen Health College Faculty, Hungary*
*e-mail: laszlo.darago@axelero.hu*

**Abstract.** Several hospital management tools are currently used by the DRG financial system. Each case is classified into a DRG group, so it is necessary to know the distribution of hospital or departmental cases into DRG groups, and to follow the variances of this distribution. The DRG's properties include the income and expenses related to each case. There are differences in the profitability of the cases, depending on their DRG. It is important to know own expenses and the recuperated costs for every case.

There are several systems for data collecting and analysis in hospitals, depending on existing hospital information systems and management. We can, however, be sure, that a DRG data collection system works in every department, because it is the basis of assessing income. The tool, which is shown in this article, facilitates an overview of the DRG, presenting the hospital's or other healthcare provider's own data. These services are supported by a platform-independent, accessible Internet application.

**Keywords:** Medical informatics, DRG, Caseview, Casemix, Hospital management, Health management, Medical economy, Health insurance.

## Introduction

The Caseview[1] was invented by Pierre Lévy (Hôpital Tenon, Assistance Publique Hôpitaux de Paris, INSERM U444, France). It is used daily as a tool for control and finance management in approximately 60 French hospitals.

The present application is based on the *Hungarian DRG*, a Hungarian version of the original idea. The original software runs in an Excel spreadsheet. Our research is an experiment aimed at achieving a platform-independent Internet-based solution. The user does not need to install any supplementary software or tools to access the service. The application can visualise the DRG, and DRG-based data in two dimensions. The main DRG groups are regrouped for easier overview.

## 1. Materials and Methods

The Caseview_HUN has inherited the original French structure fundamentals to allow a comparison with the native version. The DRG is contained in 12 table columns. These columns are created by contractions of DRG main groups. The table header shows the names of the contracted groups. A horizontal line splits the table. Medical groups are placed above that line, while surgical groups are placed underneath it. The half-columns (that is, upper and lower sections, divided by the horizontal line) contain the DRGs in a decreasing order, by weight number. A geometric criterion has been employed to render the

[1] The Caseview name given by Pierre P. Lévy

picture "as full as possible": by sorting the columns from left to the right in a decreasing order of surgical column length.

In this manner, one can create the impression of a three-dimension sight by using colours. Clicking on the content of the cell (if the cell contains data) displays the given DRG's properties in a message window (see Fig. 1.).

The language of the application can be selected by clicking on a national flag, then on the *Refresh* button. The *weight number limits* determine the background colour of the data containing the cell background colour of the DRG, whose weight number is in the appropriate range. The *inner limits* determine the background colour of the table content, which fits the selected range (viewing the DRG weight numbers and codes has no effect).

Some pre-defined views can also be selected in a combo box. These views show the structure of the DRG, and they also give information on how to use Caseview_HUN. D-DRG illustrates a possible new version of the Hungarian DRG, which regroups the so-called *hidden costs* from general costs to direct costs[2] (this is just an example and suggestion).

### *1.1 Analysing the Institute's Own Data*

There are general DRG properties which are worth analysing. There are also countrywide DRG databases to analyze and recognise trends, but it is always most important to clearly display the hospital's or department's own data and history related to the DRG. That data must be structured in a simple, two-field text file, where the first field contains the DRG code, while the second one includes corresponding data values.

This application serves to facilitate viewing of own files. Its data will not be shared with others, because it is deleted from the server's temporary folder immediately after first use.

The present application operates on the Hungarian DRG. However, since all the national DRGs originate from the same fundamentals, they are comparable and can be integrated into a European DRG. In addition to a joint economy, the Community also requires a uniform health finance system.

### *1.2 Accessibility*

The application can be accessed on 3 servers at the present time:

- University of Debrecen Health College Faculty:
  *http://mail.de-efk.hu/~darago/caseview/caseview.php*
- GYOGYINFOK (The Hungarian Casemix institute)
  *http://www.gyogyinfok.hu/darago/caseview/caseview.php*
- MEDINFO (The Hungarian medical information center)
  *http://www.medinfo.hu/darago/caseview.php*

[2] Laszlo Darago: Improving the DRG system in Hungary

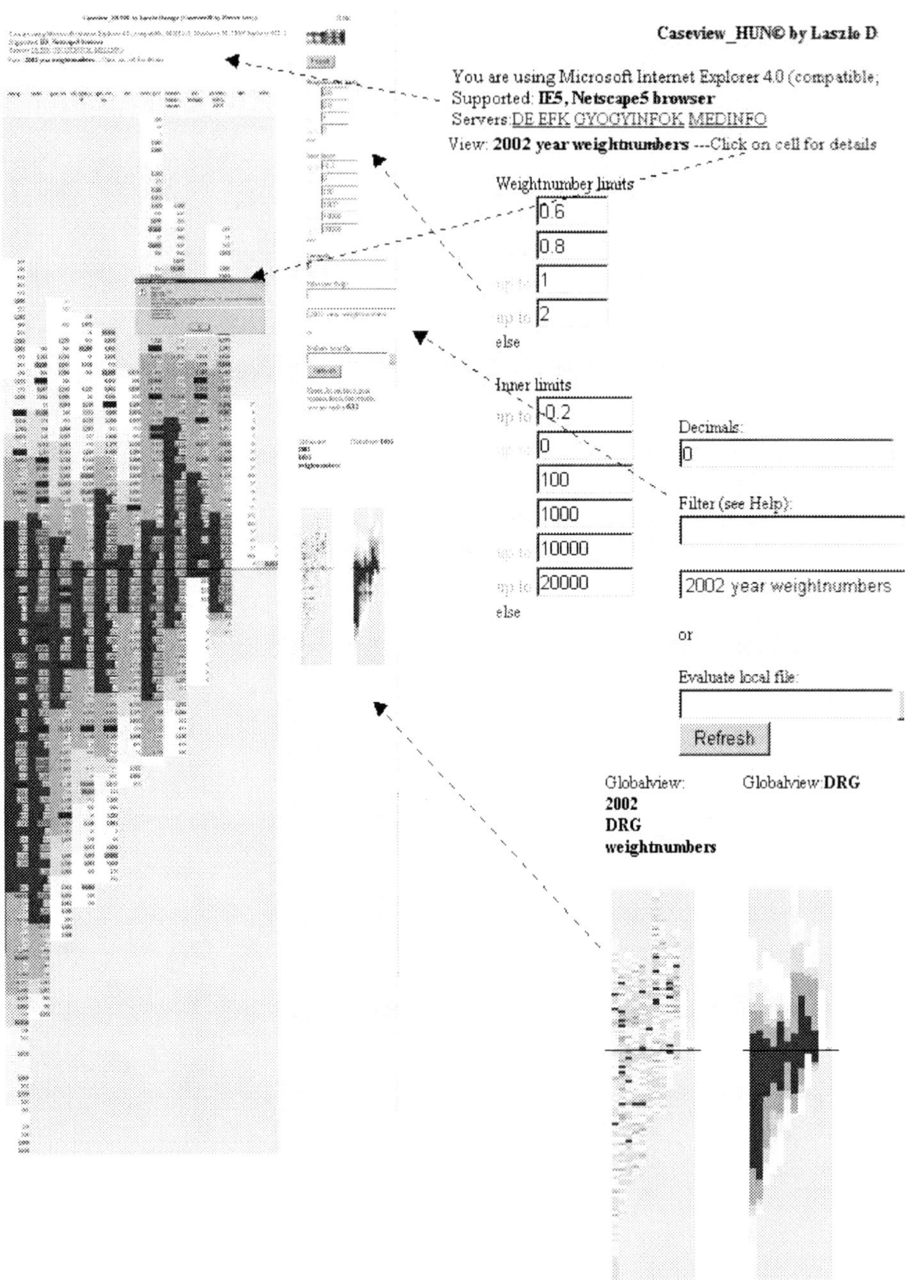


**Fig. 1**. A view of Caseview_HUN

## 2. Results

The next set of figures demonstrates the fields of application of the tool. The figures contain global views, their inner limits and areas of detailed sheets.

## 2.1 Number of Cases

The global view shows that the number of cases decreases (changes into yellow in color) for heavier DRGs.

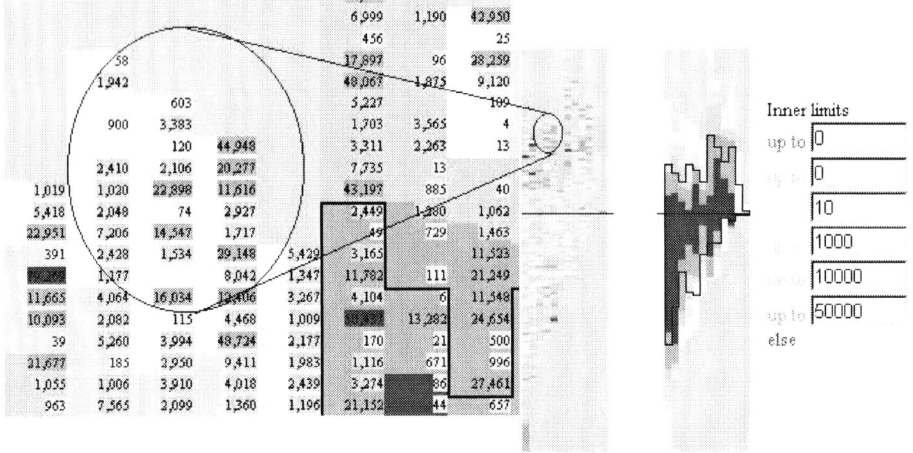


**Fig. 2.** Number of cases

The sheet on the left is a zoomed part of the global view. It shows that there are groups, which have no corresponding cases in a full year. A question can therefore arise: do we need to use such a classification? Is this a very rare group, or do the hospitals classify its cases as belonging to other groups?

Another question is, if we have too many cases in a group, should we try to discover a finer substructure of this classification? Such groups must be examined individually.

Another point of view can be to examine concurrent professions or departments (outside analogy), or the same department's cases in different periods (inside analogy).

We can also analyse the number of DRG cases for several departments representing the same, or similar professions in different hospitals. Comparing the relative frequency of cases in the DRGs can show us the differences between patient compounds of the department. Assuming that the patient compounds are the same, this can highlight the differences between diagnostics or therapy methods and their results.

We can compare the numbers and frequencies of DRG cases of several departments at the same hospital. In this way, we can discover parallelisms of care structures at each hospital, if several departments exhibit the same or similar patterns in the case view window.

## 2.2 Observing the Structure of the DRG

We can observe the DRG itself too. The weighting factor of the DRG is proportional to the cost of an acute hospital case; such a weighting factor can be divided into indirect and direct cost elements. We name as indirect those cost elements, which cannot be assigned, or which we don't want to assign directly to any case. Figure 3 shows the daily indirect cost component of the DRG. We can see that the pattern is similar to the weight number distribution of the DRG, which means that expensive infrastructure is generally needed to treat more complicated cases. The small dark patch in the left square marks some very complicated cases (brain surgery, onco-radiology, intensive care).

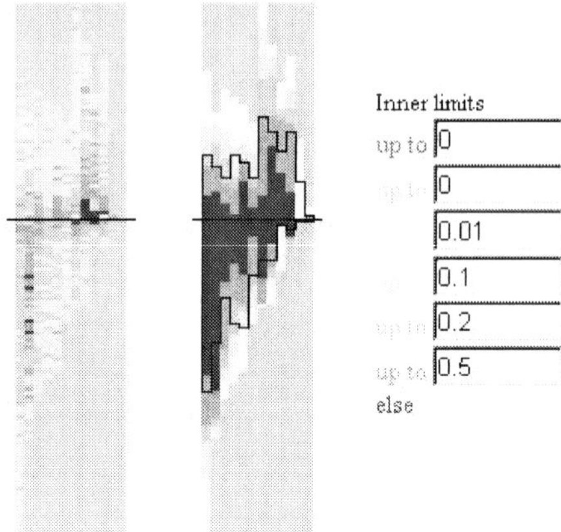


**Fig. 3.** Daily indirect costs

### *2.3 Bed Usage, Nursing Days*

Another possible examination can involve nursing days. In the global view, the upper half of the sheet is darker than the lower half. This means that there are significantly more nursing days for each surgical case than for each medical case.

The zoomed section shows the groups which incurred the greatest amount of nursing days. These include spinal and bone diseases, heart diseases, psychological cases and rehabilitation. Knowing the nursing day claims of each case, bed capacity can be adjusted to better match real needs.

We can analyze the nursing days as a matter of fact ($D_i$), but we also can analyze the normative (or standard) nursing days:

$$D_i^{st} = n_i * N_i \tag{1}$$

where $n_i$ is the number of cases in the $i^{th}$ DRG, while $N_i$ is the length of stay in the $i^{th}$ DRG.

By comparing the factual and normative nursing days we can discover overnursed and undernursed DRGs. Continuing the observation, the departments, cases, and even individual persons can be traced.

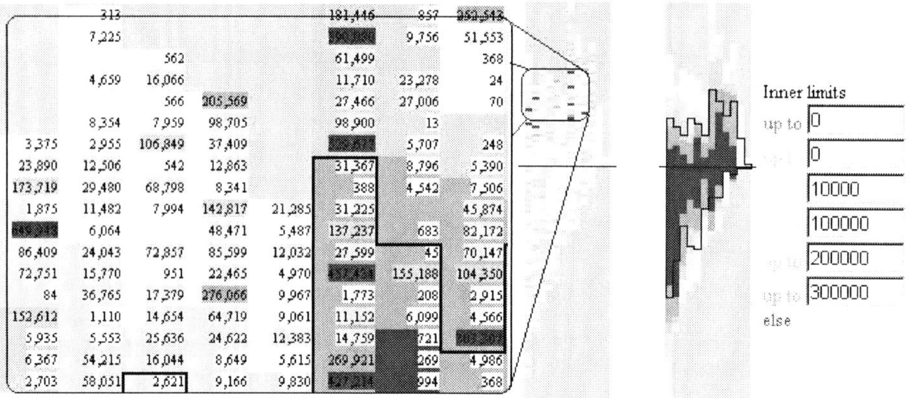


**Fig. 4.** Nursing days

## *2.4 Using the Filter*

Among the 3066975 inpatient cases in Hungary in 2002, there were 234196 cases in which diabetes[3] appeared as the main or conjoined diagnosis. There were 43376 cases where the patient's basic disease was identified as some kind of diabetes. This means that the primary reason could be any diagnosis, but that diabetes is in the background. Here, we have examined only some DRGs, especially for circulatory diseases and the AMI. The following figures show the differences between diabetic and non diabetic patients' DRG cases (see Fig. 5. and Fig. 6.) The numbers of cases are divided by their sum, then multiplied by 1000.

It can be recognized, that while the AMI rate is higher for diabetic patients, when compared to non-diabetics, the rate of amputations are about 8 times higher in the diabetic base disease cases. This result does not mean that diabetic patients are immune to hearth attacks – it merely shows that they are under continuous medical control, which helps reduce the risk of catastrophic heart failure. This article does not, however, advocate any medical course or procedure.

Because there is a facility to upload the users' own data, the user can decide for which department, doctor and period the cases are to be analysed. Filters are another possibility to hide unneeded data. The filter condition is a logical expression on the DRG code, which the row must satisfy, lest it be ignored. Filters can involve subsets of DRGs and their unions.

[3] Diagnoses between E1000 and E1999. ICD 10 version

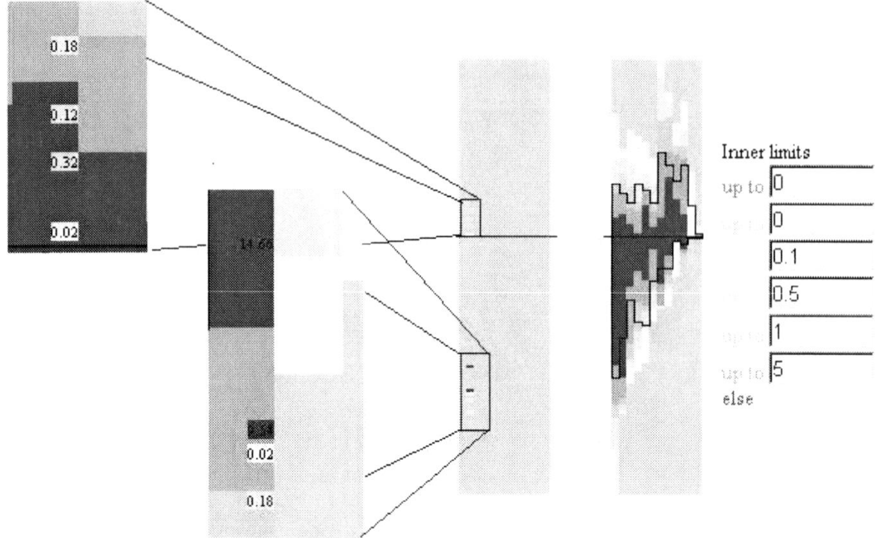


**Fig. 5.** Amputations (lower square) and AMI (upper square) rates for diabetes cases

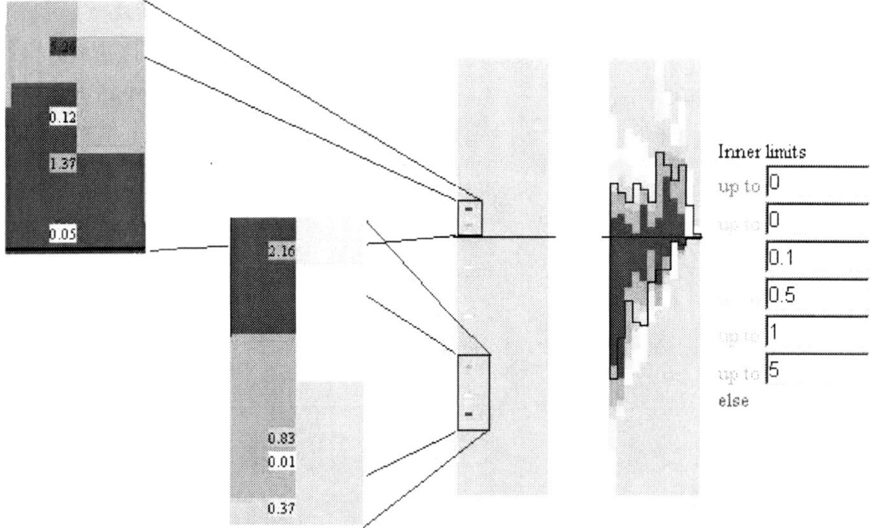


**Fig. 6.** Amputations (lower square) and AMI (upper square) rates for all cases

## 3. Conclusions

The figures above are just examples demonstrating the usefulness of the Caseview tool. Because it is a free application, hospitals and other users can use it freely. They can analyse their own data without publishing them – the application draws tables from each user's own data and deletes them immediately from the Internet server.

The Caseview tool can highlight and mark the subsets of the DRG and identify pertinent information, to be analyzed from the medical or economical standpoint. DRGs which are not conspicuous are not displayed at the forefront.

The use of filters can help sharpen the analyses. Consequently, the marked set can be divided into subsets by using a filter. This helps regroup the marked DRG cases.

The Caseview helps compare national Casemixes and interchange experience and knowledge about the DRGs and Casemix. It is easy to adopt on any national DRG reference set.

**Acknowledgement.** I would like to thank Pierre Lévy (France) for his advice and cooperation in developing the Caseview_HUN, the first Internet-based Caseview application. I also wish to thank István Bordás (Hungary) for his support, and the technical help from the GYOGYINFOK and the MEDINFO. I am grateful to György Surján (Hungary) for his ideas, which led me to build in the filtering mechanism, and to Mario Gonzalez (USA) for his help in correcting and improving the English version article.

## References

[1] Bordás István: Mit fejeznek ki a HBCs súlyszámok?, *Egészségügyi Gazdasági Szemle*, 1999:37,1

[2] Lévy P.P.: Le case view, une méthode de visualisation du case mix, Journal d'Economie médicale, mars 2002, vol 20, n°2 , pp.118-

[3] László Daragó: Javaslat a HBCs rendszer korrekciójára, Egészségügyi gazdasági szemle, 41/3. 2003 május. 35-38.o.

[4] Laszló Daragó: Improving the DRG system in Hungary, The new navigators: from Professionals to Patients. Proceedings of MIE2003, St. Malo, France, IOS Press Nieuwe Hemweg 6b 1013 BG Amsterdam, 818-823.

[5] László Daragó, Pierry Lévy: Caseview_hun: un outil internet pour appréhender les DRG hongrois, Journal d'Économie Médicale, 2003. Vol 21. no 7-8, 451-454.

[6] László Daragó: Caseview_hun: eszköz a homogén betegségcsoportok (HBCs) áttekintéséhez, Egészségügyi gazdasági szemle, 42/1. 2004 január.47-50. o.

# Universal Electronic Health Record MUDR

Petr HANZLICEK, Josef SPIDLEN, Miroslav NAGY
*EuroMISE Center – Cardio, Institute of Computer Science AS CR,*
*Pod Vodarenskou vezi 2, 182 07, Prague 8, Czech Republic*
*e-mail: hanzlicek@euromise.czpeople*

**Abstract.** One of the important research tasks of the European Centre for Medical Informatics, Statistics and Epidemiology – Cardio (EuroMISE Centre – Cardio) is the applied research in the field of electronic health record design including electronic medical guidelines and intelligent systems for data mining and decision support. The research in the field of data storage and data acquisition was inspired by several European projects and standards, mostly by the I4C and TripleC projects. Based on experience gathered during cooperation in the TripleC project we have proposed a description of a flexible information storage model. The motivation for this effort was the large variability of the set of collected features in different departments - including temporal variability. Therefore, a dynamically extensible and modifiable structure of items is needed. In our model we use two basic structures called the knowledge base and data files. The main function of the knowledge base is to express the hierarchy of collectable features – medical concepts, their characteristics and relations among them. The data files structure is used to store the patient's data itself. These two structures can be described using graph theory expressions. Based on this model, a three-layer system architecture named "Multimedia Distributed Record" (MUDR) has been proposed and implemented. During the implementation, modern technologies such as Web Services, SOAP and XML were used.

For the practical usage of EHR MUDR, an intelligent application called MUDRc (MUDR Client) was created. It enables physicians to use EHR MUDR in a flexible way. During the development process, maximum emphasis was placed on user-friendliness and comfortable usage of this application. Several methods of data entry can be used: pre-defined forms, direct entry into the tree data structure of the EHR MUDR, or automatic unstructured free-text report parsing and data retrieval. The system enables fast and simple importing and exporting of data as well. The system integrates modern multimedia formats (X-ray photos, sonography and other pictures, video-sequences, audio records) as well as progressive methods of decision support systems realized by medical guidelines and other modules

## Introduction

The electronic health record systems, used nowadays as part of hospital information systems in the Czech Republic, are mostly free text-based and offer only a limited set of structured data for further automatic processing. The information stored in a free text-based system can be used by the physician during the examination of the patient; the systematic processing of stored free text is, however, very complicated. A modern electronic health record system should offer the possibility to use the stored information for statistical processing or as a data source for decision support systems. The applied research at the EuroMISE Center in the field of electronic health records (EHR), electronic medical guidelines and intelligent systems for decision support has been inspired by several European projects and standards, mostly by the I4C and TripleC projects [1]. The analysis of existing solutions, experience of experts in the field of medical informatics and statistics, as well as cooperation and discussions with physicians has resulted in the following list of requirements, which the proposed advanced electronic health record (EHR) should fulfill.

*Structured Way of Data Storage Combined with Free Text*

The usability of free text for automated data processing and conclusion drawing is very limited. To be able to process the collected data automatically, to conduct statistical analyses or simply to present a progression of some symptom in time, the data has to be collected in a structured way. On the other side, free text is the natural way of expressing physicians' findings. Physicians are not forced to change the way they think during patient examination when searching for a correct term in a set of medical concepts. To avoid entering the same data twice into separate systems, one for clinical and one for statistical purposes, the electronic health record should combine both approaches in a single form. The automatic extraction of structured data from free text is a difficult task, yet several approaches based on regular analysis exist [2], benefiting from the simple structure of the standard medical reporting language.

*Dynamically Extensible and Modifiable Set of Collectable Data*

The needs of different departments and groups of users with regard to the set of required data are very diverse and subject to frequent changes and modifications. It becomes even more difficult to come to an agreement on the set of data to be collected when dealing with a large group of potential users. New discoveries in the field of medicine and new diagnostic methods also lead to modifications of the collected data structure. The electronic health record system should therefore be easily adaptable to these changing requirements with as little labour as possible. The classical solution – to change the application and database structure when any changes in the data collection process are perceived – is very ineffective.

*Verification of the Data – Decision Support System*

The potential advantage of an electronic health record is the possibility of scanning the data entered for internal inconsistencies. Verification can be extended from simple bounds checking (maximal and minimal value) to advanced checks of conformance with medical guidelines. Such verification can also be used for evaluation of a physician's work, comparing his data with recommendations provided by medical guidelines. The system should e.g. warn the physician about possible counterindications for a given medication or recommend an adequate investigation to minimize the potential risk of complication implied from the existing data. The physician, however, should be able to enter any data even if it is contrary to the recommendations of medical guidelines. The responsibility for a given treatment lies always with the physician.

*Multilinguality*

The structured way of data storage carries the advantages of language-independent data representation. The stored data then can be presented in any language supported by the EHR system. Thus, the exchange of structured electronic documentation between different countries becomes much easier.

*Pedigree Information*

The ability of the system to express the family relations of examined persons can be very useful for research in the field of genetics or to track some hereditary diseases in the family history. Personal data security must be well maintained and respected in this case.

*Registration of all Changes of Data*

As mentioned before, health-related information is one of the most sensitive data types. Therefore it is necessary to keep a detailed, automatically-generated log of every change – including information on who (and when) accesses the data, adds, modifies or deletes any part of the patient record. In the case of modification or deletion, old data versions must remain stored in the system for legislative purposes, to be able to restore the state of the health documentation at any point in its history.

*Multimedia Information as Part of EHR*

Many modern methods of medical examination produce large amounts of multimedia data – such as high-resolution pictures (X-ray reports, sonography, computer tomography) and videos (angiography). To make all this data accessible from one place in a unified way, it is necessary to include such kinds of information in the electronic health documentation of a patient.

## 1. Architecture of MUDR EHR

Following these requirements, a modular structure of a system called MUDR (Multimedia distributed health record) has been defined. The main architecture of the electronic health record is developed using a three-layer architecture – the database layer, the application layer and the user interface layer. This approach separates physical data storage, application intelligence and the user interface, minimizes the requirements for client-side software and enables developers to create various types of client applications according to requirements of a particular user, without changing the rest of the system. The database layer is implemented using the Oracle 9i Enterprise Edition ver. 9.0.1.1 database server. The main reason for this decision is to achieve maximum flexibility, robustness and capability among other products currently being marketed. The application logic offers basic commands for knowledge base editing, storing and recalling the patient data, modifying access rights, etc.

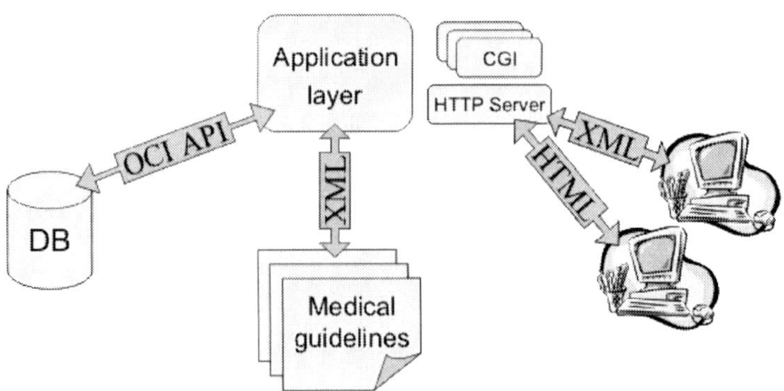


**Fig. 1.** The architecture of the MUDR EHR system

Communication between the client application and the application layer is implemented by an XML-based communications protocol. The communication syntax between the client and the application layer is defined by an XML Schema – recommended by W3C in May 2001 (see Appendix 1). XML documents are transported by the HTTP protocol between the client application and an HTTP server. The CGI scripts executed by the HTTP server provide the interface for the application layer running as a Windows NT service. This solution makes it possible to create different communication interfaces for the application layer. The XML commands and responses can be transformed to dynamic HTML or WML, enabling the use of web browsers or mobile phones for EHR access. An important part of an application layer is the decision support module, realized as a set of DLL libraries, used for conformance analysis to medical guidelines or as a decision support tool during patient examination. For the pilot application, a library based on "1999 WHO/ISH Guidelines for the Management of Hypertension" has been implemented.

## 2. Data Representation

The set of collected features – medical concepts – varies in different departments and organizations, also from a temporal viewpoint. Therefore, we need a dynamically extensible and modifiable structure of items allowing a reorganization of the database structure. The set of features and their relations named "knowledge base" is described by a directed graph $G = (V, E)$. Graph vertices $v \in V$ are defined by quaternions (id, name, dtype, validity), where *id* is the unique identifier of a vertex, *name* is the internal name of the vertex, *dtype* describes the data type of the vertex and *validity* contains identifications of the user who created the vertex and the user who possibly deleted the vertex. This quaternion is also referenced as a "semantic type". Edges $e \in E$ are defined by quaternions ($v_1$, $v_2$, etype, validity), where $v_1$ is the starting vertex, $v_2$ – the ending vertex, *etype* describes the type of edge and *validity* contains information about users entering and modifying the edge, similarly to vertices. The physical data type can be chosen from a set of basic data types – number, boolean, string, multimedia (picture, audio, video, generic binary) and reference (data reference or knowledge base reference). The dominant edge has the "inferior" type. An edge of this type is used to build the hierarchical tree structure of the knowledge base, so that the knowledge base can be described by a directed forest with several trees. These trees are also called "knowledge base domains". Other edge types are used mostly to describe other relations between vertices like equivalence or contraindications of drugs.

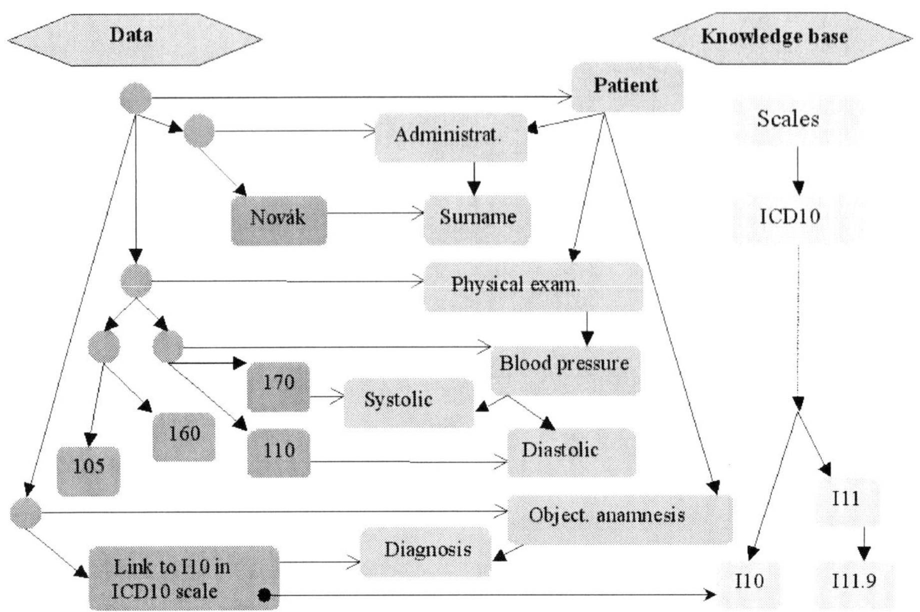


**Fig. 2.** Example of a knowledge base and real data in MUDR

To prepare the knowledge base content for the pilot project implementation in cardiology, a set of important medical concepts for the diagnosis of cardiology patients has been defined basing on a consensus of many physicians, cooperating in multidisciplinary research at the EuroMISE Center – Cardio [3]. The mentioned set of medical concepts – the minimal data model for cardiology patients is being prepared for approval by the Czech Society of Cardiology. Other knowledge base domains contain e.g. the international classification of diseases, ICD10 and ATC classifications, SI units or sets of usable drugs.

The collected data is stored using a directed graph (directed forest) $F=(D, E)$. Each tree in the forest describes the data of one patient. Vertices are represented by quaternions (id, semantic type, value, administrative data). Each vertex in the tree describes one instance of the medical concept from the knowledge base through an identification of the concept in question (internal name of the vertex), its value (with the possibility of specifying a range of values), date and time of examination, valid datetime range for the entered data, certainty of the determined data and identification of the user who entered, confirmed (doesn't have to be the same as the person who entered the data) and possibly marked the instance as deleted. The values are physically stored in separate tables according to their physical data types described by the semantic types.

## 3. The Application Layer

The application layer consists of four basic components – an HTTP server used for communication with client applications, an EHR-AppL service implementing the main application logic, a CGI script (potentially more than one), serving as an interface between the HTTP server and the EHR-AppL service and, possibly, medical guideline modules. The application layer realizes a set of functions provided to the client application and implements the functionality of the EHR system on a more abstract level by isolating clients from database implementation details. This solution enables future changes in the database without influencing client applications and helps achieve a higher level of safety and security. The EHR-AppL service is internally structured into 4 sublayers – database connection, database services, output generator and input analyzer. The database connection sublayer implements and encapsulates communication using the Oracle Call Interface API (OCI API), keeps the database connection and stores the necessary system variables. The database services sublayer is responsible for SQL or PL/SQL commands, command execution, converting C++ variables and MFC classes to Oracle variables, error handling, etc. The output generator initiates commands required by the client and transforms the responses of the database layer into the XML format using Microsoft XML Core Services 4.0. The input analyser validates the syntax of incoming XML documents through the Microsoft XML Parser and uses the output generator to provide responses.

Communication between clients and the application layer is performed by the secure HTTPS protocol (Hypertext Transfer Protocol). An HTTP server is therefore a necessary part of the application layer. Nevertheless, it is not necessary to build one's own HTTP server, many free products exist. The Apache HTTP server has been used as a testing platform. Communication between the client and the application layer proceeds in the following manner: the HTTP server (configured to run CGI scripts) waits for a client connection by "listening" on a specified port (usually port number 80). When a client wants to communicate with the server, it opens the TCP connection and, using the HTTPS protocol, requests the HTTP server to run a specified CGI script. The HTTP server then receives the data from the client in the form of an HTTP POST request and forwards this data to the CGI script – a special program run in multiple instances according to client's requests by the HTTP server. The CGI script connects to the EHR-AppL service, sends the request, waits for the response and outputs the response back to the HTTP server, which ensures the transport of the output XML document to the client application. This approach opens the possibility of creating special CGI scripts for communication with lightweight clients, such as web or wap browsers, enabling the use of mobile devices to connect to the EHR.

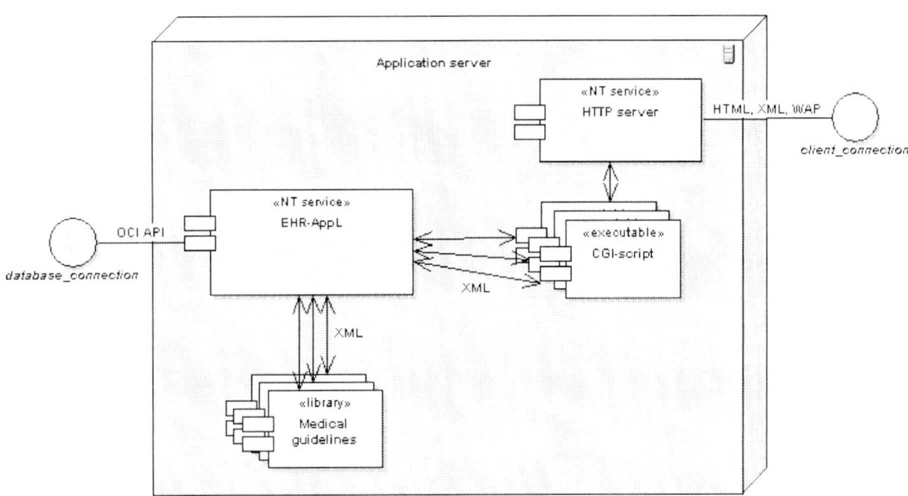


**Fig. 3.** Application layer structure

## 4. Other Features

### *4.1 Pedigree Information*

The patient is represented by the instance a root vertex of main knowledge base domain in the real data tree. Therefore, the graph structure can be used to express relations between patients in the database, e.g. pedigree information by using edges of type "parent". The information about relatives of the patient can be expressed by creating new "virtual" patients or by creating a new edge of type "parent" when the relative is already present in the database. The main reason for this solution is the intention to avoid inconsistencies in family anamnesis, when provided by different people (siblings, parents and children, etc.) This type of information can be utilized for research in the field of genetics or epidemiological examination and it is a necessary step towards the Electronic Family Health Record. However, it can be a bit controversial from the point of view of personal data security, so security should be well maintained.

### *4.2 Uncertainty of the Data*

The data collected by physicians can be often inaccurate or somewhat unreliable. Two types of data uncertainty can be recognized. The first type is caused by limited precision of the measuring devices or data sources. The system helps express this type of uncertainty of numeric or date values representing them as value intervals. The precision of dates can be specified by possible formats of date representation: "dd.mm.yyyy", "mm/yyyy" or "yyyy". Boolean values use three-value logic with the logical values of "true", "false" and "unknown".

The second type of uncertainty expresses the physician's doubt about the correctness of the data. It can be found out at the diagnosis determination stage or when asking a patient for the information he cannot remember precisely, like e.g. diseases of his grandparents. Support for this type of uncertainty in the system is included in the reliability item, in the appropriate vertex. Reliability is represented by a numeric value between 0 and 100.

### *4.3 Expression of Time and Validity of Values*

A particular value of a symptom is often valid only within the frame of specified time period. A formalized specification of such a time period is very important for the physician to draw the correct conclusions. One possible way of expressing time periods is the explicit definition of a concept of type “date”, where necessary. However, it can be difficult to judge the necessity of date specification during knowledge base modelling. In the MUDR EHR a new system is introduced. During the entry of each data item, the beginning and the end of the validity of the entered value can be specified. The date can be entered in various formats (“dd.mm.yyyy”, “mm/yyyy” or just “yyyy”), thus specifying the precision of the date. A date interval can also be used to specify the validity threshold. Using this capability, we can formally express sentences, such as e.g. “The abdominal pain had started when he was 20-22 years old and ended after successful pancreatolithectomy in May 1998”. This approach provides a generic way of expressing the evolution of a value of any concept from the knowledge base.

### *4.4 Multilinguality*

The structured data, stored in the EHR, provides a language-independent source of information. Expression of this information in various languages is a relatively easy task – the meanings of concepts in the knowledge base can be easily translated into different languages and stored in the system vocabulary. Each vertex in the knowledge base has a unique name, used only internally and not shown to the user. Therefore, vocabulary containing the translations of names of concepts has been implemented in the system. The information stored in the EHR can then be displayed in user applications in a selected language version, using this predefined vocabulary.

### *4.5 Multimedia Information*

The physical data type of a knowledge base vertex can be chosen from basic data types – number, boolean, string, multimedia (picture, audio, video, generic binary) and reference (data reference or knowledge base reference). Multimedia data are stored directly in the database, which is not optimal for very large multimedia files such as angiography videos, but it can have several advantages for graphical data like X-ray pictures or ECGs. The planned future version of the system will support external storage of binary files and communication with PACS.

## 5. Decision Support

An important attribute of an EHR, improving the effectiveness and quality of a physician's work during data entry, is the decision support capability. If we focus on decision support during data entry or consultation, the concept of so-called reminders appears helpful. The reminder is a result of a verification of a logical rule set, defining restrictions for instances of medical concepts (real patient data). Using the above-mentioned hierarchical structure of medical concepts in MUDR, we can come up with a set of rules defining – for example – counterindications for a specified drug due to other medications prescribed before, which could be overlooked by the examining physician. Dangerous violations of rules should then raise a warning – the reminder – to the physician. Less important warnings, like the unknown value of some medical concept possibly causing a risk, can be hidden until the physician asks the system for consultation. The set of rules should be based on medical guidelines for a specific medical area. These capabilities of the EHR should be smoothly integrated into the user interface to provide good support for the physician's work.

In the EHR MUDR, an algorithm described in "1999 WHO/ISH Guidelines for the Management of Hypertension" [4] has been formalized and implemented as part of the system. The decision support system in the proposed EHR is implemented as a set of loadable DLL libraries. Each library communicates with the rest of the application layer in a similar way as the client application and uses the same XML format (see Appendix 1), to speed up the communication process. An internal communication interface based on Win32 layer with DLL library exports is used. According to the specified procedure, the hypertension grade is computed and the potential risk of a cardiovascular event in the coming 10 years (based on Framingham's study) is derived. Subsequently, usable drug groups are sorted according to their applicability – drug groups with counterindications are discarded first, while drugs with indications are preferred. The approximate price of the drug group in question is also taken into account. If some information, needed to determine the counterindications, is missing, a warning is shown, notifying the physician about potential risk. General information about dosage and drug group combinations is also displayed.

## 6. User Interface

Nowadays, an important task is to motivate the potential users of EHR – namely the physicians – to use a modern system providing structured data entry, storage and processing instead of a free text-based system. The functionality, combined with a good user interface, is crucial for the physicians' acceptance. The most successful strategy is based on providing as many benefits for physicians as possible with as little effort as possible [5]. Universal access to patient data coming from different sources is the most frequently offered functionality of EHR systems. When designing a system, two types of its usage should be taken into account – consultation and data entry. Consultation requires minimal search time, presenting information as an inquiry, problem-oriented grouping of findings and patient visits. Data entry requires maximum ease and speed of entering the data into the system. However, the designs of EHR systems often focus too much on data entry and neglect the consultation part. The main principles for the consultation part of an EHR should involve overviews and a predictable and clinically-relevant presentation. The overview should present a combination of data from different sources in one predictable view relevant to the patient's state. The importance of the presented information should be emphasized; a graphical view of time progress of important quantitative data can be very helpful. A simple link to more detailed information from parts of the overview is also important. A problem- or organ group-oriented view of the patient's history can help physicians find the information they need much faster than they would otherwise. The possibility of viewing historical data in different ways can improve the effectiveness of the physician's decisionmaking process.

The simple pilot implementation of the MUDR EHR user interface is created as an MS Windows application, providing only structured data entry, based on the above-mentioned hierarchical structure of medical concepts (knowledge base). The decision support system implements the "1999 WHO/ISH Guidelines for the Management of Hypertension" and can be used as a consultation tool for testing the entered data's conformance with medical guidelines.

Analysis of the physician's work during patient examination have shown that the physician often requires consultation of historical data even during the process of data entry. Therefore, the idea of a more advanced user interface, providing both historical data and the possibility to enter new items in one form has been studied. The main form is thus divided into several areas; each of them used to display a specific type of information in various ways. These ideas are currently being implemented in a new version of the client part of the MUDR electronic health record, developed in the Java 2 programming language. The developed application implements the functionality of structured data entry combined with free text including tools for formalization of such text. The structured data can be entered either directly by selecting the appropriate items from the tree structure of the knowledge base, or by using dynamically-created forms. Printable reports and user entry forms are created dynamically following the definitions in XML documents. Multimedia data items are processed using the functionality of the Java Media Framework API. The performance of communication between the client application and the application layer of the MUDR EHR system has been considerably improved by the implementation of a caching mechanism.

### 6.1 Predefined Forms

The knowledge base of the MUDR can contain a lot of medical concepts from different parts of the medical domain. During a routine examination of a patient only part of this information is examined and stored in the EHR. To simplify the process of routine data entry, the user can prepare forms containing only the information needed during the examination. A graphical WYSIWYG form editor is part of the MUDRc application. A similar editor is also used to create the output reports, enabling the presentation of data in the form of discharge letters or medicine prescriptions.

### 6.2 Tree View

The basic method of data entry involves splitting the screen in two parts. The left-hand part shows the knowledge base, containing the hierarchical structure of all the medical concepts that can be stored in the EHR in a structured way. Detailed information on the selected node is shown in the lower section of the screen. The right-hand part of the screen shows data belonging to the selected patient in a structured way, reflecting the structure of the knowledge base. Finally, the lower part of the screen shows detailed information on the selected node – the value, the validity range, reliability and the users who entered, confirmed or eventually deleted the node.

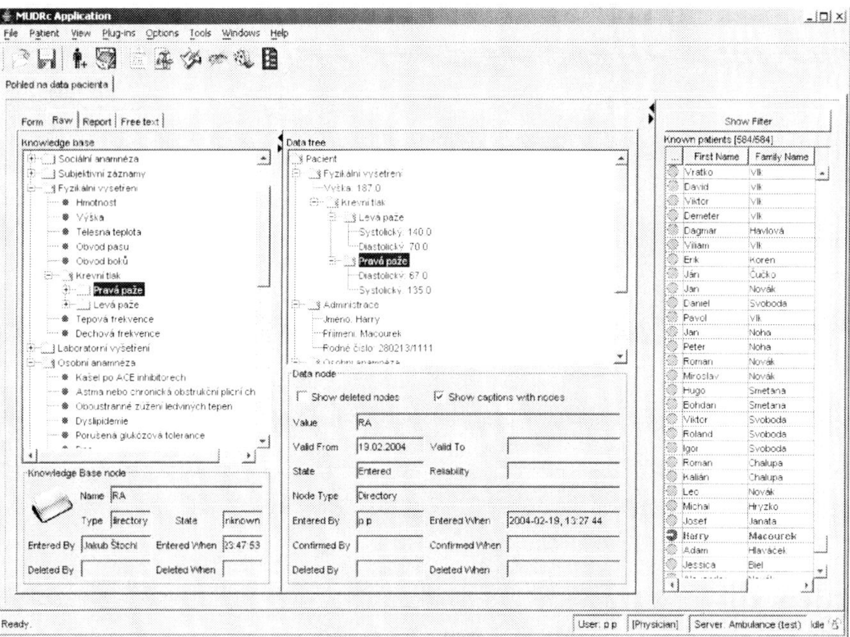


**Fig. 4.** Data entry using a tree view

### 6.3 Free Text Entry

The last method of data entry is the formalisation of a free text report. The editor allows the user to write the report in free text form and then links parts of the text to the terms in the knowledge base. This functionality allows storing both the textual report and the structured data. A semiautomatic analyser of the entered text based on regular analysis [2] has been implemented in the system, so that the manual marking of the text can be considerably reduced. The implemented system contains a set of rules created manually through analysis of anonymous Czech medical reports of patients from several institutions.

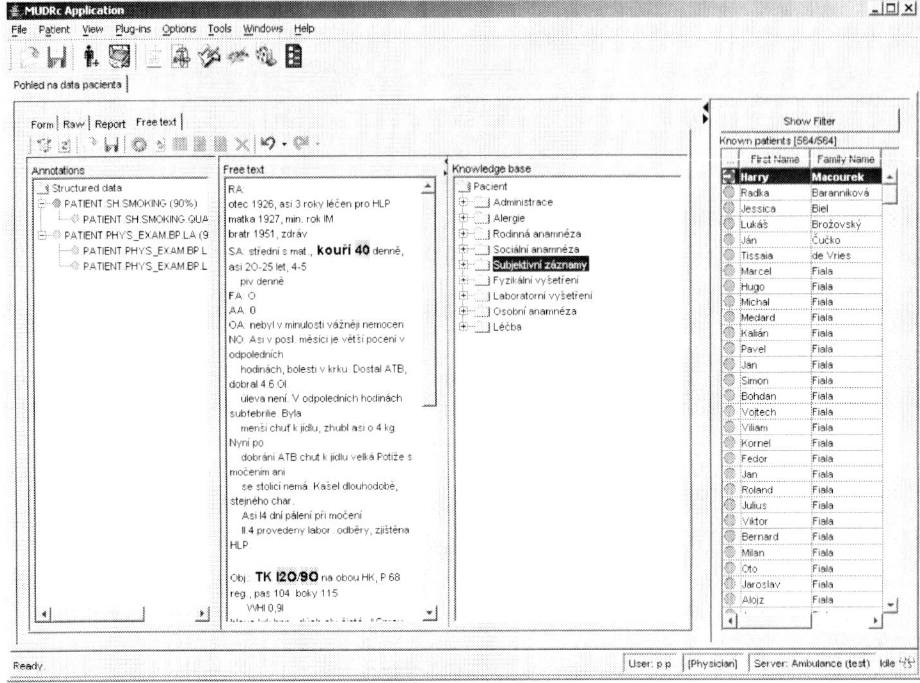


**Fig. 5.** Data entry done by free text analysis

## 6.4 *Consistency of the Entered Data*

The consistency of the entered data can be checked by a separate mechanism, controlled by the consistency rules. This functionality allows the user to specify different formats or limits of values for particular medical concepts or even the relations between those concepts. The system contains a simple set of rules for checking several basic formatting conventions and relations. Consistency can be checked on demand of the user or automatically, depending on settings.

The application utilizes the guideline module part of the MUDR EHR application layer and either shows the text of a selected guideline or starts the process of consultation of the selected patient's data with the guideline module. The module thus computes the hypertension grade and the potential risk of a cardiovascular event in the following 10 years is derived. Subsequently, usable drug groups are sorted according to their applicability. The potential risk of counterindications resulting from missing data is also mentioned.

## 7. Conclusion

The new architecture of the electronic health record, inspired by European and international standards has been proposed and partially implemented. A modern three-layer architecture provides advantages for system developers (by separating physical data storage, application logic and user interface), minimizes the requirements for client-side software and enables the creation of various types of client applications according to the requirements of particular users without changing the rest of the system. The system offers very robust and configurable functionality for managing the mostly hierarchically-organized medical data by representing sets of collectable symptoms and investigations through a directed graph with a dominant tree structure. The system is adaptable to virtually any medical domain, by creating a knowledge base and describing the hierarchy of symptoms to be collected. The set of symptoms, represented by the knowledge base, can be easily and effectively modified and adapted to changing requirements. Any change of the knowledge base structure results in the previous structure being cached, thus no historical data can be lost by changing the way data items are collected and stored. The client application (MUDR Client) offers a wide range of possible user interactions with the system and open access to the decision support system based on medical guidelines. The MUDR Client provides a user-friendly, functional and powerful interface to the information stored in the electronic health record MUDR.

**Acknowledgments.** The research is supported by the project LN00B107 of the Ministry of Education of the Czech Republic.

## References

[1] van Ginneken AM. The computerized patient record: balancing effort and benefit, International Journal of Medical Informatics 65 (2002), 97-119

[2] Semecký J, Zvárová J. On Regular Analysis of Medical Reports, Proceedings of Workshop on Natural Language Processing in Biomedical Applications, March 8-9, 2002, edited by R. Baud and P. Ruch, Nicosia, Cyprus 2002, pp. 13-16.

[3] Tomeckova M. Minimalni datovy model kardiologickeho pacienta – vyber dat. – in Czech, Cor et Vasa, Vol. 44, 2002, No. 4 Suppl., pp. 123 (ISSN: 0010-8650)

[4] 1999 WHO/ISH Hypertension Guidelines for the Management of Hypertension, 1999, Journal of Hypertension 17, 151-183.

[5] van Ginneken AM, Verkoien MJ. A multi-disciplinary approach to a user interface for structured data entry. Medinfo 2001;10(Pt 1):693-7

[6] Hanzlicek P. Development of Universal Electronic Health Record in Cardiology. MIE 2002. Proceedings of MIE 2002. IOS Press 2002, Amsterdam. ISBN 1-58603-279-8, ISSN 0926-9630

[7] Spidlen J, Hanzlicek P, Implementace formalizovanych lekarskych doporuceni v elektronickem zdravotnim záznamu MUDR. [Implementation of the Formalized Medical Guidelines in the MUDR Electronic Health Record.], Znalosti 2003. (Ed.: Svátek V.) – Ostrava, FEI – VSB 2003, pp. 386-391 (ISBN: 80-248-0229-5)

[8] World Wide Web Consortium: XML Schema Part 0: Primer, Part 1: Structures, Part 2: Datatypes; *http://www.w3.org/XML/Schema#dev.*

[9] ENV13606 Parts 1-4, CEN/TC251

[10] Petr Hanzlicek, Josef Spidlen, Jana Zvarova; The Internet in Connecting Electronic Health Record Mobile Clients – Technology and Health Care, Vol. 10, 2002, No.6, pp. 502-503 (ISSN: 0928-7329)

# MUDRLite – Health Record Tailored to Your Particular Needs

Josef SPIDLEN, Petr HANZLICEK, Jana ZVAROVA
*EuroMISE Centre – Cardio, Institute of Computer Science AS CR*
*Pod Vodarenskou vezi 2, 182 07 Prague 8, Czech Republic*
*e-mail: spidlen@euromise.cz*

**Abstract.** Nowadays most hospitals use electronic health records as part of their hospital information systems. However, these systems are more suitable for hospital management than for physicians. The health record is not sufficiently structured; it includes a lot of free-text information, and the set of collected attributes is fixed and practically impossible to extend. Physicians, gathering information for the purpose of medical studies, often use varied proprietary solutions based on MS Access databases or MS Excel Sheets.

The EuroMISE Centre – Cardio is developing an electronic health record (EHR) application called MUDRLite, which could easily fill the gap between existing EHRs. MUDRLite is the result of applied research in the field of EHR design, which is based on experience gathered during cooperation in the TripleC project. MUDRLite development is an extra branch in the MUDR (MUltimedia Distributed Record) development; it simplifies both the MUDR architecture and the MUDR data storage principles.

MUDRLite itself is an empty body, which has to be filled in with an XML configuration file. This file completely describes the visual aspects and the behavior of the EHR application. It includes simple 4GL-like constructs written in the MUDRLite Language (MLL). This enables - using the event-oriented programming principles - to program various handling procedures for a range of actions, e.g. clicking a button fills a form with the result of an SQL statement. MUDRLite can be tailored to particular needs of any healthcare provider. This makes the MUDRLite application easy to use in specific environments. In the first instance, we are testing it at the Neurovascular Department of the Central Military Hospital in Prague.

## Introduction

The European Centre for Medical Informatics, Statistics and Epidemiology – Cardio (EuroMISE Centre – Cardio) focuses on new approaches to electronic health record (EHR) design, including electronic medical guidelines and intelligent systems for data mining and decision support [1]. Participation in the I4C-TripleC project [2, 3, 4] of the 4th Framework Program of the European Commission as well as the CEN TC 251 standards and cooperation with physicians has produced significant experience, which resulted in formulating a list of 15 requirements for EHR systems [5].

To create an EHR system which would fulfill these requirements, the EuroMISE Centre is developing an EHR application called MUDR (MUltimedia Distributed Record) [6, 7, 8, 9, 10]. Following the requirements stated before, a modular structure of the system has been defined. It is based on a 3-tier architecture, using a database layer, an application layer and a user interface layer, which enables the separation of physical data storage, application intelligence and client applications.

The set of collectable attributes varies at different departments and in different organizations (also over time). MUDR uses a dynamically extensible and modifiable structure of items based on a so-called knowledge base and data-file principles. This approach allows the reorganization (without change) of the database structure. It makes the system absolutely universal, but it also raises complications. It is quite difficult to develop universal user interfaces which would be sufficiently friendly and comfortable. Deploying the MUDR health record in a particular environment demands some effort; the knowledge base must first be modeled and built, and all the MUDR components must be installed and configured.

Currently most hospitals have some form of electronics health records included into their clinical information systems. Yet, these systems are often more suitable for hospital management than for physicians. The health record is not sufficiently structured; it includes a lot of free-text information, and the set of collected attributes is fixed and practically impossible to extend. Physicians gathering information for the purpose of medical studies often use varied proprietary solutions based on MS Access databases or MS Excel Sheets. MUDR usage in such cases is possible, but this solution may be too complicated and tedious. Furthermore, the result may not be as user-friendly as that of a special application, intended for the particular user's needs.

## 1. MUDRLite

The use of the MUDRLite heath record would be an easier solution. MUDRLite is a result of applied research in the field of EHR design and it constitutes a spin-off of original MUDR development. MURDLite simplifies both the MUDR architecture and the MUDR data-storing principles.

### *1.1 MUDRLite Architecture*

MUDRLite architecture is based on two layers. The first one is a relational database. Currently, MS SQL server versions 7 and 2000 are supported. The second layer is a MUDRLite User Interface running on a Windows-based operating system.

The database schema corresponds to particular needs and varies in different environments, as opposed to the fixed database schema in the MUDR data layer. MUDRLite universality is based on a different approach. The database schema can be designed using standard data modeling techniques, e.g. E-R Modeling [11]. The MUDRLite User Interface is able to handle varied database schemas. This feature often simplifies the process of importing old data stored in different databases or files.

### *1.2 MUDRLite User Interface*

All the visual aspects and behavior of the MUDRLite User Interface are completely described by an XML file. The end user observes a set of forms. A form can be defined by a form element, as follows:

```
<form name="new_hosp_form" label="New Hospitalization" author="JS"
date="27.1.2004" language="en" sizeX="420" sizeY="410"> … </form>
```

The attributes describe the internal name of the form; the label, which will be presented to the user; who and when created the form; which language is used in the form and the visual size of the form. Form controls are described using various sub-elements like `<button>`, `<combobox>`, `<groupbox>`, `<textbox>`, `<datagrid>`, `<checkbox>` etc.

A control is placed in the form through the following syntax:

```
<label name="but_del_hosp" label="Delete..." posX="200" posY="315"
sizeX="80" sizeY="23" tabIndex="2" color="indigo" />
```

The attributes name, label, posX, posY, sizeX, sizeY, tabIndex and color are used in all elements describing the various controls in a form. They describe the internal name of the control; the label presented to the user; the position and size of the control; the tab index and the color of the control. A new localized MUDRLite User Interface can be created very fast, just by translating labels in the configuration file. A choice of over 160 color names is at the user's disposal. The names are defined in the GDI+ library of the .NET Framework [12]. They cover the usual colors as well as system-defined colors, e.g. the application workspace color, the window color, the window frame color etc. There are some simple elements, e.g. <groupbox> or <label>, which use only these attributes. Another attribute, called readonly, is very often used to determine the possibility of editing a value. Other elements use more attributes that will be described in detail.

The most typical control is a textbox, defined by the <textbox> element. Additional attributes acceptsReturn and acceptsTab determine whether the user can enter line breaks and tabulators. Through the multiline attribute, the form designer enables viewing more than one line of text in the textbox. Scrollbars are placed using the scrollbars attribute, which can assume the none, horizontal, vertical and both values.

A data grid is also a common control element in database applications. In MUDRLite the <datagrid> element uses the colwidth attribute to set the preferred column width. Other visual aspects, such as the columns' titles, can be set by similar techniques. These will be described later.

Enumerative variables are often bound with combo or list box controls. The <combobox> element uses the maxDropDownItems numeric attribute to specify how many items can be shown together. The sorted attribute determines whether the items should be alphabetically sorted. There are two different styles of the combo box control: a list style, where the user can select a value from a fixed list, and an editable style, which enables adding new values to the list. Style is set by the dropDownStyle attribute. There are two ways of filling in the combo box with values. The first one is by using the <item> sub-elements, which define an item by its value and display attributes. The value stored in database doesn't have to be the same as the one the user sees in the form. This property helps maintain the 3$^{rd}$ normal form [13] of the database while keeping the form user-friendly. The second way to fill in the combo box is by using an SQL statement. This statement is processed while loading the form. It should return two columns: a value member and a display member; or just one column if the value and display members are identical. Technically this is realized by the <items> sub-element with the command attribute.

There are some more controls being prepared, such as tree views, tab panels, image boxes, scroll bars, progress bars, status bars, tool bars and tool tips, but they aren't completely finished yet. Their full description will be included in the MUDRLite Designer's Manual after they have been completed. A small example of a user-defined form can be seen in Figure 1. It is defined as follows:

```
<form name="edit_patient" label="Edit patient details" author="JS"
 language="en" date="18.2.2004" sizeX="320" sizeY="290">
  <label label="Name:" name="lbl_patient" posX="20" posY="38"
     sizeX="80" sizeY="25" color="indigo"/>
  <label label="Address:" name="lbl_address" posX="20" posY="98"
     sizeX="80" sizeY="25" color="indigo"/>
  <label label="Gender:" name="lbl_gender" posX="20" posY="168"
     sizeX="80" sizeY="25" color="indigo"/>
  <textbox name="e_nm" posX="100" posY="35" sizeX="200" sizeY="15"/>
```

```
    <textbox name="e_ad" posX="100" posY="65" sizeX="200" sizeY="60"
       acceptsReturn="true" multiline="true"/>
    <combobox name="c_g" posX="100" posY="135" sizeX="200" sizeY="21"
       sorted="true" maxDropDownItems="2" dropDownStyle="list">
     <item value="1" display="man"/><item value="2" display="woman"/>
    </combobox>
    <label label="" name="l_id" posX="0" posY="0" visible="false"/>
    <groupbox name="g_p" label="Patient details" posX="10" posY="10"
       sizeX="300" sizeY="190" color="red"/>
    <button label="Save" name="bs" posX="20" posY="250" sizeX="120"
       sizeY="23" tabIndex="0" color="blue"/>
    <button label="Cancel" name="bc" posX="180" posY="250" sizeX="120"
       sizeY="23" tabIndex="1" color="blue"/>
</form>
```

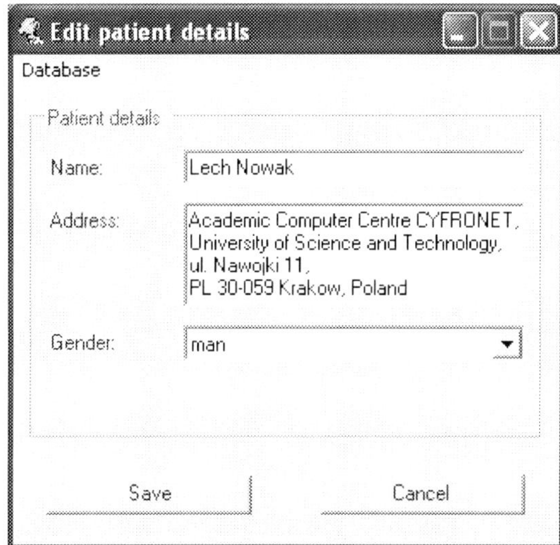


**Fig. 1.** Example of a simple user-defined form

The definition above creates a form as seen in Figure 1, but there are two problems left: there is no action connected with pressing each of the two buttons, so no matter how many times the user clicks, nothing happens. The other problem is that even though the form should load the details of selected patient upon startup, it always opens empty. Both problems can be solved using the MUDRLite Language.

### *1.3 MUDRLite Language*

The MUDRLite Language (MLL) is a simple event-based language used to describe the behavior of the MUDRLite User Interface. It contains 4GL-like constructs, which allow the processing of database operations.

The MLL constructs are included in the XML configuration file through the `<action>` element. This element can be placed as a sub-element under a form or under a control element, thus determining whether the action should be bound to the entire form or just to a control element in the form. Each action starts with an event and various event types exist. The most typical events involving controls are a click and a double click. With forms, a typical event is loading a form, closing a form, etc. Starting events are bound to actions by the `invoke` attribute.

There are also various action types. Action content is always described in the contents of the `<action>` element. Simple actions work with form controls. The user can, for example, clear, hide or show a control using the `<clear>`, `<hide>` and `<show>` sub-elements. Target controls are specified by the `result` attribute and identified by their names. Typically, more target controls can be specified simply by separating their names with commas. Sometimes a reference to a control placed in another form is needed. In this case, a dot-connected full name is used. It is constructed from the form name connected by a dot to the control name. The reserved name `parent` is used to reference the parent form, i.e. the form, which had been active before the current form was opened. Therefore, no form can be named "parent". The dot-connected full name can be more complicated in case one needs to address a special part of a control instead of the whole control. A typical example is addressing a column of a data grid. In this case, a dot is used to connect the control name to the control part name, e.g. the column name of a data grid. The full name of a column can look like this: `parent.patients_grid.patient_id`.

Other action types allow working with entire forms. A form can be closed by the `<exit_form>` action element. A new form can be opened by the `<new_form>` element with the `name` attribute, which specifies the form to be opened. For example a form for editing patient details can be started by the following code:

```
<action invoke="click">
    <new_form name="edit_patient"/>
</action>
```

The most powerful actions involve using the MLL Language to communicate with the database and to set/get values into/from controls. An extended variant of SQL is used in the contents of these actions, in the `command` attribute. The control names in these commands are joined by pairs of colons. Result controls are specified by their names in the `result` attribute. Again, more result controls can be addressed by separating their names (or dot-separated full names) with commas. Hence, a select action can be executed by the following code:

```
<action invoke="load">
  <select
    command="select full_name as 'Name', address as 'Address',
                    sex_id as 'Gender', patient_id as 'Patient ID'
             from   patient
             where  patient_id = ':parent.patients_grid.patient ID:'"
    result ="e_nm, e_ad, c_g, l_id"/>
</action>
```

This example shows how the "Edit patient details" form is filled with details of the patient currently selected in the patients' grid of the parent form. It also demonstrates a simple trick: the patient's identifier is stored in an invisible label, which plays the role of an internal temporary variable. When the user presses the "Save" button, this variable is used to specify the user who should be updated with the MLL update action. Typically, the count of values returned by the select command should correspond to the count of controls specified in the `result` attribute. An exception is using a data grid as a result control. In this case, the column names of the data grid are specified by the "as" SQL expression. Insert, update and delete operations are performed by the `<insert>`, `<update>` and `<delete>` elements using the same principles as with the `<select>` element.

There is one additional action included in the first MUDRLite version. Text can be read by the computer through the `<speak>` action, which uses the `text` attribute. So far, only English pronunciation can be used.

Of course, many different actions can be performed at the same time. Figure 2 shows a more complex scenario – a form designed for the Neurovascular Department of the Central Military Hospital in Prague (English translation).

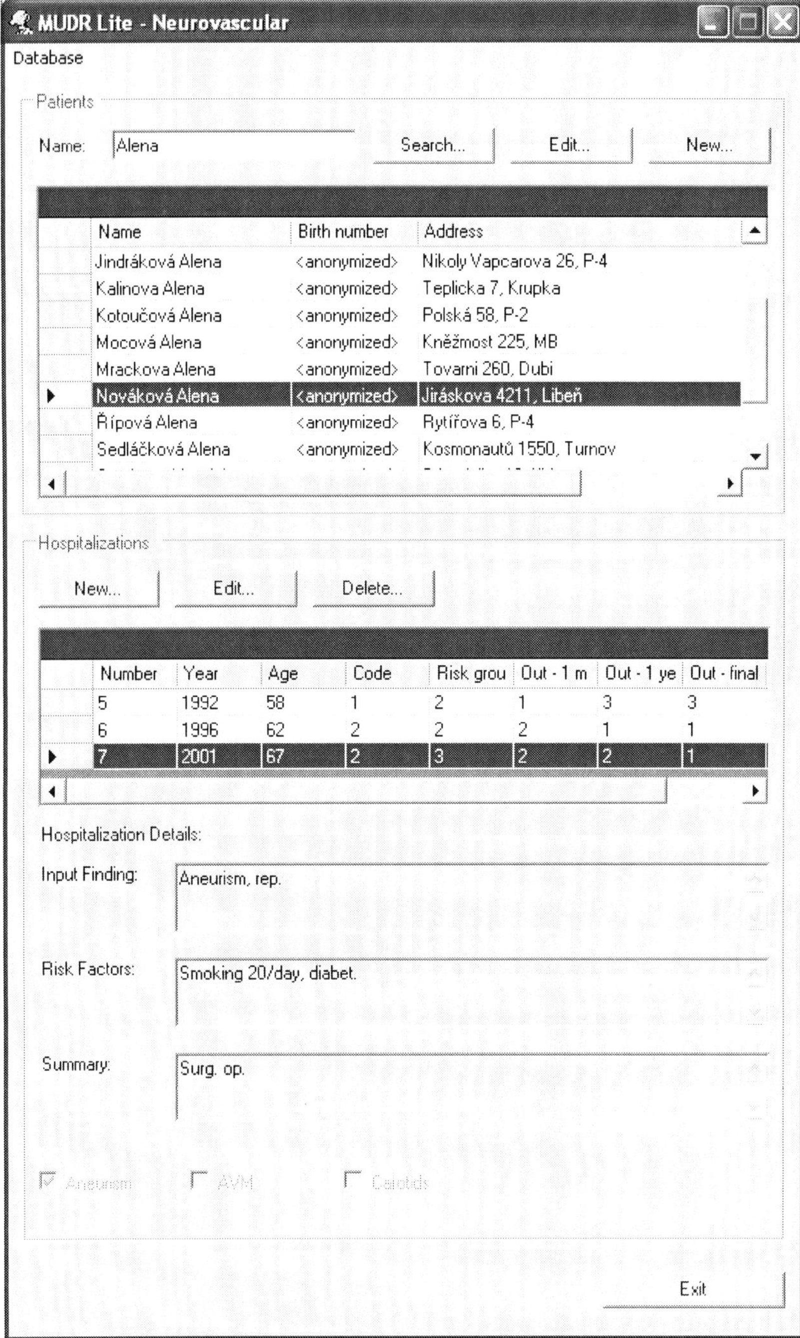


**Fig. 2.** MUDRLite form – Neurovascular Department of the Central Military Hospital in Prague

## 2. MUDRLite Deployment

MUDRLite deployment in a particular environment involves preparation phases. First of all, physicians must specify what information should be stored. This must be done precisely. A model including all attributes to be collected must be built. It must include attribute types as well as relationships among them, units of measurement, specifications of numerical attributes' precisions etc. Together with data engineers, an entity-relationship model (E-R Model [11]) is built.

Two more phases follow in parallel. One of them involves data migration from an existing system (MUDRLite is seldom deployed in an environment, where no data had been collected preciously). This is done using various techniques and SQL Server Data Transformation Services. The result of the second phase is the definition of MUDRLite user-defined forms and MUDRLite application behaviour using the MLL Language. Various XML editors can help create the XML configuration file. To simplify this phase, a special application called "MUDRLite Forms Designer" is being prepared. After the XML configuration file is finalized, MUDRLite should be tested. Subsequently, the application is fine-tuned according to the physicians' comments.

## 3. Results

MUDRLite testing has confirmed that this health record is flexible enough to allow dynamic changes of the database structure, with just small alterations in the XML configuration file. The XML file can be constructed using various XML editors, but we are preparing a special MUDRLite Forms Designer to make this process much simpler. The two-tier architecture separates the user interface from the data storage system. This enables remote access to health records. To make remote access more flexible, we plan to develop a Pocket PC version of the MUDRLite User Interface, which should run on various portable devices.

We have also verified the functionality and simplicity of the MLL Language. It is useful and sufficient for many applications; mostly thanks to the power of SQL. However, we would still like to increase the power of the language. We plan to do this by including arithmetical expressions and logical conditions into the language. We are aware of the fact that we also have to keep it as simple as possible.

## 4. Conclusion

Our interest is in increasing the quality of EHR systems, in simplifying data sharing and data migration among various EHR systems and in helping overcome the limitations of classical free-text-based health records. This way, quality of healthcare can be increased, benefiting the patient. Most healthcare providers already use some kind of an EHR system. However, the health record is often insufficiently structured. Physicians gathering information for the purpose of medical studies often use varied proprietary methods.

We thus present the MUDRLite universal solution. It is an easy way to build an electronic health record tailored exactly to one's needs. In the first instance, we are deploying MUDRLite at the Neurovascular Department of the Central Military Hospital in Prague. We have also started cooperation with the Dental Medicine Department of the Charles University, 1$^{st}$ Faculty of Medicine, which should result in spreading MUDRLite among Czech stomatology ambulatories. We hope this will introduce our solutions into real, practical use, which should bring advantages for healthcare in the Czech Republic.

**Acknowledgment.** The work was partially supported by grant number LN00B107 of the Ministry of Education of the Czech Republic.

## References

[1] Rauch J.: Mining for Statistical Association Rules. In: Fong J., Ng M.K. (eds.): The Fifth Pacific/Asia Conference on Knowledge Discovery and Data Mining, University of Hong Kong (2001) 149-158

[2] Iakovidis I.: Towards Personal Health Record: Current Situation, Obstacles and Trends in Implementation of Electronic Healthcare Record in Europe. Int J Med Inform 52, Nos. 1-3 (1998) 105-115

[3] Pierik F. H., Ginneken A. M., Timmers T., Stam H., Weber R. F.: Restructuring Routinely Collected Patient Data: ORCA Applied to Andrology. In: Bemmel J. H., McCray A. T. (eds.): Yearbook of Medical Informatics 98, Health Informatics and the Internet, Schattauer, Stuttgart (1998) 257-263

[4] Ginneken A. M. The Computerized Patient Record: Balancing Efort and Benefit, Int J Med Inform 65, (2002) 97-119

[5] Hanzlicek P.: Development of Universal Electronic Health Record in Cardiology. In: Surján G., Engelbrecht R., McNair P. (eds.): Health Data in the Information Society. Amsterdam, IOS Press (2002) 356-360

[6] Zvarova J., Hanzlicek P., Spidlen J.: Electronic Health Record in Cardiology: Pilot Application in the Czech Republic. In: MIST2002 Proceedings, Taiwan, John Wiley & Sons Pte Ltd. (2002) 10-13

[7] Spidlen J., Adaskova J., Heroutova H., Zvarova J., Mazura I.: Statistical Processing of Genetic Information in the MUDR Health Record. In: Vignerova J., Riedlova J., Blaha P. (eds.): Anthropology and Society, Charles University, Prague (2003) 190

[8] Hanzlicek P., Spidlen J., Heroutova H.: User interface of MUDR Electronic Health Record, Medical Informatics Europe Proceedings CD (2003)

[9] Hanzlicek P., Spidlen J., Zvarova J.: The Internet in Connecting Electronic Health Record Mobile Clients, Technology and Health Care, Vol. 10, Num 6, IOS Press (2002) 502-503

[10] Spidlen J., Hanzlicek P.: Implementace formalizovaných lékařských doporučení v elektronickém zdravotním záznamu MUDR. In: Svatek V. (ed.): Znalosti 2003 proceedings of the 2nd annual conference, VŠB-TU Ostrava (2003) 386-391

[11] Reingruber M. C., William W. G.: The Data Modeling Handbook : A Best-Practice Approach to Building Quality Data Models, John Wiley & Sons, Inc. (1994), ISBN: 0-471-05290-6

[12] Microsoft Corporation: Microsoft® .NET Framework 1.1 Class Library Reference Volume 7: System.Windows.Forms, System.Drawing, and System.ComponentModel, Microsoft Press® (2003), ISBN: 0-7356-1818-6

[13] Piattini M., Diaz O.: Advanced Database Technology and Design, Artech House, Inc. (2000), ISBN: 0-89006-395-8

*Transformation of Health Care with Information Technologies*
*M. Duplaga et al. (Eds.)*
*IOS Press, 2004*

# Access Control Mechanisms for Distributed Healthcare Environments

Marita SERGL-POMMERENING
*International Health Care Management Institute, University of Trier*
*Sickingen Str. 98, 54296 Trier, Germany*
*e-mail: sergl@uni-trier.de*

**Abstract.** Today's IT-infrastructure provides more and more possibilities to share electronic patient data across several healthcare organizations and hospital departments. A strong requirement is sufficient data protection and security measures complying with the medical confidentiality and the data protection laws of each state or country like the European directive on data protection or the U.S. HIPAA privacy rule. In essence, the access control mechanisms and authorization structures of information systems must be able to realize the *Need-To-Access* principle. This principle can be understood as a set of context-sensitive access rules, regarding the patient's path across the organizations. The access control mechanisms of today's health information systems do not sufficiently satisfy this requirement, because information about participation of persons or organizations is not available within each system in a distributed environment. This problem could be solved by appropriate security services. The CORBA healthcare domain standard contains such a service for obtaining authorization decisions and administrating access decision policies (RAD). At the university hospital of Mainz we have developed an access control system (MACS), which includes the main functionality of the RAD specification and the access control logic that is needed for such a service. The basic design principles of our approach are role-based authorization, user rights with static and dynamic authorization data, context rules and the separation of three cooperating servers that provide up-to-date knowledge about users, roles and responsibilities. This paper introduces the design principles and the system design and critically evaluates the concepts based on practical experience.

## Introduction

Within the last ten years we have observed that the electronic information processing in healthcare has achieved a new dimension. The past was characterized by standalone specialized information systems in hospital departments or healthcare centers e.g. for the needs of administration, lab, radiology or intensive care monitoring. Nowadays, we find information systems at nearly all departments and organizations. Data and functionality of systems are available from everywhere via intranets or the Internet. Runaway healthcare costs require the use of efficient communication mechanisms and data sharing among organizations in order to ensure high quality of care.

Most importantly, the flow of healthcare information requires mechanisms that properly protect data from unauthorized notice and manipulation complying with the medical confidentiality and data protection laws of each state or country. Privacy requirements are for example established by the European directive on data protection as well as the privacy rule issued by the USA as part of the Health Insurance Portability and Accountability Act (HIPAA) [1]. One aspect of these requirements is the access policy – required by each organization – defining which persons may access a patient's data in a particular mode at a given time. This policy has to regard organizational and structural requirements as well as existing and future infrastructure and resources. The advantages of electronic information processing shouldn't be reduced by unnecessary restrictions. Unfortunately, today's clinical information systems still lack sufficient access control mechanisms to fulfill these requirements. The most important reasons are missing information about the responsibility of persons and organizational units during the treatment process and missing consideration of causal contexts. Therefore, we need information about responsibility and participation relations as well as rules that represent the (time-dependent) "Need-To-Access" relations for patient data. With regard to the heterogeneous, distributed nature of information systems in healthcare, we can achieve satisfactory access control only by providing the needed functionality and authorization information to all hospital systems by means of appropriate services. Thus, we have developed an access control system, called the *Master Access Control System* (MACS), at the university hospital of Mainz [2]. The MACS is designed as a central service, consisting of various other services that allow to define a complex access control policy (able to comply with the "Need-To-Access" principle) and to appropriately provide information about the permissibility of patient data accesses to a distributed healthcare information system. Related work is discussed in section 9.

## 1. The Access Control Policy

The main question an access policy has to answer is: "Which person or system is allowed to access which part of a particular patient's data in which way at a given time?" According to the medical confidentiality principles, only persons who participate in the treatment or patient care, or their assistants, may access the patient's data.

When a patient is admitted or transferred to a hospital department, the physicians of the department, the nurses of the care unit and all persons performing diagnostic or therapeutic procedures, like laboratory assistants, radiologists, or anesthetists, participate in the treatment in the above sense. Billing is also part of the treatment context, therefore administrative staff is permitted to access the relevant data. In large hospitals accessing a particular patient's data cannot be allowed for all of the medical staff. Only the physicians at the entire department level such as urology, gynecology or pediatric department may be considered as a working team.

The permitted access mode and data set depends on the accessing person's responsibilities according to the "*Need-To-Access*" principle. For instance, the physician on duty needs to know all results and therapeutic measures that have been taken – *also in other departments or health centers* – from the patient's admission to a hospital up until the present time. He also has to document the patient's state and diagnoses, as well as orders and prescriptions issued *during the patient's stay in his department or unit.*

All these informal requirements have to be laid down in the form of access rules as described below, considering the specific organizational structures and processes.

### *1.1 Structure of Access Rules*

Treatment periods belong together with different access operations in particular situations. We call a rule that defines such a set of treatment periods *a context rule*. For example, the *treatment context rule* of a hospital unit covers all clinical treatment episodes of patients that actually stay in the unit, beginning with their first visits to one of the hospital departments relative to a particular illness, including all visits or transfers to other departments, intermittent absences from the hospital, discharges and further visits after a readmission. Figure 2 in section 3 shows an example of another context rule that determines the set of patient records a particular unit or organization is authorized to get updated information for by the communication system.

By means of context rule definitions, we can derive which part of the patient record needs to be accessed at a time within the treatment process. An access rule includes – apart from the context rule – the authorized *access operation* and the *accessing subject* (typically a person) or, instead, for a defined person – their *membership in a healthcare organization or unit* and *responsibility* within the unit. These parameters depend on organizational structures such as relations between the organization's facilities or the composition of professional groups.

## *1.2 Structures Influencing Access Rules*

### *1.2.1 Organization-Specific Structures*

In order to know which persons are involved in a treatment period, we have to check the patient's location and the service providing facilities, as well as the people who are working in these facilities and their responsibilities:

*Organizational structure:* In hospitals, for example, the facilities are hierarchically-ordered. Thereby the hospital is divided into various domain-specific departments and institutes that either consist of further sub-departments or of care units, outpatient units and service facilities.

*Professional groups:* The medical staff belongs to various hierarchically-ordered professional groups. Each hospital department, for example, has one *medical director* and several *assistant medical directors* who are responsible for particular subdepartments and supervise a number *of ward physicians* who work together in teams that are responsible for patients at one or more care units. Members of a particular group have identical tasks that are (partially) contained in the set of tasks of the superior group. The departmental schedule determines which persons are on duty for a particular organizational unit at a given time and in a particular function.

*The treatment process:* The treatment process can be described as a sequence of treatment periods associated with persons, facilities or organizations. Various medical or administrative events, such as admission, transfer, discharge, order entry and observation reporting, mark the beginnings and ends of the periods. Each association is uniquely identified by a patient identifier, an admission identifier, the participant's identifier and role and the beginning – as well as end – of the period.

### *1.2.2 Structures of Information Processing*

The information-processing model determines the nature of *access to patient data*. The electronic patient record is the basic concept of patient-based information processing. It includes various kinds of electronical patient data, such as structured data, reports, graphs and images, ever acquired for a particular patient. The patient record is distributed over various organizations, departments and information systems, and its contents can be subdivided according to different treatment periods and types of data or documents. Each data manipulation can be described as a specific operation on the electronic patient record. The set of information processing operations is determined by the functionality of every single information system.

While building the model, we have paid special attention to two important aspects of specific structures in health environments: the time-dependency of assignments and the hierarchical structure of professional groups and facilities. Due to the time-dependency, individual access rights can be ascertained by rule evaluation only at access time. Due to the hierarchy of professional groups and facilities, access rules implicitly apply to subfacilities as well as higher-level professional groups.

## 2. The Information Model

### *2.1 A Model of Access Rights*

Access rights have to implement the access policy (the access rules) and are assigned to persons or other subjects (such as systems) for the purpose of authorization in various healthcare organizations or hospital units. In order to enable authorization without exact knowledge of data objects and persons, the representation of access rights must refer to *abstract classes of data objects* (including appropriate access operations) *and subjects*. Because of the time-dependency of participation and responsibility relations, such a representation has to contain dynamic parts that are interpreted at access time. We therefore chose a representation of access rights that fulfills this requirement by dividing the information into *general parameterized context rules* and *individual abstract access rights*, made up of a context rule instance (a context rule with fixed parameter values e.g. a particular hospital unit) and static attributes referring to object classes. Processing an access right at runtime determines the specific set of treatment periods that define the accessible part of the patient record and the kind of data operations the accessing subject may perform at this time.

### *2.2 Role-based Authorization*

As described in [3, 4, 5] in detail, *role models* are ideal for the representation of *subject classes* in healthcare. They support mandatory access control by mapping hierarchical responsibilities to sets of access rights. Every role represents the responsibilities of one subject or a group of subjects – mostly within a particular organization or department – like the "ward doctor of children's intensive care unit".

Apart from the mapping of hierarchical responsibilities, role hierarchies facilitate authorization because they offer a kind of a construction kit. Each role (except the initial root role) inherits its assigned access rights from another role and adds further access rights. A role represents a particular set of functions by its assigned access rights, and groups the subjects who possess these functions. Authorization can also be limited to a time interval.

We have specified the following hierarchy of hospital roles: One root-role groups all subjects of the hospital. The root-role by itself has no access permissions for patient data. Roles for different professional groups (*functional roles*) and clinical departments (*department roles*) derive from this root-role. Each further role derives from an appropriate functional and department role and thus inherits the assigned permissions of both. Not all of the possible combinations of professional groups and organizational units result in meaningful roles. We create roles only for those combinations with different functions or permissions. Figure 1 shows an example extract of the role hierarchy.

The inheritance structure of roles reduces the implementation effort of the access policy and allows decentralized administration of access permissions and authorization of users.

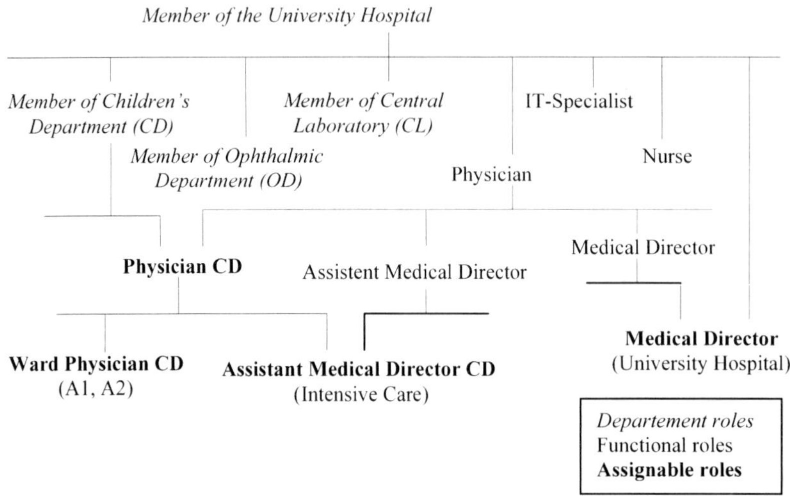


**Fig. 1.** Extract of the role hierarchy at the university hospital of Mainz showing some basic department roles, functional roles and the inherited roles that can be assigned to a subject.

### 2.3 *User-based Authorization*

In addition to the concept of abstract access rights we define a class of user-and-patient-based access rights (*user-specific rights*). This allows simply authorizing a specific subject (e.g. a consulted physician of another hospital department) to access a particular patient record. Instead of a context rule instance as contained in the abstract access rights, the user-specific rights contain a patient record reference, defining the patient record part that relates to a particular treatment period by means of the hospital-wide valid and unique identifier for the patient and the admission and, optionally, the start and the end of the treatment period. Additionally, the user permission refers to the hospital-wide valid and unique user identifier of the authorized subject.

### 2.4 *The Controlled Vocabulary – Semantically Linking Distributed Systems with the Access Control Service*

The classification of objects requires an agreement covering the ontology mapped to keywords and their meaning in terms of access control policy. These requirements are laid down in a controlled vocabulary that consists of separate sections for different attribute types, such as *data operation*, *data class*, *information source* and *organizational unit.* Names of *context rules* are also registered as vocabulary terms in form of function prototypes enclosing a type declaration for each existing rule parameter. Thus a policy definition tool can look up all terms and structures that may be used to define the object class of an abstract access right.

Every section of the vocabulary (except the context prototypes) is hierarchically arranged in order to represent semantic inclusions of terms (e. g. "GetPatientRecord" includes "GetPatientObservations"). Several independent terminologies such as standardized and self-defined terminologies or different terminology versions can be used concurrently by defining named vocabulary subsections.

### 2.5 Context Rules and the Treatment Process Model

As mentioned above, context rules allow the definition of access rights that relate to temporarily changing sets of health record sections. For this purpose, rules must operate on a knowledge base containing all relations between treatment periods and participating organizations or organizational units. A treatment period is exactly determined by the time interval and the responsible organizational unit, and it corresponds to a section of the electronic health record. In our information model, we distinguish between two basic knowledge concepts: a) different kinds of patient visits in hospital units (in- and outpatient visits and some more Germany-specific kinds of visits) and health center and b) different types of participations during the visit involving further organizational units or persons. Both concepts are regarded as treatment relations. Each treatment relation belongs to a medical case. At each time, a context rule instance defines a subset of relations contained in the knowledge base. These subsets are defined with set-theoretic methods such as classification of elements by required attributes values, the use of quantifiers (e.g. the existence of elements with particular properties) and logic links of subsets. We have limited the variety of possible rule structures to two types that could express all context rules of the current access. Figure 2 shows an example of the more complicated type.

$$\texttt{UPDATE\_CONTEXT(UnitT } \textit{particp}\texttt{)} := \left\{ \mathbf{r}\in\mathbf{R} \;\middle|\; \bigvee_{\text{ind}\in\mathbf{R}} \bigwedge_{\text{r}\in\mathbf{R}} \begin{array}{l} \textbf{ind}\texttt{.unit=}\textit{particp}\texttt{,} \\ \textbf{r}\texttt{.admID=}\textbf{ind}\texttt{.admID,} \\ \textbf{r}\texttt{.begin<=}\textbf{ind}\texttt{.end} \end{array} \right\}$$

**Fig. 2.** Parameterized context rule defined by the existence of special "indicator" relations and dependent relation properties: „If the organizational unit *particp* participates in a patient's treatment period, all concurrent and following relations of the same case belong to the defined set."

### 2.6 Information Retrieval Structures

Due to the need to communicate current access rights or access decisions to the departmental information systems the model includes request and result structures for information retrieval. The requesting system has to specify the user's subject id, his active role and search attributes in order to define the class of requested accesses. Search attributes include a list of named values restricting the set of health record parts to a particular context and values restricting the class of requested operations, data and information sources. Context attributes include the time period, hospital department, particular treatment type and a unique patient or case identifier. The more general search values are specified the larger the result set of actual access rights. Each element consists of an operation term, the data view (if specified), an information source identifier and the related health record section defined by the patient identifier, the case identifier, the beginning and the end of the related treatment period. If access rights from the result set include each other, only the most general right remains. For an exactly-specified request including only one specific access relating to a particular health record episode, the result set will have zero or one element. This is a so-called binary access decision. The retrieval interface also allows for requesting partial information, e.g. only an identifier list of patient records or cases the user may access.

Our request model goes beyond the access decision interface specified by the Resource Access Decision Service (RADS) specification, that is part of the CORBA healthcare domain standard [6]. The RADS only supports binary access decisions, that may lead to communication overhead e.g. in a case where patient or record lists are needed.

## 3. Applying the Model to a Healthcare Environment

The model introduced here allows for consistently handling access control rules and permissions in an independent access control server that offers access decisions to each subsystem of a healthcare environment. However, many of the existing systems have their own – even though insufficient – access control mechanisms. A completely independent access control system requires specifying data objects and operations of all subsystems in order to build access rights and integrate corresponding permission requests into the subsystems.

Even though our intent was to develop a complete model that can be used in such a way, another important goal is to integrate the existing systems in order to achieve sufficient access control for distributed health information systems in the medium term. To integrate subsystems we need – besides technical solutions that handle the interoperability task – an access control service, able to separately provide all partial aspects of access control the subsystems need. Many systems have their own internal access control mechanisms, e.g. the control of different user actions on particular patient data classes assigned to different user groups. Nevertheless, hardly any system includes mechanisms for defining and controlling dynamic, context-sensitive authorizations regarding different sets of health records. Each access right equally relates to all records registered in the system or, at best, to all records belonging to a particular organization or department. The access control mechanisms of such systems can be extended in the following way: for each combination of a functional user group (subjects that are responsible for the same patients) and context (expressed by a context rule instance) we define one access right. Then we extend the internal access control routines with appropriate access decision requests.

The suitability was evaluated by applying the model to real scenarios. We have exemplarily defined the necessary permissions and designed the integration routines for three scenarios of existing systems: 1) context-sensitive transmission control via a communication server, 2) user access control for a self-developed web-based cancer documentation system and 3) extension of access control mechanisms of the local patient administration system.

## 4. Implementation

### *4.1 Architecture*

We have implemented an access control system consisting of tree basic information servers (user registry, role definitions and automatically updated treatment process information) with common relational database technology and – for the user registry – an LDAP directory server. The application layer is subdivided into three independent services: 1) the *Policy Administration Service* including acquisition of roles, permissions, context rules, data views and vocabulary, 2) the *Authorization Service* and 3) *the Master Access Control Service* providing the retrieval functionality (Figure 3). In the first version, context rules were translated into database queries. There are concepts for future work with user-controlled rule definition and dynamic rule processing. We have implemented all services with basic CORBA technology. A prototype version of all services is finished and running in a test environment.

In every subsystem that needs to request access rights or access decisions, MAC-Client functions have to be integrated. In the case of scenario 1 above (section 4) we have integrated MAC-Client functionality without any redesign of existing routines by using a type of user exits provided by the software producer. In scenario 2 existing Perl-scripts had to be extended for the communication with external MAC-Clients, and scenario 3 is a classic example where modification and recompiling of existing software components would be necessary.

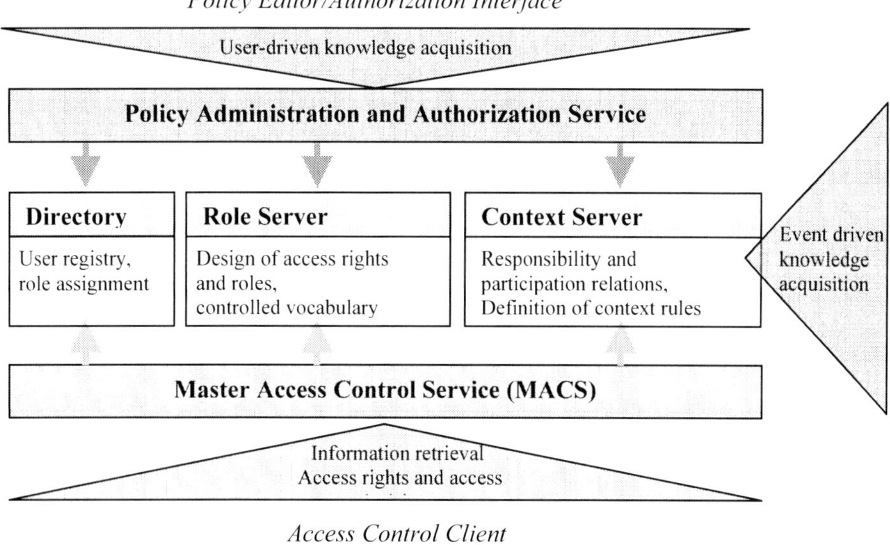


**Fig. 3.** The Master Access Control System architecture

### *4.2 Interfaces to the Environmental Data Flow*

An important goal was to integrate MACS into existing healthcare environments (in our case – the university hospital of Mainz). This requires that structural information about the environment and information about actual treatment processes is made available within the system. We have entered names of organizational units, information systems and their – partially hierarchical – relations into additional sections of the vocabulary. Unit and system names were needed for the definition of access rights and the organizational hierarchy – expressed through a hierarchical naming scheme – to derive implicit treatment relations. The vocabulary must be updated manually or, at best, automatically by an event-driven interface with information from a master system (usually an administrative information system). It is even more important to obtain information about treatment processes on time, (this includes all admissions, transfers and discharges, lab order entries etc.) Therefore, the context server is updated trough an event-driven interface that is provided with messages from the communication system of the organization (or a higher-level organization in the case of research or healthcare networks). At best, the communication system can derive all information about changing participations. Today, in most hospitals only basic information about administrative actions (such as patient movements) is available. Electronic order entry systems are exceptions rather than standards.

### 4.3 Security

Authorization in a healthcare environment is a critical task, and so a system dealing with access rights needs appropriate security features and architecture. Communication between the MACS-Services and between MACS-Services and Clients uses secure channels based on the secure socket layer protocol (SSL), which are included in the basic CORBA functions. To this end, all MACS-Clients and Servers need valid certificates for authentication. Authentication of users is not within the responsibility of the MACS.

## 5. Experiences

We have performed tests with test data separately for each server – particularly for the context server. Tuning issues have been identified concerning the server performance in the case of large quantities of participation relations. The whole system was tested with a preproduction version of our cancer documentation system.

The cancer documentation system only needs to know about participation of hospital departments in treatment processes, because functions and data views do not vary for different roles. Hence, we had to define one role with one appropriate access right for each hospital department. The following example shows the relevant part of an access right:

```
cdoc_derma.dataview = "Cancerreport"
cdoc_derma.dataop.term = "OP->MedDoku->ExtRegistration"
cdoc_derma.dataop.voc = "INTERNALVOC"
cdoc_derma.context.rulename = "TreatetCases(2)"
cdoc_derma.context.arguments = {{UNIT, "DE"},{DAYS, -1}}
```

The context rule named "`TreatetCases(2)`" returns all treatment periods of patients treated in the dermatological department ("`DE`") without any time limit ("`DAYS after discharge or transfer = -1`") – not just the currently treated patients, because cancer documentation should be compiled when all information about the patient's disease is available. The specific functional requirements of the cancer documentation system allowed us to implement control requests as binary access decisions by limiting the requests to single patients or medical cases (instead of departmental patient lists). Because of the small size of the search space, these requests performed very well.

## 6. Related Work

There are some other articles describing solutions for particular aspects of authorization and access control in hospitals or networked institutions of public health.

One example of comprehensive access control in institutions of public health is represented by the approach of the British Medical Association [7]. The model uses access control lists – one for each patient record – containing authorized users and access modes. Different points of view on patient information are represented by separate records. This approach shifts the dynamic and context-sensitive right components into the (likely manual) authorization task. That's why it is manageable only in domains with few, rarely changing authorizations per record (which does not include large hospitals).

Role-based access control models are the subject of many papers, e.g. [3, 4, 5, 8, 9, 10]. The National Institute of Standards and Technology reported a demonstration project that proved the suitability of role-based access control within public health [3]. They defined permissions by referencing data object methods and predefined data views. Dynamical aspects or context-sensitivity have not been considered in this approach. Ravi Sandhu has developed a general and comprehensive model of role-based access control

(RBAC) including a role-based administration model [8]. Access rights are defined using controlled vocabularies, whose terms are interpreted by the participating applications. Our model bases on Sandhu's approach and was extended for the given requirements.

Ultes-Nietsche, Teufel [11] and Stacchini et al. [12] have described dynamical and context-sensitive access control. Stacchini et al. has designed so-called "working lists", where each list defines current "need-to" relations between treating persons and patients. An event-driven mechanism updates the working lists according to a set of confidentiality rules based on the user's relation to functional domains, care units or on current orders or emergency situations. Access decisions depend on the user's identity and the hospital unit the workstation is located in. Thus, the access control mechanism can be supported by access control mechanisms of the computer network.

The context-sensitive access control model introduced by Ultes-Nietsche and Teufel was designed for accessing a particular database system and uses a workflow management system. Every treatment process state was associated with a tuple containing the usergroup, the datafields and the access mode. The access control mechanism evaluates the current workflow together with user information and the user's access rights. In case of an affirming result, the user is temporarily assigned to a database usergroup with unrestricted access permissions in order to enable the demanded access.

Another approach, the CORBAmed Resource Access Decision Service [6], defines a framework and generic naming schemes for resources and operations that can be used for context-sensitive access control in a CORBA-based environment, but the concrete design of access rights, the vocabulary and the structure of rules and dynamic information for the specific needs of the health area is not determined within the RAD specification or related work [13]. Information exchange between the RAD service and the client is limited to binary access decisions. No detailed information about up-to-date access rights is provided.

## 7. Discussion

None of the approaches found in literature represents an all-encompassing solution for access control in heterogeneous distributed health information systems. The information structure of access rights is mostly adapted to the particular data model and architecture of a particular information system. Environment-specific dependencies and context-sensitive aspects are scarcely considered by the more general approaches.

### *7.1 Advantages of the Approach*

Our model fulfills the needs of authorization and access control in heterogeneous distributed information systems. The information model permits an a-priori definition of who may access which patient record in which way, considering the environment-specific dependencies. Data classes, access operations, context rules and basic environmental structures are designed to be flexible and thus can also be extended after starting with the access control service. Flexibility is achieved by using a controlled vocabulary, by the variety of possible context rules and by using named-value lists as flexible data structures for information retrieval. Thus, it is possible to adapt the system to different healthcare environments.

At first sight, this model looks complex and extensive. In reality, however, it is just as possible to implement simple partial aspects or coarse access rules as to completely implement complex and detailed access rules. Appropriate external access rights and built-in decision requests can compensate the information systems' lack of sufficient access control mechanisms or context information in order to provide decision support. Also, if there is a set of detailed and complex access rights, requests should be specified in a way that makes the result set small and easy to process (by restricting the search space, using wildcards and requesting only partial information).

With this approach, we propose an extensive, flexible and integrating solution for access control in distributed heterogeneous hospital information systems.

### *7.2 Further Questions*

#### *7.2.1 Interoperability*

If we want to create a robust central access control system, we especially have to consider standards for the electronic healthcare record by building up vocabulary in order to achieve homogeneity and decrease complexity. Nevertheless, this requires strong cooperation between system developers and policy administrators. Other important requirements would be a detailed common model of access classes and standardized vocabularies (e. g. based on the HL7 terminology or on classification of clinical documents [14, 15]). The development of such a detailed model raises a number of questions regarding the standardization of electronic health records and information systems that have not yet been answered.

#### *7.2.2 Availability*

Another important aspect is the availability of the access control system, i.e. to make sure that all components and the real-time acquisition of the relevant treatment process information perform very well. Therefore we need immediate documentation of medical treatment and electronically supported order entry and scheduling. As long as the infrastructure is incomplete, missing information has to be completed by manual authorization (see also section 3.3 *User-based authorization*).

Even if we can ensure high availability, each client system of the master access control service has to provide fallback procedures for exceptional situations. The treating physician should be able to enforce unrestricted access on the patient's record, if needed. In this case each access has to be logged in detail.

#### *7.2.3 Performance*

As mentioned above, the performance of rule processing by the context server is of critical importance. Binary access decisions have performed well, but insufficiently-limited requests, for example involving all periods of the last month, have taken too much time to process. Therefore we have analyzed the queries and designed an alternative mechanism based on rule preprocessing.

**Acknowledgements.** The project was supported by a research award of the Boehringer-Ingelheim foundation.

## References

[1] U.S. Department of Health & Human Services. Health Insurance Portability and Accountability Act. [on-line]. Available *http://www.hhs.gov/ocr/hipaa/*, [cited: 3.3.2004].

[2] Sergl M. Konzepte und Komponenten für die Zugriffskontrolle in verteilten heterogenen Krankenhausinformationssystemen am Beispiel des Mainzer Universitätsklinikums. Dissertation, Fachbereich Medizin der Johannes Gutenberg-Universität Mainz [online]. Available: *http://ArchiMeD.uni-mainz.de/pub/2002/0043/diss.pdf*, 2002, [cited: 3.3.2004]

[3] Poole J, Barkeley J, Brady K, Cincotta A, Salamon W. Distributed Communication Methods and Role-Based Access Control for Use in Health Care Applications [online]. Technical report, National Institute of Standards and Technonlogy, 1996 [cited: 3.3.2004].

[4] Hayden M, Prichard J. Role-Based Access Control Techniques for Open Medical Information Systems [online]. In Proceedings of the Decision Sciences Institute Conference. East Carolina University, 1998.

[5] Potamias G, Tsiknakis M, Katehakis D, Karabela E, Moustakis V, Orphanoudakis S. Role-Based Access To Patients Clinical Data: The InterCare Approach in the Region of Crete. In Medical Infobahn for Europe, Proceedings of MIE2000 and GMDS2000 Amsterdam: IOS Press, 2000: 1074-1079.

[6] Object Mangement Group. Resource Access Decision (RADS) [online]. Technical report, OMG and CORBAmed DTF, 1999 [cited: 3.3.2004].

[7] Anderson R. Security in clinical information systems [online]. Available: *http://www.cl.cam.ac.uk/users/rja14/policy11/policy11.html*, 1996 [cited: 3.3.2004].

[8] Sandhu RS. Role-Based Access Control. Advances in Computers 1998, 46: 237-286.

[9] Goh C, Baldwin A. Towards a more Complete Model of Role [online]. Available: *http://www.hpl.hp.com/techreports/98/HPL-98-92.pdf*, 1998 [cited: 3.3.2004].

[10] Barkley J, Beznosov K, Uppal J. Supporting Relationships in Access Control Using Role Based Access Control. In Proceedings of the Fourth ACM Workshop on Role-Based Access Control, Fairfax 1999; 55-65.

[11] Ultes-Nitsche U and Teufel S. Secure Access to Medical Data over the Internet. In: Trends in Information and Communication Systems for the 21st Century - Proceedings of the 8th European Conference on Information Systems, Wirtschaftsuniversität Wien 2000; 2: 1331-1337.

[12] Staccini P, Joubert M, Fieschi D, Fieschi M. Confidentiality Issues within a Clinical Information System: Moving from Data-driven to Event-driven Design. Methods of Information in Medicine 1999; 298-302.

[13] Beznosov K, Deng Y, Blakly B, Burt C, Barkley J. A Resource Access Decision Service for CORBA-based Distributed Systems [online]. Available: *http://www.acsac.org/1999/abstracts/fri-b-0830-beznosov.html*, 1999 [cited: 3.3.2004].

[14] Inc. Health Level Seven. HL7 Version 2.3 (ballot draft) [online]. Available: *http://www.hl7.org*, 1996 [cited: 3.3.2004].

[15] Document Ontology Task Force DOTF. Proposal for an Ontology for Exchange of Clinical Documents [online]. Available: *http://www.hl7.org/Special/dotf/docs/DocumentOntologyProposalJuly00.doc*, 2000 [cited: 3.3.2004].

[16] Rector A and Horrocks I. Experience building a large, re-usable medical ontology using a description logic with transitivity and concept inclusions. In: Proceedings of AAAI'97. AAAI Press, 1997.

[17] SNOMED International: The Systemized Nomenclature of Medicine [online]. Available: *http://www.snomed.org*, 2001 [cited: 3.3.2004].

*Transformation of Health Care with Information Technologies*
*M. Duplaga et al. (Eds.)*
*IOS Press, 2004*

# The Performance of Information Technology in a Cardiovascular System

Liana Gabriela BERA[1], Ioan MANITIU[2]
[1] *University "Lucian Blaga" Sibiu, Faculty of Medicine, Medical Informatics Department, Sibiu, Romania*
[2] *University "Lucian Blaga" Sibiu, Faculty of Medicine, Cardiology Department, Sibiu, Romania*

**Abstract.** Our paper presents the results of a research study concerning the accuracy of the diagnosis and/or therapy for a cardiovascular patient. From the electronic patient records we have built a special database. The structure of this database offers possibilities for performing research studies on: cardiovascular pathology, risk factors action, medical treatment action, efficiency programs for primary and secondary prevention of diseases. The patient's data can be introduced from all intranet workstations of the cardiology department. The database structure is established to permit: optimal allocation of disk space, robust statistical analyses.

The coding scheme can be explained as follows: if the information can have two or more values which exclude each other, the information is represented by a character; if the information can have more values which don't exclude each other, the field contains many characters representing possible values.

Our paper shows that this database structure makes it possible to analyze every data piece that is stored. This system makes it possible to obtain a comprehensive summary of the cardiovascular population in real time by using standard reports and graphics, drill-down and roll-up on hierarchical dimensions, and analysis of temporal indicators. The database now contains information on 4000 patients undergoing effort tests as well as 2500 patients in the recovery program, and the system is being tested for all registered patients. We hope that field tests can begin in the near future, in the framework of a national cardiovascular infrastructure program.

## Introduction

Nowadays, medical applications need to be connected to an increasing number of information sources that are likely to be hosted by heterogeneous and distributed data management systems. Cooperation among different medical information systems is required to improve patient healthcare [1].

As the patient's medical data is disseminated in different health structures, developing a medical patient-oriented data warehouse has some specific requirements compared to intra-healthcare data warehousing projects [2].

The quality of data limits the ability of the end user to make the correct decisions, which can have fatal consequences, especially in a domain such a healthcare provider's environment. There is a number of indicators for the quality of data: accuracy, integrity, consistency, timeliness and completeness (among others) [3].

Computer science, with its methods, can make substantial contributions to effective storage, analysis, and visualization of complex correlations between data pieces [4].

The art of diagnosis is based on a correct application of data storage.

Our work includes research for an accurate diagnose and/or therapy for a cardiovascular patient. The project presented in this paper shows that an intranet for a cardiology department is necessary. It must be integrated with hospitals and communicate with other cardiovascular centers (recovery, cardiovascular surgery).

## 1. The Problem Area

In our region, the information system for a cardiovascular patient is illustrated in Fig. 1.

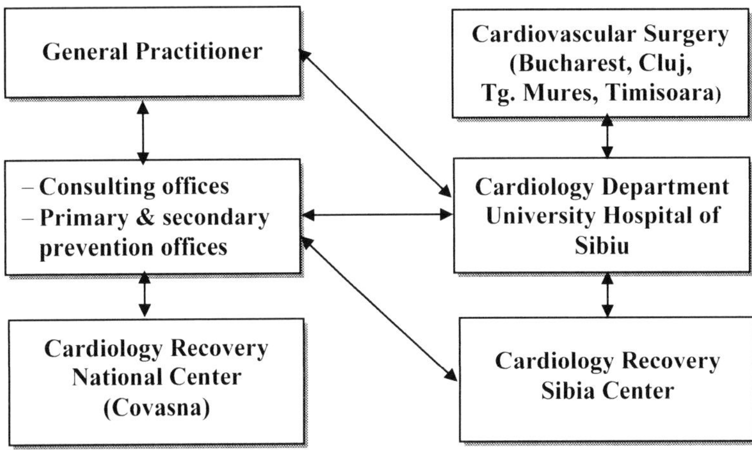


**Fig. 1.** The information system for a cardiovascular patient

Cooperation in the healthcare area concerns many partners. These partners often use different classifications systems to encode their data. A possible solution to this problem involves regrouping data issued from different sources into a centralized data warehouse, that is periodically updated according to the collaborative conventions.

## 2. Overview of the Design of the System

The art of establishing a diagnosis depends heavily on correct information. The information system for diagnosis and/or therapy is shown in Fig.2.

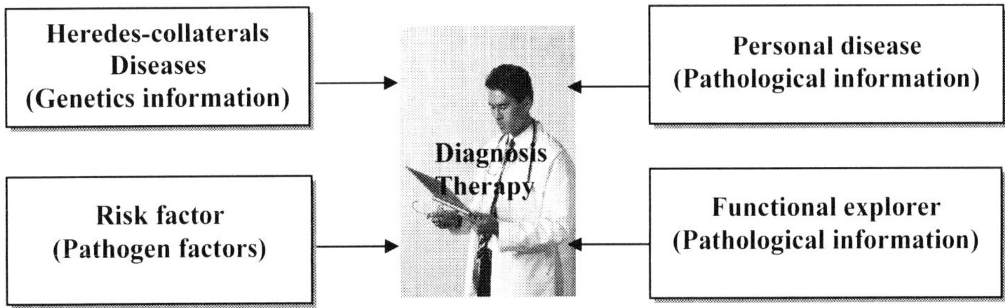


**Fig. 2.** The information system for diagnosis/therapy

Our cardiology database is built on top of the existing information flow for cardiovascular patients at the Cardiology Department, University Hospital of Sibiu, Romania (Fig.3).

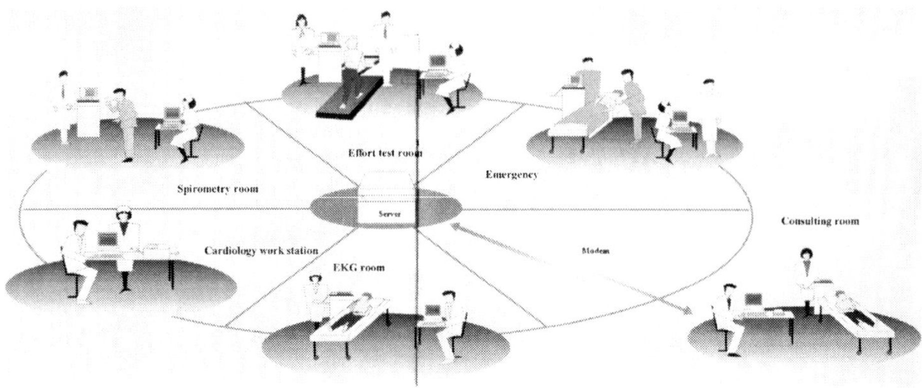


**Fig. 3.** Information flow for a cardiovascular patient

The patient's data is introduced from all stations of the intranet.

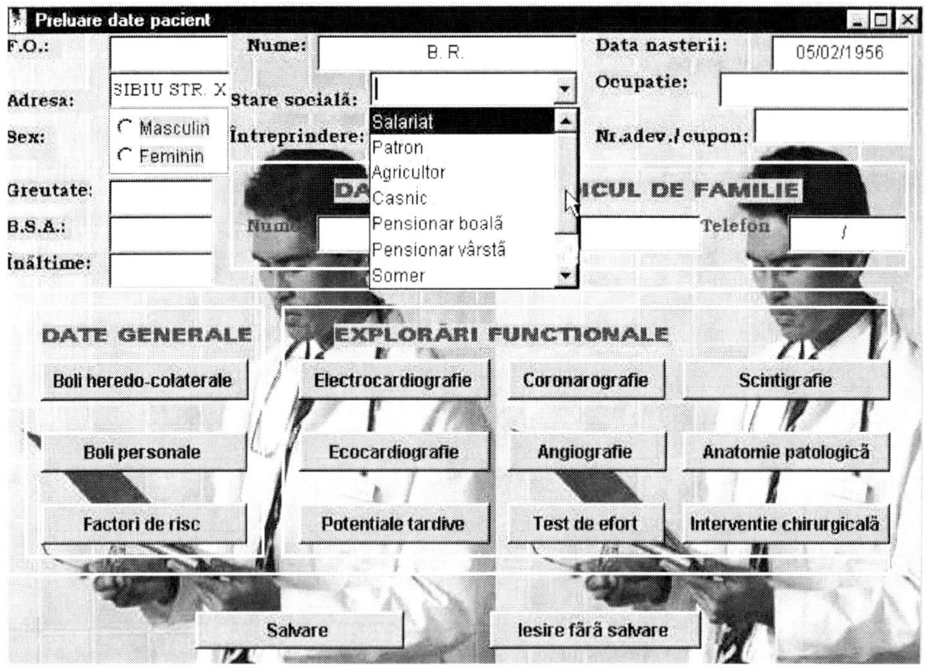


**Fig. 4.** General patient medical information

The cardiovascular data consists of the following main entities: patient data (Fig. 4), patient's diseases, cardiovascular risk factors (Fig. 5), drugs and hereditary conditions (Fig. 6), EKG and Eco changes (Figs. 5, 6), involvement of the patient and effort test evolution

(Fig. 7), the choices of exercises, objective data (blood pressure and AV), subjective exercises, the symptoms which appear during recovery or during effort tests (Fig. 8), etc.

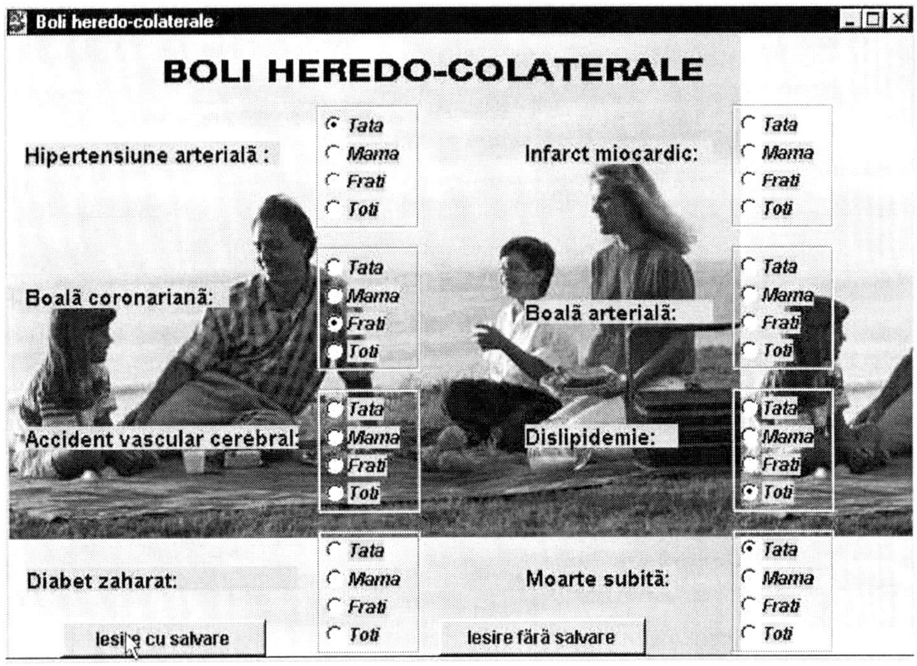


**Fig. 5.** Hereditary (collateral) diseases

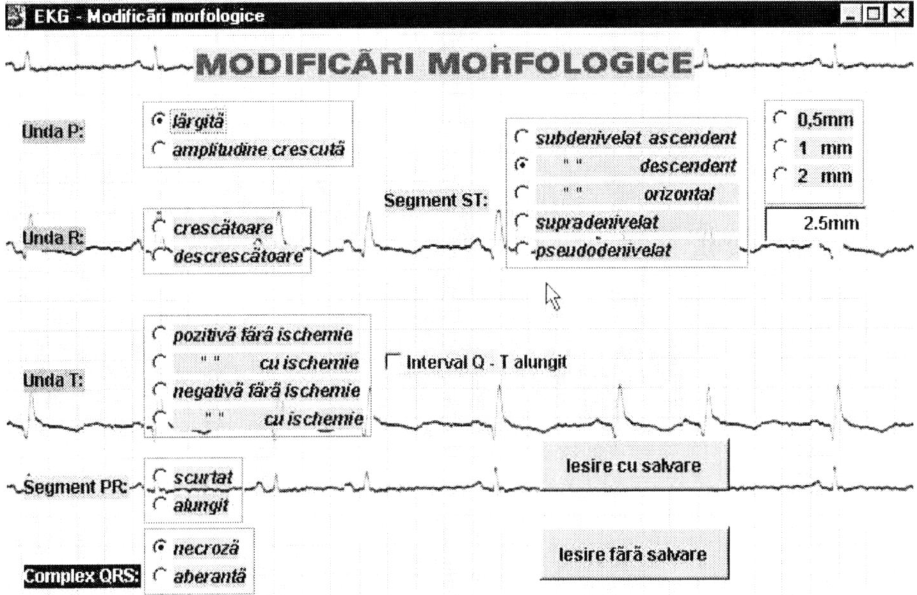


**Fig. 6.** EKG – morphological modification

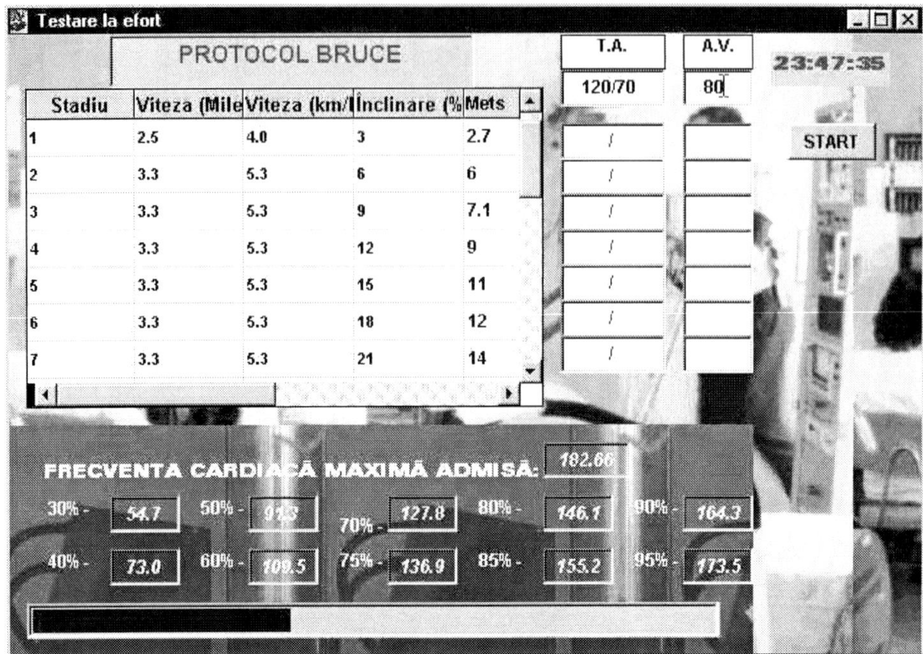


**Fig. 7.** The effort test

This project enables us to estimate the correct effort accommodation, the clinical evolution and the changing of risk factors for each patient. The structure of the database files offers the possibility to conduct research studies on [5]:

- cardiovascular pathology,
- risk factors action,
- medical treatment action,
- efficiency programs for primary and secondary prevention of diseases.

The medical information is used by the physician for:

- diagnosis and therapy,
- statistical analyses.

The database structure is established in order to permit:

- optimal allocation of disk space,
- robust statistical analyses.

We attempted to attain these objectives with a custom encoding method.

## 3. The Encoding Method

The encoding can be explained as follows [6]:

- if the information can have 2 or more values which exclude each other, the information is represented by a character (each person suffering from a particular disease will be represented by a character),
- if the information can take more values which aren't mutually-exclusive (i.e. hereditary conditions), the field will contain one character for each value.

**Table 1.** Personal diseases field

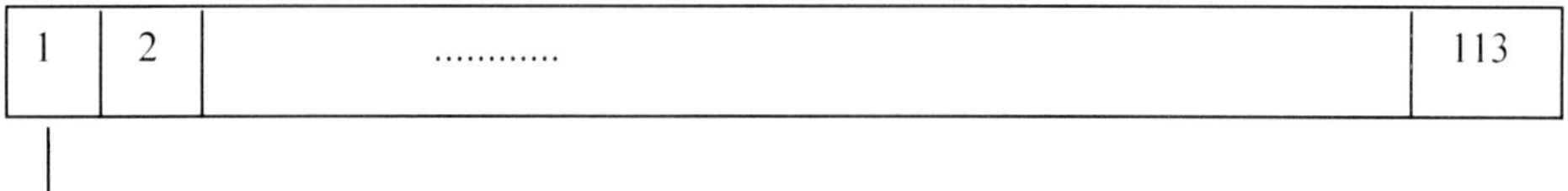

IMA inferior 0 – doesn't have the disease/1 – has the disease

An example is shown in Table 2:

**Table 2.** Hereditary/collateral diseases

| Field position | The disease which is represented | The meaning of the byte (i.e. who suffer s from that disease) |
|---|---|---|
| 1 | Arterial hipertension | 1 – father 2 – mother 3 – brother 4 – all family |
| 2 | Myocardial infarction | 1 – father 2 – mother 3 – brother 4 – all family |
| 3 | Coronary disease | 1 – father 2 – mother 3 – brother 4 – all family |
| 4 | Arterial disease | 1 – father 2 – mother 3 – brother 4 – all family |
| 5 | Sudden death | 1 – father 2 – mother 3 – brother 4 – all family |
| 6 | Stroke attack | 1 – father 2 – mother 3 – brother 4 – all family |
| 7 | Dislipidemia | 1 – father 2 – mother 3 – brother 4 – all family |
| 8 | Diabetes | 1 – father 2 – mother 3 – brother 4 – all family |

Our cardiology recovery center treats common heart diseases. It takes into account the first phase and the second/third phase of recovery for myocardial infarction. The recovery application permits easy control of: effort intensity and the evolution of recovery.

The patients can learn the maximum effort they can undertake (resulting from effort tests).

The recovery application draws a lot of files from the common cardiology database: patient files, myocardial infaction files, paraclinic files, etc.

## 4. Patient Use of the Internet

With the spreading availability and use of the Internet, the general public has easy access to online health information. Aside from actual diagnoses, it is possible for patients to explore this medium, searching in information regarding their conditions. Definitions of "good practice" may include a provision to ensure that the patient has more information than is currently provided on their condition, or perhaps direction from the practitioner to online resources that are accepted and qualified by the practitioner. The general public. whilst having the ability to receive information, only select appropriate and useful information [19]. For our patients, we consider it important to create a website with a guide of exercises taking into account the level of the effort, specific symptoms and the attitude of each patient.

## 5. Results

The instruments described are adequate for further research studies regarding [5]:

- cardiovascular pathology,
- risk factors action,

- medical treatment action,
- efficiency programs for primary and secondary prevention of diseases.

The database now holds information on 4000 patients undergoing effort tests along with 2500 patients in the recovery program. The system is still being tested and the developed database structure allows for in-depth analyses of stored data [7].

Further work will include integration with the intranet at the Clinical Hospital of Sibiu. We hope that field tests can begin in the near future, in the framework of a national cardiovascular infrastructure program.

Information reliability in a cardiovascular system can be provided through statistical analysis.

This system makes it possible to obtain a comprehensive summary of the cardiovascular population in real time, by using standard reports and graphics (curves, charts), drop-down and roll-up of hierarchical dimensions, as well as analysis of temporal trends for indicators.

Our paper shows that the database structure makes it possible to analyze all the stored data.

**Repartiția testelor de efort la pacienții cu obezitate**

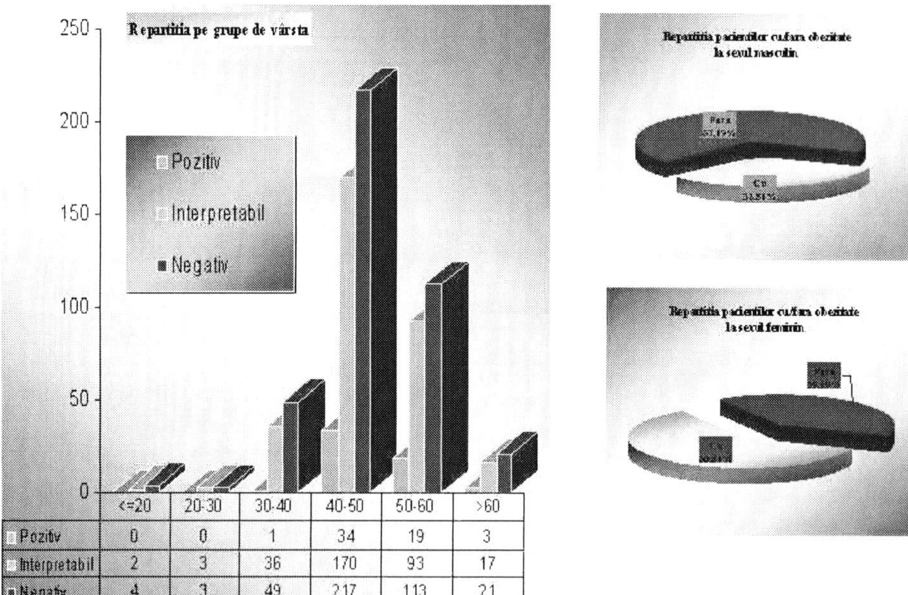


| | <=20 | 20-30 | 30-40 | 40-50 | 50-60 | >60 |
|---|---|---|---|---|---|---|
| Pozitiv | 0 | 0 | 1 | 34 | 19 | 3 |
| Interpretabil | 2 | 3 | 36 | 170 | 93 | 17 |
| Negativ | 4 | 3 | 49 | 217 | 113 | 21 |

**Fig. 8.** The distribution of the effort test results for a selected risk factor

**Repartiția /număr factori de risc**

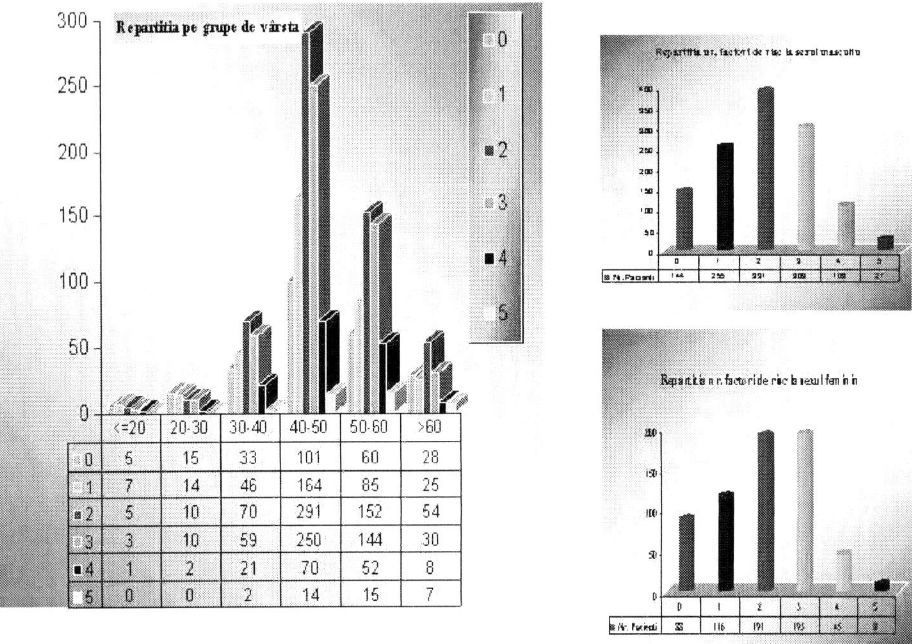


**Fig. 9.** The distribution of the effort test results for a number of risk factors

## 6. Conclusion and Future Work

We propose adopting the concept of data warehousing technology, including a Virtual Intranet, to ensure the confidentiality of patients' data, provided by various healthcare structures at regional levels.

The main features of the Virtual Intranet are: enabling secure cooperation between the project partners by ensuring the security of their respective data pieces and access to data warehouses for each partner according to specific project protocols. Each organization can use the Virtual Intranet structure to offer access to some of its data to other partners, in which case the Virtual Intranet enables Extranet services.

The creation of a website serves as a guide to:

- the exercises for cardiovascular diseases recovery,
- the hypocaloric and/or hypolipidic diet,
- the attitude to various symptoms.

**Acknowledgments.** We would like to thank the physicians of the Cardiology Department of the University Hospital of Sibiu who implemented the computer application, and we would especially like to acknowledge the help of Professor Ligia Blag, professor in the Recovery Center.

## References


[1] Yigang Xu, Ludovic D'Alessio, Marie-Christine Jaulent, Dominique Sauquest, Stephane Spahni, Patrice Degoulet, *Integrating Medical Applications in an Open Architecture Through Generic and Reusable Components*, Medinfo 2001, London

[2] El Mostafa Kerkri, Catherine Quantin, Thierry Grison, Francois André Allaert, Anne Tchounikine, Kokou Yétongnon, *A Virtual Intranet and Data/warehousing for Healthcare Co-operation*, Medinfo 2001, London

[3] Tatjiana Welzer, Izidor Golob, Marjan Druzovec, Smiljana Slavec, Boštjan Brumen, Iztok Takac, *Data Quality in Clinical Information Systems*, The Second International ICSC Symposium , pp: 261-264

[4] Ralf Kauert, Thoralf Topel, Uwe Scholz, Ralf Hofestadt, Information System for the Support of Research, Diagnosis and Therapy of Inborn Metabolic Diseases, Medinfo 2001, London, pp:353-356

[5] Manițiu, I., Bera L., *Progrese în recuperarea secundară a bolilor cardiovasculare*, Ed. Universitatea "Lucian Blaga", Sibiu, 1997

[6] Liana Bera, Fiabilitatea informației în explorări funcționale cardiologice, PhD., Sibiu, Romania, 2001

[7] Manițiu I., Blaga L., Bera L., Bălan C., Moldovan M., Băcilă E., Crișu M, Cojan R, Draia M., Icușcă G., Moga V.V., Moga Rodica., Lazăr D *Rezultatele programelor de recuperare a bolilor cardiovasculare în Centrul de Recuperare cardiologie Sibiu*, A IX-a Conferință Națională a Secției de Cardiologie Preventivă și Recuperare, Iași, 200

[8] Williams, P.A.H., Maj, S.P., Shaw D. *Does Your Doctor Supprot Your Use of the Internet as a Decision Support System?- An Australian Perspective*, International NAISO Congress on Information Science Innovations (ISI'2001)

*Transformation of Health Care with Information Technologies*
*M. Duplaga et al. (Eds.)*
*IOS Press, 2004*


# Diagnosis and Improvement of Oral Development of Polish Children with an Impaired Hearing System

Jolanta ZIELIŃSKA
*Academy of Pedagogy, Kraków, Poland*
*e-mail: jzielin@wsp.krakow.pl*

**Abstract.** The experimental research presented in this paper concerning the evaluation and the development of oral abilities of Polish children with impaired hearing systems has been conducted with the use of two digital modules: the PCLX Laryngograph Processor and Nosality, connected to a PC computer. The aim of the research was the assessment, evaluation and determining positive changes in the level of oral development of Polish children with impaired hearing systems. The obtained results and following practical conclusions can serve as guidelines in clinical and logopedical applications in voice rehabilitation and communication development of groups of non-hearing children whose native language is not necessarily Polish.

**Keywords:** impaired hearing system, oral ability, communication development rehabilitation

## 1. Research Background

The basic task facing a child with an impaired hearing system is to acquire the ability of oral language communication in order to better communicate with the hearing environment. Existing hearing impairments largely limit the child's possibilities. Early revalidation activities, ensuring the child's contact with oral speech in its critical period, namely in the first years of its life, seem to be the most fundamental. If hearing problems appear before year 6-8 of the child's life, then language abilities which are not properly strengthened, will decline (T. Gałkowski, 1993). At present, activities aiming at the development of a language system which enables a non-hearing child to communicate with the hearing population are largely aided by rapid developments in computer technology. Its use in diagnostics and rehabilitation of the voice of a child who has problems with achieving proper phonic speech substance covers both computer software and specialized equipment (B. Siemieniecki, 1996). This development is being stimulated by significant didactic-educational results, that have been obtained thus far. Computers are used comprehensively in this field, enabling the withdrawal of development disorders, development of intellectual abilities, assistance for individual development and acquaintance with new learning and rehabilitation tools. The experimental research presented in this paper concerning the evaluation and development of oral abilities of Polish children with impaired hearing systems has been conducted with the use of two computer attachments: the PCLX Laryngograph Processor and Nosality, connected to a PC computer. This kind of computer research is the first and unique in its scope. It fully accounts for the specific character of the Polish language, including the large number of difficult to articulate dental phonemes, digraphs and prosodic features of speech, mainly the flow of the melodic waveform, which largely influences the understanding of speech in Slavonic languages (B. Wierzchowska,

1967). Hence, the research results can be applied not only to diagnosis and rehabilitation of children with oral problems, for whom the verbal language is often not a natural language (K. Krakowiak, 1998), i.e. those children who cannot hear, but also for those, who have cleft palates or other defects. They can also help teach Polish to foreign students.

## 2. Aim of the Research

The aim of the research was the assessment, evaluation and inducing positive changes in the level of oral development of Polish children with impaired reception hearing systems attending grades 1-6 of special elementary schools (aged 7-13), but it also included younger (6 year-olds) and older (14-15 years) children. Individual cases of transmission deafness were also considered. The research was based on the possibilities of applying multimedia computer technology to the evaluation of speech events through the use of a computer-operated research post in the diagnosis and rehabilitation of children's voices. The post was based on two PC computer attachments: Laryngograph and Nosality (E. Abberton, 1998), which monitored the work of the voice route as a speaking-breathing organ. The following research problems have been stated:

1. What is the oral level of Polish children with impaired hearing systems and which representative criteria should be adopted?
2. What is the sound expression level in the examined groups of children?
3. What difficulties related to oral development do children with impaired hearing systems face; how can their voice and speech be characterized?
4. In what way and to what extent can computer technology aid the oral development of non-hearing children?
5. Which factors influence the effectiveness of computer-aided work on the voice quality of a child with an impaired hearing system?
6. Which basic features of the Polish language make its proper articulation, including oral expression, difficult to achieve, and how to exercise them?

## 3. Methods and Procedures of the Research

The research was conducted using a pedagogical experiment method, following all the necessary procedures. A multimedia research post, enabling computer presentation and evaluation of basic speech event parameters for communication processes has been specially designed for this purpose.

### *3.1 Characteristics of the Computer-Operated Research Post*

The computer-operated research post was created by connecting the two aforementioned digital modules to a computer. The first one, Laryngograph, is based on electro-glottography. Two electrodes are placed on both sides of the throat at the larynx level. The electrical impendence between them is the function of their mutual location, which changes during larynx vibrations. It is smaller when vocal folds are close and larger when they are separated. The voltage on the speaker's neck is about 20MW (at a 1 MHz frequency). The upper frequency limit is ca. 5 kHz. In the case of a typical male voice, the signal-to-noise ratio is ca 40 dB. In the case of small children and babies the relative noise is more significant, although satisfactory results can be obtained even for newborn babies. The computer screen shows vibrations of vocal folds (waveform Lx in Figure 1) and the basic frequency of this process (waveform Fx in Figure 1).

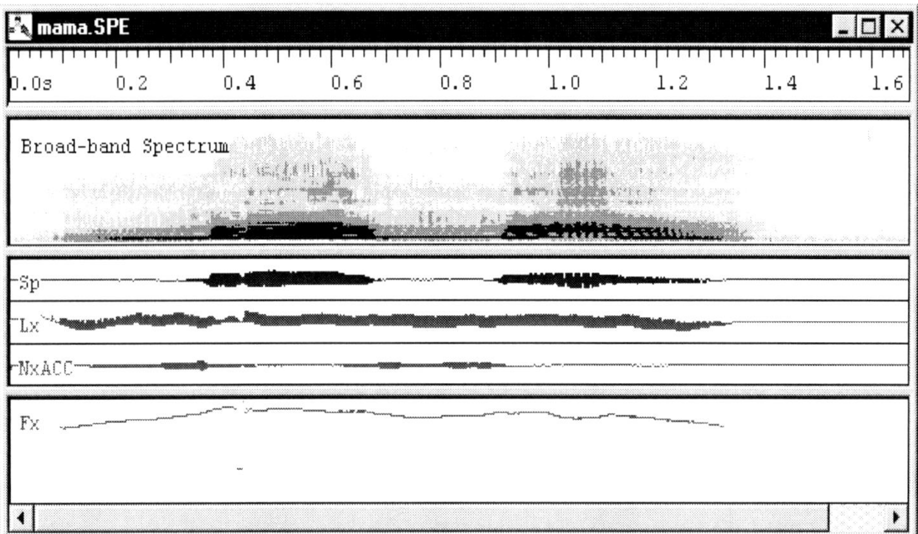


**Fig. 1.** Computer presentation of the signal 'mama'

The measuring results depend not only on vocal fold movements but also on larynx size and vibrating muscles. Thus, the whole phonic structure is evaluated. A separate part of the Laryngograph, namely a microphone, provides the signal which shows changes in the acoustic wave over time (lines Sp in Fig. 1) on the computer screen. These are oscillograms from which, through the analysis of visible changes of the vocal wave amplitude in time, its basic acoustic properties, including sound and nasality can be derived. However, this method of presentation, does not provide full information about the proper articulation of nasal phonemes by the examined person, the possible nasality process and its character, as well as the dynamics of air flow through the nose channel, which influences the quality, including the colour of the voice. All these possibilities are offered by the computer attachment called Nosality, which is a second part of the research post equipment. An electrode placed on the nostrils is its inlet. The waveform generated by this electrode and displayed on the computer screen shows the dynamics of air flow through the nose of the examined person, by measuring nostril vibrations through an accelerator, which measures changes of speed in time, i.e. the acceleration of nostril movements (lines NxACC in Fig. 1). Figure 1 shows a computer presentation made by a therapist working with a child under examination. The first waveform is a dynamic spectrograph called the sonograph, which is a broadband spectrum, used for acoustic evaluation of normal and pathological phonation, which is one of the speech parameters in the segment plane, including the voiced/voiceless differentiation. The picture shows frequency changes in time, and, through the level of darkening, the level (amplitude) of the signal. The amplitude maximum can be seen as visible, darkened stripes. The lowest stripe corresponds to the basic frequency Fx; subsequent stripes correspond to the respective resonance frequencies in the voice channel. Precise maximum amplitude values can be specified by creating a two-dimensional amplitude-frequency spectrum, and the PCLX Laryngograph software has these capabilities. Maximum values, visible on the computer screen are called formants. Their frequency and amplitude characterize a phoneme and are closely related to the articulator configuration that has appeared during its creation. Figure 2 is a deliberately transformed picture for fuller analysis of oral efficiency.

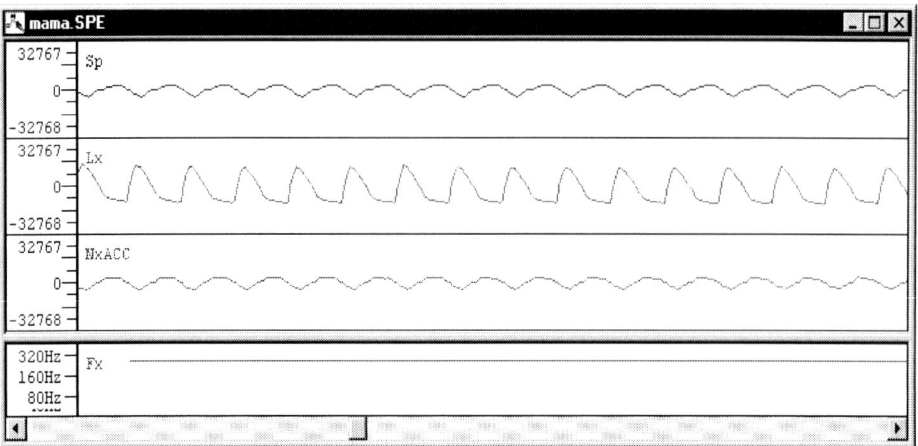


**Fig. 2.** Computer presentation of the signal 'mama', enabling the evaluation of the child's oral efficiency

The initial signal of the laryngograph Lx (the second waveform in Fig. 2) reflects the work of vocal folds and is the base for determination of basic frequency Fx (waveform in Figure 2). Analysis of the signal cycle Lx helps separate its three phases. The first phase is a quick signal growth, corresponding to the quick closing of the vocal folds. The second phase corresponds to the slightly slower signal fall and is connected with their opening. The third phase, which is a flat waveform, correspond to the state, when the vocal folds are open. Frequency Fx is calculated while measuring each work cycle length in the middle of the Lx signal amplitude value (in practice, the measurement of time intervals between transitions of the signal through that level is conducted). The sought Fx value is the reverse of the Lx signal cycle length. The shape of the Lx signal provides information about any abnormality of vocal route action, especially the work of vocal folds. Signal Sp (the first waveform in Figure 2), which is obtained from the microphone inlet, enables a dynamic visualization of signal timing, an evaluation of its volume, loudness and exercising dentalized phonemes, i.e. pairs s – sz, z – rz, which are very often misused and mistaken by children having oral problems, including lisping. The analysis of signal Fx gives information about all parts of the proper signal, which are easily evaluated even by a child. They are: proper dynamic breathing, economical breathing, work of vocal chords, proper articulation, prosodic features, such as pace, rhythm, accent or melody, i.e. these elements, which decide about signal expression and, additionally show the level of phoneme voicing (no voicing – no picture). Signal NxACC (third waveform in Fig. 2) enables to determine proper nasal phones production, including the work of glottis. Such analysis of voice parameters enables drawing many practical diagnostic-therapeutic conclusions.

### *3.2 Pedagogical Experiment Method*

The 6-month research covered 88 children from a special elementary school in Krakow. They experienced either serious (70-90 dB, 23 % of the group) or deep (above 90 dB, 77% of the group) reception hearing impairments. The pedagogical experiment method of parallel groups was applied. During research, the following research tools were used: a research chart of the child's voice using words and sentences and a questionnaire, interviewing psychologists and teachers. Group equivalence was checked by comparing selected features of children's voices, such as dynamic breathing, work of vocal cords, nasality, voice pitch, articulation and prosodic features. Accompanying variables which could influence voice rehabilitation progress were also taken into consideration when evaluating the equivalence. These were: pace of learning, operational memory capacity, a constant characterizing the process of forgetting, intellect, sight-movement coordination, age, time and level of hearing loss, family conditions, notes at school, method of communication while using oral speech and the way revalidation had taken place. Calculated mean values, variants, mean tests t and variant F, and validity coefficients for the variables mentioned above have shown statistically unimportant differences between the groups. The evaluation of group selection equivalence in relation to selected features of children's voice quality in categories 0, 1, i.e. proper/improper, is shown in table 1. Only articulation was evaluated as a percentage of properly-articulated language material, being a quantity variable.

**Table 1.** Evaluation of the equivalence of experimental and control groups (for selected features of voice quality).

| Group | Experimental | Control |
|---|---|---|
| Dynamic breathing | 0,13 | 0,18 |
| Work of vocal cords | 0,49 | 0,50 |
| Nasality | 0,50 | 0,49 |
| Voice pitch | 0,21 | 0,26 |
| Articulation | 1,67 | 1,48 |
| Prosodic features | 0,03 | 0,05 |

The global statistic mean calculated for those variables was 3.03 for the experimental group and 2.96 for the control group. Statistically unimportant differences of the calculated total means pointed at the equivalence of the examined groups in relation to voice quality as well. Pretest, actual, post and distance research tests were also conducted. The language material for rehabilitation exercises held as part of actual research was chosen on the basis of practical, phonetic, audio and communication criteria. The selected material was characteristic for the Polish language mainly in phonetic terms, since it comprised an adequate amount of dentalized or nasal phones as well as diphthongs. Forms of control were connected with the research tools mentioned earlier, child's observation sheets during actual research and computer diagnostic-rehabilitation equipment. Both the samples of speech of hearing children of equivalent age and all the speech of the non-hearing children covered by the pedagogical experiment were stored in computer memory.

### *3.3 Procedures of Actual Research*

Actual research covered voice rehabilitation of children with impaired hearing systems from the experimental group. It lasted six months. A multimedia research post was used for that purpose. Meetings with children took place regularly twice a week and lasted 30 minutes each. The exercises were divided into breathing, phonation, articulation, prosodic, removing nasality, voice complex and self-improvement of the child's pronunciation. The exercises were chosen to suit each individual child's voice needs, depending on earlier diagnosis and were aimed at achieving the proper ortophonic form of speech. Breathing exercises were very important and thus they were conducted in parallel. Computer presentations were selected for each type of the exercises in a way which would be characteristic of the exercise's aims, understood by the revalidated child and, at the same time, easy to interpret for the therapist. The efficiency of the assumed therapeutic procedure depended mostly on the language material, selected for the exercises. Those included: logotomes, onomatopoeias, two- and multi-syllabic words and sentences, including affirmatives, questions and ejaculations, which show speech expressiveness. At the beginning, the material contained mostly vowels, successively linked with nasal consonants such as 'm' or 'n'. This helped achieve and maintain proper voice pitch. In the end, 'r' as well as dentalized and nasal labial phones were introduced. Self-improvement of the child's speech exercises was achieved through language entities and the PC Pitch Target computer. Two identical windows were shown on the computer screen. One showed the model speech of a hearing child of the same age as the examined one, the other one showed the real speech of the child with impaired hearing. Computer logs of the results and notes about the child's behaviour were included in each child's observation sheet by the therapist.

## 4. Results of the Research

During the pretest, oral ability in selected categories for all the subjects with impaired hearing was evaluated (Table 1). The results of this pretest are shown in Table 2.

**Table 2.** Percentage results of the pretest analysing oral ability of children with impaired hearing, n = 88

| Category | Evaluation | | |
|---|---|---|---|
| | Proper | Partially proper | Improper |
| Breathing | 13% | 11% | 76% |
| Work of vocal cords | 16% | 7% | 77% |
| Phonation | 24% | 3% | 73% |
| Prosodic features | 1% | 2% | 97% |
| Nasality | proper | 5% | |
| | closed | 42% | |
| | mixed | 46% | |
| | open | 2% | |
| | No evaluation | 5% | |
| Articulation | (75%, 100%> | 5% | |
| | (50%, 75%> | 23% | |
| | (25%), 50%> | 26% | |
| | (0%, 25%> | 41% | |
| | No evaluation | 5% | |

As the data in table 2 shows, similar results of the pretest evaluation of oral ability were obtained in the following categories: dynamic breathing, work of vocal cords and phonation. Around 70% of the children showed abnormalities in these categories. Prosodic feature testing gave the worst results. Only ca. 1% of the children showed proper prosodic features. Ca. 5% of the children obtained proper results for nasality and articulation. It should be stressed here that only 2% of the children showed open nasality. Mixed or closed nasality appeared in the remaining group in more or less equal proportions (ca 45%). 5% of the children did not make any articulated voice, therefore evaluation was impossible. The research enabled some conclusions about the features of non-hearing children's voices, which will be referred to later. According to the research procedure of the pedagogical experiment, experimental and control groups were selected on the basis of pretest results. Subsequently, only in the experimental group the specially-designed therapeutic procedure was used. The procedure improved the voice route which was treated as a breathing-phonation organ of the rehabilitated children The results of both pretests and posttests which make the evaluation of the effectiveness of activities possible, are shown in Table 3.

**Table 3.** The effectiveness of the diagnostic-therapeutic procedure, testing increases in practice. Experimental group pretest and posttest, n = 44.

| | Increase mean d | Standard deviation $S_d$ | Student's test t | Level of confidence | Number of increases | Test $\chi^2$ | Level of confidence p |
|---|---|---|---|---|---|---|---|
| Total | 2,727 | 2,003 | 8,93 | 0,001 | 26 | | |
| Articulation | 4,05 | 2,33 | 11,40 | 0,001 | 20 | | |
| Breathing | | | | | 14 | 9,624 | $<0,01$ |
| Work of vocal cords | | | | | 26 | 30,788 | $<0,001$ |
| Nasality | | | | | 16 | 16,56 | $<0,01$ |
| Phonation | | | | | 26 | 31,31 | $<0,001$ |
| Prosodic features | | | | | 17 | 19,398 | $<0,01$ |

Statistic research showed that practice increased in all categories of the children's oral ability and the adopted diagnostic-therapeutic procedure proved very successful. The retention of practice in time was specified on the base of distance test results, conducted three months after the actual tests. The comparison of post- and distance tests results are shown in Table 4.

**Table 4.** Posttest (% of the subjects who made progress in the evaluated oral category in relation to the pretest research) and distance test (% of the subjects who suffered regression compared to the posttest research) results. Experimental group, n = 44.

| Research | | Posttest | Distance |
|---|---|---|---|
| Breathing | | 31.8% | 7.1% |
| Work of vocal cords | | 59.1% | 11.5% |
| Phonation | | 59.1% | 34.9% |
| Nasality | | 36.4% | 12.5% |
| Articulation | | 45.5% | 35.0% |
| Prosodic features | Accent | 4.5% | 5.9% |
| | Rhythm | 34.1% | |

Distance tests showed that a visible regression took place only in two categories of oral ability evaluation, namely in phonation and articulation. The regression was about 35% and meant the comeback of the observed abnormalities from the period before the actual tests. In the remaining categories, the drop was relatively small and ranged from 6 to 10%. Such behaviour could result from the fact that those categories which showed regression were typically trainable and habitual. Hence, the children returned to their earlier habits. The remaining categories were more physiological and their therapy, considering difficulties resulting from the specifics of the Polish language, followed the muscular-aerodynamic theory of voice formation. Therefore changes in those areas lasted longer.

## 5. Conclusions

Computer analysis of selected children's speech samples with significant or deep impairment of hearing proved that the majority show symptoms characteristic of hyperfunctional dysphonia with mixed or closed nasality. Nasality is functional and is caused by the improper work of the soft palate and glottis. The tests showed improper, mostly collar bone-rib breathing channels and harsh voice (too low or to high, generally with lessened sonority). Additionally, the following phenomena were observed: shorter phonation time, disturbed prosodic features and voice tone with nasality features.

The tests and following statistical conclusions showed very high efficiency of the diagnostic-rehabilitation method suggested here. The comparison of all the progress (number of people who improved) of the experimental and control groups in a general category, i.e. with no improvement, is shown in Table 5.

**Table 5.** The comparison of all the progress of the experimental and control groups as an evaluation of method effectiveness

| Group | Experimental | Control |
|---|---|---|
| Increase mean d | 2,727 | 0,624 |
| Standard deviation $S_d$ | 2,003 | 0,74 |
| Student test t | 6,554 | |
| Level of confidence p | 0,001 | |

The tests of the oral ability of children with significant or deep hearing impairment enabled us to specify the pathology of changes characteristic for this group in some selected evaluation categories, and they also provided preliminary possibilities for removing them on the basis of voice breathing rehabilitation connected with the release of larynx muscle tonus and the work of soft palate muscles and glottis. The fact that the research was made on a statistically valid group of children makes it possible to generalize the presented conclusions and compare them with clinical tests performed in this area (A. Obrębowski, 1992). The analysis of the efficiency of the diagnostic-therapeutic procedure (data shown in Table 4 as posttest results) showed that the therapy aiming at achieving proper dynamic breathing is connected with the work on nasality and prosodic features of speech, while the work of vocal cords is connected with proper voice pitch. The research gave unique, physiological results. Dynamic breathing, the work of vocal cords, voice pitch, and dynamic breathing with nasality behave according to the rules of mathematical implication, which was confirmed by practical tests on a statistically valid group of children. For example, if dynamic breathing is proper, then the work of vocal cords must be proper, too, whereas improper breathing does not have to cause improper work of vocal cords. Many diagnostically practical conclusions, useful for the planning of the rehabilitation process, can thus be formed.

Other statistic conclusions from the tests, shown in Table 6, specify the influence of the assumed accompanying variables on the efficiency of the therapeutic process by testing their impact on the increase of practice in general. It can be assumed that they play a very important role during the child's work with the computer, aiming at the achievement of the correct phonic speech substance. Other accompanying variables mentioned earlier did not exercise any influence on rehabilitation procedures.

**Table 6.** The efficiency of the therapeutic process vs accompanying variables (increase of practice in general).

| Accompanying variables | Mean value x | Standard deviation S | Pearson's correlation coefficient r | Level of confidence P |
|---|---|---|---|---|
| Capacity of operation memory | 0,447 | 0,174 | 0,196 | n.i. |
| Pace of learning | 0,537 | 0,203 | 0,620 | <0,01 |
| Forgetting constant | 0,0897 | 0,214 | 0,423 | <0,01 |
| Motivation | 0,705 | 0,456 | 0,259 | <0,1 |
| Intellect | 0,818 | 0,386 | 0,406 | <0,01 |
| Sight-movement coordination | 0,705 | 0,456 | 0,434 | <0,01 |
| Social environment | 0,413 | 0,212 | 0,314 | <0,05 |

As the data in Table 6 shows, a statistically-important influence on improving the efficiency of voice quality in children with impaired hearing (with the use of computer) is exerted by the pace of learning, the forgetting constant, intellect and sight-movement coordination. The influence of the family environment was smaller (though still statistically important); motivation was not statistically important. The capacity of operation memory played a statistically unimportant role in the process. It should be stressed here that there was no influence on the therapeutic activities of the child's age, the course of previous rehabilitation, earlier preferences of oral speech in the communication process, time and level of hearing loss and notes at school. The contribution of the pace of learning and the forgetting constant, characterizing the time during which a child keeps information in memory, was obvious in the discussed progress, since they characterize the child's mental speed, i.e. formal properties of information processing. The lack of such influence from operational memory seems surprising, but it could result form connecting computer work on voice quality to repeated exercises imposed by the researcher. Therefore, the subjects based their improvement strategy not on memory scope but on methods of accelerating the learning curve. The influence of other variables, i.e. intellect seen as mental power with its own contribution to the learning process, and sight-movement coordination, which is connected to perception, seems to be obvious. Disorders of coordination are usually related to disorders of perception and movement, e.g. during speaking. Teaching correct speech phonic substance using the multimedia research post during the experiment involved a perception-motor character, so the motor level influenced the level of learning. It can be stated then, that if the coordination disorder is deep, work on oral efficiency using a computer will not be possible. When interpreting statistical results one should consider justification of the weak influence of the social environment on the obtained therapeutic results. The same procedure should be applied to justify the even weaker influence of motivation. This is due to the fact that they were specified by the school pedagogues and Polish language teachers, and not, like the other variables, with the use of special tests by the researcher, which would make them more objective. It was difficult to contact the children's homes because they attended a boarding school, and motivation referred only to their general inclination to undertake the effort connected with learning, which was largely disturbed in the non-hearing children.

The experimental research tests filled the methodology and application gap in the process of using computer technology for diagnosis and development of oral efficiency of Polish children with impaired hearing systems. Their results and following practical conclusions can serve as guidelines in clinical and logopedical applications in voice rehabilitation and communication development of groups of non-hearing children whose native language is not necessarily Polish. At the same time, they also provide some directions on how to effectively use a computer in teaching Polish to foreigners, since such students often have similar difficulties in learning correct oral speech as the children who cannot fully control speech using hearing.

## References


[1] Abberton E., Fourcin A., 1971, First application of a new Laryngograph, Medical and Biological Illustration 21, 123-134.

[2] Abberton E., Howard D., Fourcin A., 1989, Latyngographic assessment of normal voice: a tutorial, Clinical Linguistic and Fonetics 3, 243-259.

[3] Basztura Cz., 1988, Źródła, sygnały i obrazy akustyczne (Warszawam, PWN).

[4] Carlson E., Miller D., 1998, Aspects of voice quality: display, measurement and therapy, International Journal of Language and Communication Disorders 33, 304-309.

[5] Grzanka At., Hatzopoulos S., 1998, Przegląd metod czasowo-częstotliwościowych w odniesieniu do analiz sygnałów otoemisji akustycznych, Biuletyn Audiofonologia, t. XIII, 41-53.

[6] Higgins M.B., Comey A.E., Schulte L., 1994, Physiological assessment of speech and voice production of adults with hearing loss, J. Speech Hea. Res. 37, 510-521.

[7] Jassem W., 1973, Podstawy fonetyki akustycznej (Warszawa, PWN).

[8] Jassem W., 1974, Mowa a nauka o łączności (Warszawa, PWN).

[9] Kuniszyk-Jóżkowiak W., 1996, Akustyczna analiza i stymulacja płynności mówienia (Lublin, WN UMCS).

[10] Kusznik – Jóżkowiak W., Suszyński W., Warchoł J., 1998, Spektrograficzna analiza niepłynności mowy, Logopedia 25, 37-47.

[11] Maniecka-Aleksandrowicz B., Kołodziej A., Szkiełkowska A., 1998, Zastosowanie systemów analizy dźwięku w badaniu głosu, (in) Zaburzenia głosu-badanie-diagnozowanie-metody usprawnianie, (ed.) Mierzejewska H., Przybysz-Piwkowa M. (Warszawa, Wyd. DIG).

[12] Maniecka-Aleksandrowicz B., Szkiełkowska A., 1998, Zaburzenia głosu irehabilitacja osób z uszkodzonym narządem słuchu, (in) Zaburzenia głosu-badanie-diagnozowanie-metody usprawnianie, (ed.) Mierzejewska H., Przybysz-Piwkowa M. (Warszawa, Wyd. DIG).

[13] Moczadłowski T., Grzanka A., Pawłowski Z., 1998, Przegląd metod wizualizacji drgań fałdów głosowych, Biuletyn Adiofonologia XIII, 305-319.

[14] Moczko J., Kramer L., 2001, Cyfrowe metody przetwarzania sygnałów biomedycznych (Poznań, WN UAM).

[15] Pruszewicz A., 1992, Foniatria kliniczna (Warszawa, PZWL).

[16] Szkiełkowska A., Ratyńska J., Grzanka A., Markowska R., Ocena krtani i głosu dziecka niesłyszącego, Biuletyn Audiofonologia XVIII, 161-168.

[17] Szuchnik J., Słodownik-Rycaj E., 2000, Wykorzystanie „Onomatopei" w terapii pacjentów implantowanych, Biuletyn Audiofonologia, XVIII, 49-56.

[18] Tadeusiewicz R., 1988, Sygnał mowy, (Warszawa, Wyd K i Ł).

[19] Zielińska J., 2001, Ocena skuteczności zastosowania laryngograficzno-komputerowej metody wizualizacji sygnału mowy w rozwoju oralnym dzieci z wadą słuch, (in) Komunikacja – mowa – język w diagnozie i terapii zaburzeń rozwoju u dzieci i młodzieży niepełnosprawnej, (ed.). Minczakiewicz E.M. (Kraków; WN AP).

[20] Zielińska J., Kulinowski W., Zagólski O., 2000, The use of laryngograph in assessing phonatory disfunctions of the larynx, Journal of Medical Informatics and Technolgies, 5, 111-120.

[21] Zielińska J., Kulinowski W., Zagólski O., Składzień J., 2001, The role % irregularity in electroglottographic assessment of laryngeal phonatory function in patients with vocal fold paresis-preliminary report, Journal of Medical Informatics and Technologies 2, 33-39.

[22] Zielińska J., Lisiecka-Bielanowicz M., 2000, Efficacy of physiotherapy of breathing in children using cochlear implants. Pilot study, European Congress of Oto-Rhono-Laryngology Head and Neck Surgery, Berlin, 125-129.

[23] Van Lierede K., Moerman M., Cauwenberge P., 1996, Comment on the results of voice analysis, Acta Otorhinolaryngol. Belg. 50, 349-354.

*Transformation of Health Care with Information Technologies*
*M. Duplaga et al. (Eds.)*
*IOS Press, 2004*



# Artificial Neural Network in Pharmacoeconomics

Sebastian POLAK[1], Agnieszka SKOWRON[1], Aleksander MENDYK[2], Jerzy BRANDYS[1]
[1]*Department of Pharmacoepidemiology and Pharmacoeconomics,*
*Faculty of Pharmacy, Collegium Medicum, Jagiellonian University,*
*Medyczna 9 Str., 30-688 Kraków*
*e-mail: {mfpolak, mfskowro}@cyf-kr.edu.pl*
[2]*Department of Pharmaceutical Technology and Biopharmaceutics,*
*Faculty of Pharmacy, Collegium Medicum, Jagiellonian University,*
*Medyczna 9 Str., 30-688 Kraków*
*e-mail: mfmendyk@cyf-kr.edu.pl*

**Abstract.** Pharmacoeconomics research identifies, measures, and compares the costs (resources consumed) and consequences of medical products and services, where at least one of the compared alternatives is pharmacotherapy. Pharmacoeconomics has been designed to enable the decisionmaker to identify the preferred choice among existing alternatives. The decisions are often important for the patients' lives on the one hand, and for payers on the other (where the payer is understood as the institution responsible for financial resources allocation).

One of the most commonly used types of pharmacoeconomic analysis is cost-effectiveness analysis. Two different alternatives can be compared using cost-effectiveness analysis if only their medical and clinical consequences could be measured in similar units (clinical or physical parameters).

The aim of the project is to use an artificial neural network (ANN) for medical effect prediction, which could help in the extrapolation of pharmaco-economic analysis' results. To depict neural data analysis tools, a database containing 100 non-small cell lung cancer (NSCLC) patients in non-operative IIIB and IV stage has been used. Each patient was described using 30 factors (i.e. sex, age, anticancer drugs dosage) and, as an output value, the expected survival time was established. The role of the ANN system was to predict the patient's survival time based on the above mentioned information. Binary values were tested as outcomes. Positive values (coded as 1) meant that patient survival time would be equal to or longer than 35 weeks. Negative values (coded as 0) meant that the patient survival time would be shorter than 35 weeks. Binary values were obtained using a threshold, which based on the mean survival time of patients derived from literature. Back-propagation as well as fuzzy-logic neural networks were applied. A 10-fold cross validation method was used to obtain the appropriate models. Final results were compared with the generic, logistic regression-based model. The best prediction score of the ANN model was 82%; higher than logistic regression prediction rate.

## Introduction

Epidemiological analysis shows that life expectancy is growing [1]. This is of course one of the major goals of healthcare. Nevertheless, results of prolonging life are not all beneficial, since this means that communities are getting older. Changes in the communities' demographic structure result in new public funds allocation structures. This means that nowadays a large amount of financial resources is devoted to health care (i.e. drugs). That's why economic analysis of medical results and comparisons between effects and costs are becoming more and more important.

## 1. Pharmacoeconomics

The economic evaluation of health-related procedures is gaining interest and it is also becoming more necessary to conduct. The cost-effectiveness of healthcare procedures is often considered in the decision making process, especially as relates to reimbursement and pricing decisions [2]. Pharmacoeconomics is the description and analysis of the cost of drug therapy to the healthcare system and society [3]. Pharmacoeconomic research identifies, measures and compares the cost and consequences of pharmaceutical products and services. Thus, pharmacoeconomic analysis can only identify all relevant costs of therapeutic and diagnostic process in cost-of-illness studies or compare two or more alternative therapeutic procedure as a cost-minimization, cost-effectiveness, cost-utility or cost-benefit analysis. All costs in comparative analysis are assessed in monetary units (dollars, euro etc..) and the factor which distinguishes the type of analysis is the key for effect measurement.

**Cost-minimization analysis** can be used if the outcomes of comparable alternatives are exactly the same. If the procedures impact the quality of life, **cost-utility analysis** should be carried out instead. The most useful type of analysis for decisionmakers is the **cost-benefit analysis**, which allows one to compare different procedures if their effects can be expressed in monetary units [3].

The most frequently used type of comparative pharmacoeconomic analysis is cost-effectiveness analysis [3]. It can be performed if only the effects of alternative approaches can be measured in the same natural unit, for example: the Life Year Saved (LYS), time to remission, etc. The outcome of the analysis is the cost-effectiveness ratio, which means the cost of one unit gained.

Cost-effectiveness analysis is a technique designed to assist the decisionmaker in identifying the preferred choice among possible alternatives. It is a series of analytical and mathematical procedures which aids in the selection of a course of action from various alternative approaches.

## 2. Artificial Neural Networks

Artificial neural networks systems belong to the general category of artificial intelligence [4]. They are defined as non-linear information processing systems designed in a manner similar to biological neural structures, expressed in the structural and the functional composition of ANNs. The structure of ANNs, called the "architecture" is usually organized in layers consisting of units, which are sometimes called "nodes". Nodes are artificial neurons responsible for information processing. Nodes from adjacent layers are usually fully interconnected through so-called "weights", representing synaptic connections between artificial neurons. Such connection-based approach has been proposed to simulate, in a very simple manner, the cognitive functions of biological neural systems.

One of the most important features of ANNs is their ability to detect complicated relationships, basing on empirical data. It is this feature that enables the use of ANNs in pharmacoeconomics, where complicated and indirect relationships are to be identified and processed. The statistical approach is frequently tedious and ineffective due to the unknown a priori model structure. ANNs are capable of creating a model automatically, without any prior knowledge, basing only on empirical data, as stated before [5]. If the learning process is performed correctly, the neural model will be able to extrapolate its knowledge beyond the available database. This feature, called generalization, is the ultimate goal in the neural model preparation. Good generalization ability guarantees the reliability of the neural model, thus enabling potential use of ANNs in the prediction area. Application of well-trained and generalizing neural models in pharmacoeconomics would be considered mainly in scenario predictions. The scenarios might be recognized as consequences of particular therapy strategies, with respect to cost-effectiveness analysis or other pharmacoeconomic factors. The role of the ANN would be to provide answers describing the outcome of a hypothetical therapy. In this way, effect estimation in the cost-effectiveness ratio would be performed. Cost calculation is just an arithmetic operation, thus full cost-effectiveness analysis could be easily performed once the outcome for the hypothetical therapy basing on the ANN model is predicted.

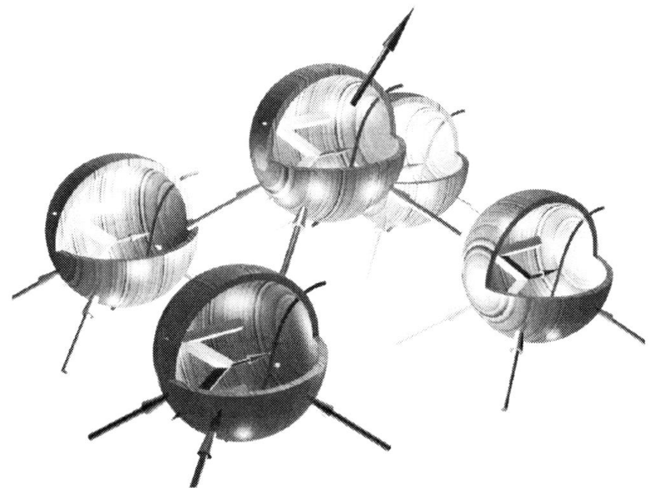

**Fig. 1.** Graphical representation of an artificial neural network

## 3. Aim of the Study

The aim of the project is the development of a tool based on artificial neural networks (ANNs) for medical effect prediction. ANNs have been chosen for this task because of their unique features allowing extrapolation of pharmacoeconomic analysis results.

## 4. Materials and Methods

### *4.1 Data*

A database containing 100 records has been obtained from three Cancer Hospitals in Poland (Gdańsk, Poznań, Warszawa). The information therein was gathered from patient hospital cards.

The inclusion criteria were:

- IIIB or IV (inoperative) stage of Non-Small Cell Lung Cancer (NSCLC)
- full schemes of anticancer therapy (adequate for every drug combination)

Every patient was described using 30 variables, as shown in Table 1:

**Table 1.** Data descriptive statistics

| Nr | Variable | Description | Min | Max | Mean | SD |
|---|---|---|---|---|---|---|
| 1 | SEX | Patient sex | .00 | 1.00 | 0.19 | .39 |
| 2 | AGE | Patient age | 41.00 | 77.00 | 62.09 | 8.98 |
| 3 | NAVELBINE | Summary dose of vinorelbine | .00 | 898.00 | 122.34 | 185.49 |
| 4 | ETOPOSIDE | Summary dose of etoposide | .00 | 4200.00 | 767.00 | 1222.89 |
| 5 | GEMCITABINE | Summary dose of gemcitabine | .00 | 100900.00 | 7182.10 | 14738.9 |
| 6 | CISPLATINE | Summary dose of cis-platine | .00 | 1380.00 | 571.87 | 3 55.54 |
| 7 | CARBOPLATINE | Summary dose of carboplatine | .00 | 3500.00 | 243.50 | 761.20 |
| 8 | ONDANSETRON | Summary dose of ondansetron | .00 | 368.00 | 46.50 | 58.50 |
| 9 | DEXAMETHASON | Summary dose of dexamethazon | .00 | 252.00 | 44.30 | 52.83 |
| 10 | TROPISETRON | Summary dose of tropisetron | .00 | 150.00 | 20.08 | 38.30 |
| 11 | FILGASTRIM300 | Summary dose of filgastrim 300 | .00 | 2400.00 | 39.00 | 251.02 |
| 12 | FILGASTRIM 480 | Summary dose of filgastrim 480 | .00 | 480.00 | 9.62 | 67.54 |
| 13 | METOCLOPRAMIDE | Summary dose of metoclopramid | .00 | 335.00 | 22.86 | 58.13 |
| 14 | AMBULATORY CARE | Total number of ambulatory visits | .00 | 27.00 | 8.72 | 7.17 |
| 15 | HOSPITALIZATION | Total number of hospitaliz. days | .00 | 129.00 | 34.22 | 30.08 |
| 16 | RTG | Total number of RTG | .00 | 13.00 | 3.35 | 2.65 |
| 17 | BONE RTG | Total number of bone RTG | .00 | 5.00 | 0.21 | 0.66 |
| 18 | MORPHOLOGY | Total number of morphology tests | 3.00 | 35.00 | 13.10 | 7.72 |
| 19 | BIOCHEMISTRY | Total number of biochemical tests | 1.00 | 19.00 | 6.38 | 3.00 |
| 20 | COAGULATION | Total number of coagulation tests | .00 | 12.00 | 1.47 | 2.56 |
| 21 | SCINTIGRAPHY | Total number of scintigraphy tests | .00 | 2.00 | .20 | .47 |
| 22 | EKG | Total number of EKG | .00 | 10.00 | 1.29 | 2.13 |
| 23 | TK CHEST | Total number of TK (chest) | .00 | 5.00 | .74 | 1.06 |
| 24 | TK HEAD | Total number of TK (head) | .00 | 2.00 | .23 | .55 |
| 25 | USG | Total number of USG | .00 | 8.00 | 1.22 | 1.82 |
| 26 | URINE | Total number of urine tests | .00 | 7.00 | 1.62 | 2.23 |
| 27 | NMR | Total number of NMR | .00 | 2.00 | .10 | 0.33 |
| 28 | HYDRATION | Total number of hydration | .00 | 18.00 | 4.70 | 3.13 |
| 29 | HOTEL | Total number hospital hotel days | .00 | 52.00 | 3.56 | 10.07 |
| 30 | RADIOTHERAPY | Total number radiotherapy units | .00 | 40.00 | 7.06 | 12.39 |
| Out | SURVIVAL | Patients survival | .00 | 1.00 | .48 | .50 |

Originally, the output value had a continuous character. Basing on the analysis of mean life duration (survival median) the output value in the database was transformed into a binary form. The threshold obtained from scientific, medical literature was set at 35 weeks [6],[7],[8],[9],[10],[11],[12],[13],[14],[15]. A positive output value (coded as 1) meant that patient's survival time was equal to or longer than 35 weeks. A negative value (coded as 0) meant that the patient's survival time was shorter than 35 weeks.

Due to the small number of learning records, a procedure based on adding noise to the learning dataset was applied: "noisy" records were thus introduced, with the amplitude of the noise falling between 5 and 10% for each particular value. ANNs were then trained for 2 million iterations (although other training periods were also applied).

### *4.2 Results Estimation System*

Neural networks were researched to find the optimal architecture. A search was performed among 32 architectures with the use of a 10-fold cross-validation scheme. This meant that the randomly-chosen 90% of the data set was used for training and then the obtained model was tested on the remaining 10% of data. This procedure was repeated ten times but each time different parts of the training data set were excluded. The estimated error rate was the average classification error rate from ten sub-samples. This was the main criterion for optimal model selection. Sensitivity analysis of best neural models was also performed. The influence of every single input (from the whole input vector) on the output value was computed using the algorithm presented in [16]. The receiver-operator curve was computed and the area bounded by it (AUROC) was used as a criterion of model comparison.

### *4.3 Notation of ANNs' Architectures*

Each time when the ANN architecture is described, it is encoded in the same way:

- numbers of nodes in subsequent hidden layers
- activation function

Example: "12_5_tanh" means that the ANN has 12 nodes in the first hidden layer and 5 nodes in the second hidden layer, and that all nodes used hyperbolic tangent as the activation function.

## 5. Results and Discussion

During the ANN architecture search phase, some optimal as well as sub-optimal architectures were identified, as shown in table 2.

**Table 2.** Best results obtained on native dataset

| Nr | ANN architecture | ALL (%) | 1 (%) | 0 (%) |
|---|---|---|---|---|
| 1 | 20_10hid sigma_30in | 82 | 76 | 86 |
| 2 | 10_7hid sigma_30in | 80 | 70 | 86 |
| 3 | 7_5_3hid sigma_30in | 79 | 68 | 86 |
| 4 | 2hid sigma_30in | 79 | 59 | 90 |
| 5 | 15_5hid sigma_30in | 79 | 70 | 84 |
| 6 | 7_5_3hid tanh_30in | 78 | 68 | 84 |
| 7 | 15_5hid fsr_30in | 78 | 70 | 83 |
| 8 | 60_20hid tanh_30in | 76 | 68 | 81 |
| 9 | 60_20hid sigma_30in | 76 | 68 | 81 |
| 10 | 20_10_2hid tanh_30in | 76 | 68 | 81 |

Notation description: All (%) – total classification rate; 1 (%) – classification rate of records with value 1; 0 (%) – classification rate of records with value 0.

The best results obtained for noisy datasets are shown in table 3.

**Table 3.** Best results obtained on noisy datasets (noise type – 2x10%)

| Nr | ANN architecture | ALL (%) | 1 (%) | 0 (%) |
|---|---|---|---|---|
| 1 | 10hid sigma_30in | 79 | 65 | 87 |
| 2 | 20_10hid sigma_30in | 79 | 70 | 84 |
| 3 | 20_18_10hid sigma_30in | 79 | 65 | 87 |
| 4 | 5_3hid sigma_30in | 79 | 70 | 84 |
| 5 | 5_3hid tanh_30in | 79 | 65 | 87 |
| 6 | 7_5_3hid tanh_30in | 79 | 68 | 86 |
| 7 | 10_7hid sigma_30in | 78 | 65 | 86 |
| 8 | 15_5hid sigma_30in | 78 | 68 | 84 |
| 9 | 7_5_3hid sigma_30in | 78 | 65 | 86 |
| 10 | 10_7hid fsr_30in | 77 | 68 | 83 |

Notation description: All (%) – total classification rate; 1 (%) – classification rate of records with value 1; 0 (%) – classification rate of records with value 0.

**Table 4.** Best results obtained on noisy datasets (noise type – 2x10%_500 000 iterations)

| Nr | ANN architecture | ALL (%) | 1 (%) | 0 (%) |
|---|---|---|---|---|
| 1 | 5_3hid tanh_30in | 79 | 68 | 86 |
| 2 | 2hid M-SLIDE_30in | 79 | 65 | 87 |
| 3 | 18_8hid sigma_30in | 79 | 70 | 84 |
| 4 | 18_8hid fsr_30in | 79 | 68 | 86 |
| 5 | 7_5_3hid sigma_30in | 78 | 68 | 84 |
| 6 | 60_20hid sigma_30in | 78 | 70 | 83 |
| 7 | 5_3hid sigma_30in | 78 | 65 | 86 |
| 8 | 2hid fsr_30in | 78 | 59 | 89 |
| 9 | 20_10hid sigma_30in | 78 | 70 | 83 |
| 10 | 20_10_2hid tanh_30in | 78 | 68 | 84 |

Notation description: All (%) – total classification rate; 1 (%) – classification rate of records with value 1; 0 (%) – classification rate of records with value 0.

**Table 5.** Best results obtained on noisy datasets (noise type – 2x5%)

| Nr | ANN architecture | ALL (%) | 1 (%) | 0 (%) |
|---|---|---|---|---|
| 1 | 7_5_3hid tanh_30in | 79 | 68 | 86 |
| 2 | 5_3hid sigma_30in | 79 | 70 | 84 |
| 3 | 20_18_10hid sigma_30in | 79 | 65 | 87 |
| 4 | 20_10hid sigma_30in | 79 | 70 | 84 |
| 5 | 10hid sigma_30in | 79 | 65 | 87 |
| 6 | 5_3hid tanh_30in | 78 | 65 | 86 |
| 7 | 15_5hid sigma_30in | 78 | 68 | 84 |
| 8 | 10_7hid sigma_30in | 78 | 65 | 86 |
| 9 | 7_5_3hid sigma_30in | 77 | 65 | 84 |
| 10 | 60_20hid sigma_30in | 77 | 70 | 81 |

Notation description: All (%) – total classification rate; 1 (%) – classification rate of records with value 1; 0 (%) – classification rate of records with value 0.

**Table 6.** Best results obtained on noisy datasets (noise type – 5x5%)

| Nr | ANN architecture | ALL (%) | 1 (%) | 0 (%) |
|---|---|---|---|---|
| 1 | 20_10hid sigma_30in | 80 | 68 | 87 |
| 2 | 18_8hid sigma_30in | 79 | 70 | 84 |
| 3 | 10_7hid sigma_30in | 79 | 68 | 86 |
| 4 | 7_5_3hid tanh_30in | 78 | 62 | 87 |
| 5 | 20_18_10hid sigma_30in | 78 | 65 | 86 |
| 6 | 2hid fsr_30in | 77 | 70 | 81 |
| 7 | 20_18_10hid tanh_30in | 77 | 65 | 84 |
| 8 | 20_18_10hid fsr_30in | 76 | 65 | 83 |
| 9 | 15_5hid fsr_30in | 76 | 65 | 83 |
| 10 | 10_7hid tanh_30in | 76 | 65 | 83 |

Notation description: All (%) – total classification rate; 1 (%) – classification rate of records with value 1; 0 (%) – classification rate of records with value 0.

## 6. Logistic Regression Comparison

Logistic regression is a classical modeling method applied when a binary outcome is observed. In this study, logistic regression analysis was used to predict survival time on the basis of 30 chosen inputs and all data sets used for ANNs training with a 10-fold cross-validation scheme. The dependent variable and independent variables entered into the analysis were the same as for ANN modeling. The comparison of results between ANNs and logistic regression favors ANNs as more accurate prediction tools (table 7).

**Table 7.** Comparison between best ANN models and logistic regression

| Nr | Data set | Modeling tool | ALL (%) | 1 (%) | 0 (%) | AUROC |
|---|---|---|---|---|---|---|
| 1 | Native | 20_10hid sigma_30in | 82 | 76 | 86 | 0.80 |
| | | Logistic regression | Covariance matrix cannot be computed. | | | |
| 2 | Noised – 2x10% | 10hid sigma_30in | 79 | 65 | 87 | 0.77 |
| | | Logistic regression | 70 | 74 | 63 | 0.75 |
| 3 | Noised – 2x10%_500 000 iter | 5_3hid tanh_30in | 79 | 68 | 86 | 0.77 |
| | | Logistic regression | 73 | 74 | 70 | 0.70 |
| 4 | Noised – 2x5% | 7_5_3hid tanh_30in | 79 | 68 | 86 | 0.77 |
| | | Logistic regression | 70 | 71 | 68 | 0.66 |
| 5 | Noised – 5x5% | 20_10hid sigma_30in | 80 | 68 | 87 | 0.79 |
| | | Logistic regression | 73 | 74 | 70 | 0.70 |

Notation description: All (%) – total classification rate; 1 (%) – classification rate of records with value 1; 0 (%) – classification rate of records with value 0; AUROC – area bounded by receiver-operator curve

## 7. Practical Application of ANNs in Pharmacoeconomics

The next step would be practical application of the best neural models in pharmacoeconomics. Using clinical and cost-related data it is possible to predict the average expected results and calculate strategy costs. The most commonly used pharmacoeconomic factor is the cost-effectiveness ratio (CER).

In NSCLC, the most common chemotherapeutic agent is cis-platin (in navelbine – cis-platine or etoposide – cis-platine scheme), due to its low price. A concurrent anticancer drug is carboplatine, which has significantly better pharmacological characteristic (lesser side effects) but its price is considerably higher. It would be valuable to know whether the use of carboplatine instead of cis-platine is beneficial to such an extent, that it might justify the related pharmacotherapy costs. It is a matter of quantified approach to assess the impact of carboplatine use on the patients' survival time and, as a consequence, to compute the CER for this procedure. However, such an experiment carried out on biological subjects (patients) would be unacceptable from the ethical point of view; therefore one is limited only to data collected from clinical cases. The original dataset was not constructed to prove or falsify the hypothesis concerning the adequacy of carboplatine treatment – rather, this is a result of accidental data acquisition, not a statistically-planned experiment (randomized, controlled trial). The ANN model provides a solution to this dilemma.

The best of the identified neural models (20_10hid sigma – native learning dataset) was used for this task. It was tested to model the effects of replacing cis-platine with carboplatine in particular patients. It is worth mentioning here, that the sensitivity analysis of the ANN model revealed that the most important factor influencing survival time was the amount of cis-platine. Therefore, any change in cis-platine use was suspected to be crucial to the patients' survival time.

The simulation was projected as follows:

1. all cases in the dataset were used to train best ANN architecture,
2. the mean survival time was computed basing on all available data,
3. a test dataset was prepared, where the records describing cases with cis-platine treatment were replaced with information about carboplatine treatment,
4. the test dataset was presented to the ANN model and the mean survival time was computed,
5. both the mean survival times from original and altered data sets were compared to reveal the impact of replacing cis-platine with carboplatine (Fig. 2).

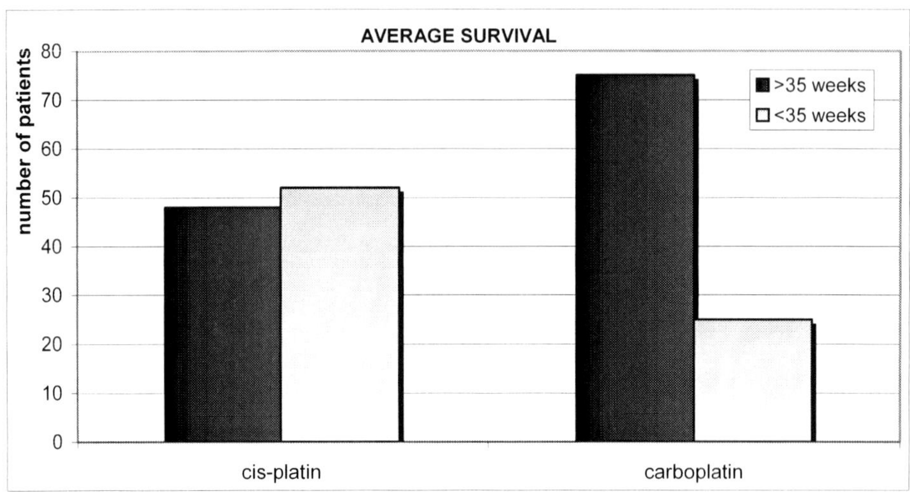


**Fig. 2.** Replacing cis-platine with carboplatine in the entire dataset

The effect understood as the proportion of patients with 35 and more weeks of survival time to patients with less than 35 weeks of survival time is better for the model carboplatine scheme. This conclusion is revealed in Fig. 2, where the bars labeled "cis-platine" represent original data and bars labeled "carboplatine" represent altered test data. Black bars representing survival time in excess 35 weeks are much higher for "carboplatine", which means that more patients have benefited from carboplatine treatment than from cis-platine. The ANN model indicates that carboplatine therapy should have better outcome than cis-platine.

Adding pricing data makes it possible to find the total price and to compute the cost-effectiveness ratio (CER) for every modeled scheme. Thus, the ANN model provides data which can be easily used by policymakers in making therapy-related decisions.

The final algorithm could be constructed as follows:

1. train ANN with data describing therapies *1*, *2*… *n* and their outcomes,
2. test trained ANN on data describing therapies *x*, *y*, *z*, where therapies *x*, *y*, *z* are not in (1…*n*),
3. for each therapy *x*, *y*, *z* collect outcomes predicted by ANN,
4. for each therapy *x*, *y*, *z* collect prices of drugs, medical procedures etc.,
5. for each therapy *x*, *y*, *z* compute CER,
6. basing on appropriate CERs decide on the optimal therapy.

## 8. Conclusions

The superior modeling abilities of ANNs are the key features, which enable their use in creating flexible and reliable tools for pharmacoeconomic analysis. An example of such an analysis proves that the use of ANNs might be considered for testing various scenarios in order to improve therapy decisions and to allocate funding resources optimally, with the greatest benefits for the patients. The application of computer simulations is strongly encouraged for ethical reasons, therefore ANNs emerge as valuable tools aiding healthcare policymakers.

It is necessary to mention here that all results obtained in this study were based on the 100 patients group, therefore a conclusion about the benefits of cis-platine replacement by carboplatine should be considered on a theoretical basis only. In this study we have merely presented a methodology to be used in pharamcoeconomics in order to benefit from the unique features of ANNs; we do not by any means advocate abandoning practical, medical guidance for cancer treatment.

## References

[1] Polish Official Statistics. *http://www.stat.gov.pl/english/index.htm*

[2] Basskin L.E. Performing a pharmacoeconomic analysis of a disease management pathway or guideline. Formulary 38, 2003 pp. 547-551.

[3] Gold R.M. (editor) Cost-Effectiveness in Health and Medicine. Oxford University Press, 1996.

[4] Hertz J., Krogh A., Palmer R.G. Introduction to the Theory of Neural Computation. WNT Warszawa 1995 (in Polish).

[5] Polak S., Mendyk A., Artificial intelligence technology as a tool for initial GDM screening. Expert Systems With Applications. 26/4 (2004) pp. 455-460.

[6] Horvath L. et all. Carboplatin and vinorelbine in untreated locally advanced and metastatic non-small cell lung cancer. Lung Cancer 32, 2001 pp. 173–178.

[7] Katakamia N. et. all. Combination chemotherapy of gemcitabine and vinorelbine for patients in stage IIIB—IV non-small cell lung cancer: a phase II study of the West Japan Thoracic Oncology Group (WJTOG) 9908. Lung Cancer 43, 2004 pp. 93—100.

[8] Laack E. Gemcitabine and vinorelbine as first-line chemotherapy for advanced non-small cell lung cancer: a phase II trial. European Journal of Cancer 37, 2001 pp. 583-590.

[9] Manegold C. Chemotherapy for advanced non-small cell lung cancer (NSCLC) Lung Cancer 38, 2002 pp. S47-S50.

[10] Manegold C. Chemotherapy for advanced non-small cell lung cancer: standards Lung Cancer 34, 2001 pp. S165–S170.

[11] Masters G.A., Hahn E.A., Shevrin D.H., Kies M.S. Phase I/II trial of vinorelbine and divided-dose carboplatin in advanced non-small cell lung cancer. Lung Cancer 39, 2003 pp. 221-226.

[12] Price A. Chemotherapy in Patients with Advanced Non-Small Cell Lung Cancer. Clinical Oncology 13, 2001 pp. 480–482.

[13] Thongprasert S., Sanguanmitra P. Juthapan W., Clinch J. Relationship between quality of life and clinical outcomes in advanced non-small cell lung cancer: best supportive care (BSC) versus BSC plus chemotherapy. Lung Cancer 24, 1999 pp. 17–24.

[14] Tjan-Heijnen V.C.G., Groen H.J.M., Schramel F.M.N.H., G. Stoter Consensus conference on palliative treatment of stage IV non-small cell lung cancer. Consensus meeting of the Netherlands Society for Medical Oncology and the Taskforce on Lung Cancer of the Dutch Society of Physicians for Lung Diseases and Tuberculosis. The Netherlands Journal of Medicine 58, 2001 pp. 52–61.

[15] Wigle D.A. et all. Molecular Profiling of Non-Small Cell Lung Cancer and Correlation with Disease-free Survival. Cancer Research 62/1, 2002 pp. 3005–3008.

[16] Osowski S. Artificial neural network in algorithmic depiction. WNT Warszawa 1996. (in Polish).

# 4. Visualisation of Medical Data

*Transformation of Health Care with Information Technologies*
*M. Duplaga et al. (Eds.)*
*IOS Press, 2004*



# Navigation Systems Based on Registration of Endoscopic and CT-derived Virtual Images for Bronchofiberoscopic Procedures

Paweł TURCZA[1], Mariusz DUPLAGA[2]
[1] *Department of Instrumentation and Measurement,*
*AGH University of Science and Technology, al. Mickiewicza 30, 30-059 Kraków, Poland,*
*e-mail: turcza@agh.edu.pl*
[2] *Department of Medicine, Jagiellonian University Medical College,*
*Skawinska Str. 8, 31-066 Kraków, Poland,*
*e-mail: mmduplag@cyf-kr.edu.pl*

**Abstract.** Bronchofiberoscopy is an essential diagnostic procedure in patients with lung cancer. Sampling methods employed during endoscopy of the respiratory tract are performed with the aim of diagnosis confirmation and staging. Transbronchial needle aspiration may be used for evaluation of lymph nodes neighbouring with trachea and bronchi. Many efforts have been undertaken to increase the sensitivity of this procedure including the application of endobronchial ultrasonography.

In recent years several research groups have proposed models of navigating systems to provide computer assistance during bronchoscopic interventions. Although they have used different techniques, their objective was the same – enabling tracking location and movement of bronchofiberoscope tip with reference to previously-acquired computed tomography (CT) images. Since a fiber-optic bronchoscope is a rather long and flexible device, determination of its tip location is not an easy task. The adoption of optical tracking methods used in neurosurgery or laparoscopic surgery to endoscopy of the tracheobronchial tree is usually not possible.

Another obstacle is related to the fact that bronchofiberoscopes usually have only one operational channel. This feature considerably limits the feasibility of navigation systems based on the use of small electromagnetic sensing devices or USG probes. The sources of positioning errors in such systems are respiratory movements and the lack of external referential coordinate system associated with the tracheobronchial tree.

A promising option for development of a bronchoscopic guidance system is the application of image registration algorithms. Such an approach encompasses registration of endoscopic images to views derived from advanced imaging methods, e.g. CT. In the first step, reconstruction of a three-dimensional, endoluminal views is performed. Next, the position of the virtual camera in a CT-derived virtual model is determined using a complex multi-level image registering algorithm. This stage is the source of the greatest differences between proposed methods and a potential field for considerable improvements.

This paper presents a review of recent as well as classical image registering methods used in navigation systems for bronchofiberoscopy. Details related to the selection of crucial elements of navigation systems based on image registering techniques, such as transformation, similarity criteria, matching and global optimization, are specified.

## Introduction

Bronchofiberoscopy is a basic diagnostic procedure used in pulmonology. It becomes nearly obligatory when lung neoplam is suspected in the patient. The procedure is usually accompanied by other diagnostic modalities enabling sampling of pathologic tissues for evaluation. Transbronchial needle aspiration allows for neoplasmatic tissue sampling as well as evaluation of lymph nodes situated outside trachea and the bronchial tree for the staging of lung cancer. Knowledge regarding the presence of cancer infiltrates in lymph nodes located in mediastinum is crucial for making the decision on whether to perform radical surgery.

From the very beginning, attempts have been undertaken to increase the sensitivity of transbronchial needle aspiration. Nowadays, this procedure is usually carried out after earlier CT examination of the thorax for visualization of potentially pathologically changed lymph nodes. However, even if transbronchial needle aspiration is performed after CT examination, it requires considerable experience and skill from bronchoscopists. They must develop good awareness of the three-dimensional topography of the chest and the ability to create a mental image of structures surrounding the bronchi after browsing two-dimensional cross-sections available from CT.

The sensitivity of transbronchial needle aspiration has meaningfully increased following the introduction of endobronchial ultrasonography. However, commonly available bronchofiberoscopic equipment does not allow for real-time visualization of the structures around the lumen of the bronchus during needle aspiration. After the examination, the ultrasonographic probe must be removed from the working channel of the endoscope, and only then may the needle be inserted into it. This shortcoming may be overcome in near future, as bronchofiberoscopes enabling simultaneous ultrasonographic examination and needle aspiration procedures are being constructed.

There is a growing interest in the use of computer-based systems enabling advanced visualization and navigation in a virtual, three-dimensional environment of anatomical structures. This trend is related to several factors including the progress of visualization abilities of the structure and function of human body, the application of advanced computing for generation of three-dimensional representations of the anatomical structure from data obtained during such imaging procedures as CT, magnetic nuclear resonance (MRI) or ultrasonography, and finally, the pressure on decreasing the invasiveness of medical procedures.

The navigation systems coupling a real operation field with virtual images produced from data obtained during imaging procedures are used with the aim of improving visualization of human body structures and pathologic lesions in the course of invasive medical procedures.

The development of an effective navigation system supporting bronchofiberoscopy poses substantial problems. Optical navigation systems applied in neurosurgery or laparoscopy rely on the use of rigid tools and they cannot be simply adopted to bronchofiberoscopy as the bronchofiberoscope is a flexible device. Attempts at applying electromagnetic methods were associated with essential problems related to attaching the sensor to a bronchofiberoscope tip and calibration of the whole navigation system.

This paper presents selected aspects of development of navigation systems for bronchofiberoscopy and solutions used to overcome technical hurdles. Particular emphasis has been put on medical image registration algorithms with potential application in modern navigation systems. The concept of a new system has also been described.

## 1. The Review of Available Navigation Systems

Initial papers, focusing on development of navigation systems coupling real environments with virtual images generated from data obtained from CT or MRI, appeared in the late nineties and continued to appear throughout that decade [1], [2], [3], [4]. Solomon et al. [1] described a system enabling determination of the endoscope tip position through the use of a miniature magnetoresistive sensor attached to it, along with three electromagnetic field sources surrounding the patient. The use of such a sensor enabled positioning the tip to within 0.5 mm of target under laboratory conditions. In real-world applications, however, this accuracy deteriorated considerably. This was related to the necessity of attaching special markers to the patient's skin prior to tomography, for system calibration. Unfortunately, the locations of markers during computed tomography scanning and endoscopy differed considerably because achieving identical patient positions during both procedures was virtually impossible. Another source of errors encountered by the authors of the paper related to distortions caused by heart contractions and respiratory movements.

Some authors, aware of the problems related to the use of sensors attached to the tip of the bronchofiberoscope, decided to develop navigation systems based on the analysis of the endoscopic images and their comparison with images produced with the use of computer tomography data. Such approach was supported by preceding research on the systems of preliminary planning and support for the biopsy procedure [5], [6], [7], corrective methods for distortions caused by the endoscopic camera itself [8], [9] and fast reconstruction algorithms, enabling the visualization of the bronchial tree from data accumulated during computer tomography [10], [11].

The first such attempt was undertaken in 1998 by Bricault [2]. He designed a method for determining the location of a bronchofiberoscope tip in relation to a virtual bronchial tree, but it could only be applied to bifurcation images. Furthermore, his method did not support fluent tracing of camera motion and could only be used in static situations. Nevertheless, it inspired other researchers to follow this track [3], [4], [12], [13].

A general diagram of the navigation system based on the registration of endoscopic images $I_A$ and views from the virtual camera $I_B$ located in the virtual representation of the trachea or bronchi (generated from CT data) is shown in the figure 1. This figure will be used for the presentation of functionalities of navigation systems, the differences between systems proposed by various teams of researchers and the authors' proposal for the improvement of such systems.

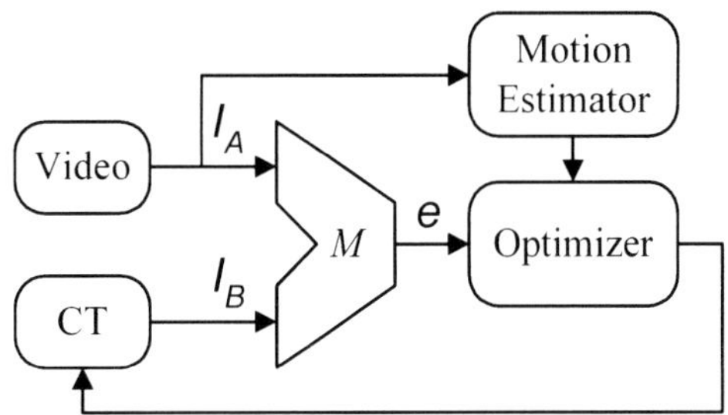


**Fig. 1.** Block diagram of an image-guided navigation system

The navigation system based on image analysis consists of a video frame grabber module which is responsible for digitalization of images obtained from the endoscopic camera; an initial estimation module for camera relocation; a virtual camera module cooperating with the image generation module (using CT data) and an optimizer module which is responsible for determining the position of the virtual camera in relation to the virtual bronchial tree in such a way that virtual image $I_B$ coming from it will be – as much as possible – similar to the image from the endoscopic camera ($I_A$) according to a chosen metric $M$.

The navigation system described above works in two stages. In the first stage, basing on analysis of the image from the endoscopic camera, relocation parameters (three vectors of translation and three rotation angles) between consecutive video frames (time stamps $T_{i-1}$ and $T_i$) are computed. In the second stage, more accurate positioning is carried out with the use of registering real and virtual endoscopic images. In order to reduce the complexity of this stage, initial estimation of camera relocation obtained in the first stage is used. The main differences between various systems depend on selection of the modules described in this diagram.

Mori et al. [3] used an optical flow algorithm [14] for initial estimation of camera relocation. However, these authors admitted that their method did not work correctly if the branching of the bronchial tree was not visible. In such a case, the angle of camera rotation could not be computed.

This problem was overcome by the same team of researchers through the application of epipolar geometry for initial estimation of camera relocation [12]. Epipolar geometry associates the coordinates of a point in relation to camera C1's coordinate system with the coordinates of the same point in relation to the coordinate system of camera *C*2. When applied to bronchofiberoscopy, cameras *C*1 and *C*2 designate the same endoscopic camera, but located in two different positions. This allows for initial determination of bronchofiberoscope tip relocation parameters between consecutive video frames (time stamps $T_{i-1}$ and $T_i$). These parameters are used in the next step for narrowing the search area in the computer-generated bronchial tree. The process is steered by the degree of similarity between real and virtual images. Unfortunately, the authors did not specify what kind of similarity measure had been used. The processing time per one image frame required by PC Pentium 1GHz was, however, shortened from 15s [3] to 6s [12]. Authors indicate that their method enables tracking of camera motion in areas without specific structural features on endoscopic views. However they only tested their methods on videotaped sequences.

Another approach has been employed by Helferty et al. [4]. The navigation system described in this paper was aimed at support of an advanced stage of the procedure – the moment of the selection of a suitable place for needle biopsy and not on tracking camera motion. It employed the method of real and virtual image registration and was used for determination of needle position in relation to the bronchial tree and lymph nodes. However modified normalized mutual information (NMI) [15] was used as a similarity measure during the image registration process. The only modification applied to NMI was the use of weighted entropy instead of standard entropy as defined by Shannon. Weighted entropy allows accounting for the fact that image registration is influenced to a greater degree by dark fragments of the image showing the branching of the bronchial tree or deformations of its walls, rather than by bright fragments of the image, typically showing walls of the bronchi. Authors have claimed that their method yields high accuracy, as the mean error was only 1.97 mm.

The extension of the system described above with the option of camera motion tracing was presented in the next paper by the same authors [13]. This time, they applied an optical flow algorithm for tracking camera (bronchofiberoscope tip) motion using only the images acquired by the camera. Parameters describing this relocation were further used for decreasing the computational complexity of the next (more accurate) positioning stage, based on NMI (analogous to papers by Mori et al. [3], [12]).

The system must possess mechanisms allowing for elimination of erroneous frames (e.g. mucus, distortions) from the registration process, if its full effectiveness and automation are to be achieved. Attempts at using faulty frames in the navigation process have led not only to positioning errors but also to a considerable increase of computing power requirements. Simple algorithms for validation of the usefulness of a particular image from the endoscopic camera for navigation based on analysis of image histograms have been described by Higgins et al. in [16].

## 2. The Review of Image Registration Methods

Methods enabling registration of images from the same or different sources have undergone extensive development through the last decades. Numerous papers have been published on this topic [17], [18], [19], [20], [21]. Such methods may be implemented both in technical applications (navigation, geographic information systems) and in medicine (tracing the progress of a disease, e.g. growth of the tumor, fusion of the images from different types of sources such as computed tomography and ultrasonography, etc.)

Image registration is the process of determining the transform $T$ that brings into spatial correspondence two images $I_A$ and $I_B$. As a measure of their spatial correspondence, a specially chosen function $S$, called the similarity measure, is used. Strictly speaking, the image registration process can be presented as a task of minimizing function $F$:

$$F\colon R^N \to R_+ : F(T) = S(I_A(p), I_B(T(p))).$$

Under the assumption that images $I_A$ and $I_B$ show structures or tissues which behave as a rigid body object, the transform $T$ can be described by the formula [19] $T(p)=Rp+t$. This assumption greatly reduces the complexity of the image registration process by reducing the number of parameters (three translation vectors $t$ and three rotation angles represented by matrix $R$) describing transform $T$, which have to be determined. In such a case, function $F$ has the following form:

$$R^6 \to R_+ : F(R,t) = S(I_A(p), I_B(Rp+t)).$$

Evaluation of function $F$, according to transformation $T$ applied to the second image, requires evaluation of image intensity at non-grid points which can easily be performed with the help of an interpolator. However, it should be stressed that the quality of interpolation process has significant impact both on computational complexity and accuracy of the whole registration process [22].

The essential issue related to image registering is the appropriate choice of function $S$ for a specific application. In the case of registration of images obtained with the same technique (mono-modality), the sum of absolute differences (SAD):

$$S_{SAD}(A,B) = \frac{1}{N}\sum_{p\in AB} \left| I_A(p) - I_B(T(p)) \right|$$

or the sum of squared differences also known as mean square error (MSE)

$$S_{MSE}(A,B) = \frac{1}{N}\sum_{p\in AB} \left( I_A(p) - I_B(T(p)) \right)^2$$

can be used. In the above equations $I_A(p)$ and $I_B(T(p))$ denote respectively the intensity of point $p$ in image $I_A$ and the intensity of point $p$ after transformation $T$ in image $I_B$. $N$ denotes the number of points in images $A$ and $B$ for which the measure is computed. Normalization (division by $N$) is justified because the use of transformation $T$ during the image registering process usually leads to partial image overlaps.

In case of registration of images obtained with different diagnostic methods (multi-modality), e.g. CT and MRI, their intensities are quite different. Of course, the choice of SAD or MSE as a similarity measure in multi-modality image registering would lead to failure.

One of the similarity measures devised especially for multi-modality image registration is called the ratio image uniformity (RIU) measure, introduced by Woods in 1992 [23]. It is based on the observation that the ratio image, calculated from intensities of images $I_A$ and $I_B$ when these two images are well registered is uniform (has near-constant brightness). If $I_A(p)$ and $I_B(p)$ are pixels with coordinates $p$ in images $A$ and $B$, the normalized standard deviation of ratio of their intensities is a good measure of such uniformity:

$$S = \frac{\sqrt{\frac{1}{N}\sum_{p}\left(R(p)-\bar{R}\right)^{2}}}{\bar{R}}, \qquad R(p) = \frac{I_A(p)}{I_B(T(p))}, \qquad \bar{R} = \frac{1}{N}\sum_{p} R(p)$$

Viola and Wells proposed another more general measure of image similarity based on information theory [24]. Their method is based on concept of joint entropy as used by Shannon for determination of the capacity of a communications channel. Viola and Wells define the following measure of image similarity:

$$I(u,v) = H(u) - H(u \mid v),$$

where $H(u)$ denotes the measure of uncertainty about the value of the random variable $u$, and $H(u|v)$ denotes the same measure but determined with the assumption that the value of the random variable $v$ is known. In this way $I(u,v)$ expresses how much the uncertainty about the value of $u$ decreases when the value of $v$ is revealed. It is obvious that if the value of conditional entropy $H(u|v)$ decreases, the value of mutual information $I(u|v)$ increases. Using the Bayesian theorem: $P(A,B)=P(A|B)P(B)$ and the definition of Shannon entropy:

$$H(u) = -\sum_{i} p_u(i)\log p_u(i), \qquad H(u,v) = -\sum_{i} p_{uv}(i)\log p_{uv}(i)$$

the equation expressing mutual information ($MI$) may be rewritten in the following form:

$$I(u,v) = H(u) + H(v) - H(u,v).$$

These equation include joint entropy $H(u,v)$, which may be determined on the basis of joint probability distribution which in turn, can be inferred from the joint histogram $h(u,v)$ after appropriate normalization.

The application of joint entropy $H(u,v)$ alone as a similarity measure in the image registering process (especially if the images are highly unregistered) may lead to false results. This can happen because such a similarity measure is determined on the basis of intensity values of overlapping parts of both images, so its value strongly depends on the size of this area. During the registration process it may happen that one of the images will be transformed in such a way that overlapping parts of images may cover a fragment with negligible information content (e.g. an area filled mainly with the background). This will lead to very low dispersion of the joint histogram and, in turn, to the conclusion of accurate image registration, where in fact the opposite is true [21]. As the mutual information measure $I(u, v)$ also includes values of marginal entropy of both images, it is much less prone to such an effect. This is associated with the fact, that when overlapping image areas decrease, both the joint entropy and the marginal entropy decrease as well.

The influence of the size of the overlapping area on the similarity measure can be further reduced by the use of normalized mutual information proposed by Studholme et al. [15]

$$NMI(u,v) = \left(H(u) + H(v)\right) / H(u,v).$$

The definitions of mutual information (MI, NMI) described above are based on first-order entropy given by Shannon. This definition assumes that probability distributions for consecutive image points are identical and independent. However, this assumption is usually false in relation to medical images. One method of adjusting for spatial interdependence occurring in registered images relies on the calculation of the intensity gradient in every point which is used for determination of mutual information. Pluim et al. have shown in their paper [25] that a combination of measures based on value and direction of the gradient vector with mutual information allows for a considerable increase in the reliability of such an extended image registration method.

Image segmentation and labeling is a more difficult method of inclusion of interdependences between neighboring points or even whole areas into the measure of registration [26].

Before the registration process, images may undergo initial processing, allowing for eradication of noise which could affect the registration process, determination of regions of particular interest, rejection of regions which could hamper the registration process and finally, exposure of features enhancing this process.

Even though the measure MI has been proposed as being global, determined by its stochastic nature, the image fragmentation and selection of the registration function for consecutive parts is possible. In this way, measure MI may be used in the registration of images showing tissues undergoing deformations (e.g. caused by heart contractions, respiratory movements or surgical interventions). In such cases, transformation $T$ bases on locally affined transformation methods [19], [27].

To decrease the computational complexity of the whole image registering process multi-resolution image representations are used. Such approach not only reduces computational complexity but also avoids many local minima, usually encountered during the optimization process. A comprehensive review of these issues may be found in the paper [28].

## 3. The Design of a New Navigation System

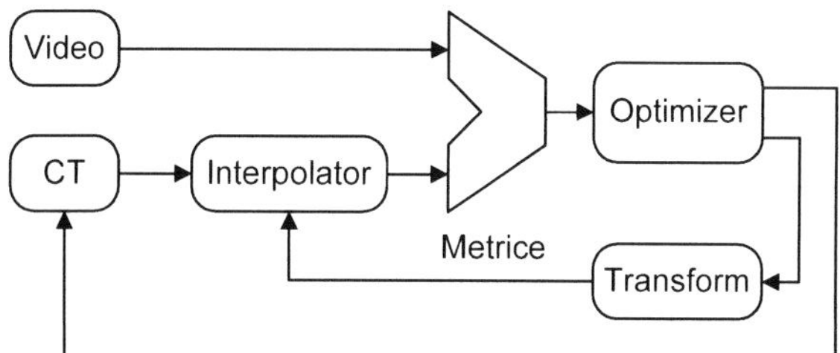


**Fig. 2.** The block diagram of a new navigation system

The design of a new navigation system for bronchofiberoscopy procedures which employs the registration of virtual bronchoscopy images and endoscopic camera images is presented in Figure 2. The main modules of this system include a video frame grabber system, a virtual camera module cooperating with the image generation system based on computer tomography data, an interpolator responsible for determination of image intensity values in non-grid points as dictated by the transformation, and an optimizer, which is responsible for determining the parameters of transforms leading to an increase in the similarity measure of virtual and endoscopic camera images, as measured by metric $M$.

The main difference in relation to earlier systems [4], [12] is the way in which the endoscopic camera position is determined with reference to the virtual bronchial tree. Previous papers utilized algorithms which changed the position of the virtual camera in relation to a virtual bronchial tree until the image obtained from it was sufficiently similar, according to an assumed similarity measure, to the image from the endoscopic camera. A disadvantage of such a solution was its high computational complexity, associated with the generation of a great number of images by the virtual bronchoscopy system.

As will be shown, the computational complexity of the algorithm used for determination of the bronchofiberoscope tip (camera) position in relation to the virtual bronchial tree may be decreased by an iterative application of a new proposed two-stage algorithm. In the first stage, each new ($T_i$) incoming image from the real endoscopic camera is compared to a previous ($T_{i-1}$) image obtained from the virtual bronchoscopy system. As a result of this process, we can obtain the parameters (scale, rotation, translation) of transformation which yield a registration. These parameters are used for determination of the new position of the virtual camera in relation to the virtual bronchial tree.

If the determined parameters of transformation differ by more than the assumed value ε from the parameters of identity transformation, a next iteration of the algorithm is executed. This algorithm reduces considerably the number of images generated by the virtual bronchoscopy system and thus decreases the computational complexity of the whole navigation process.

A further reduction in computational complexity may be achieved by the use of a different method for estimation of joint and marginal probability distribution, required for determining the value of the mutual information measure.

According to Helferty et al., this probability distribution can be derived from marginal and joint histogram, as follows [4]

$$p(k) = \frac{1}{NM}\sum_{i=1}^{N}\sum_{j=1}^{M}\delta\big(k - I(i,j)\big), \quad p_{AB}(k) = \frac{1}{NM}\sum_{i=1}^{N}\sum_{j=1}^{M}\delta\big(k - I_A(i,j)\big)\delta\big(k - I_B(i,j)\big),$$

where $\delta$ denotes the Kronecker delta.

Following Viola and Wells [24], the authors of this paper propose the usage of the Parzen window method to estimate this probability distribution:

$$p(k) = \frac{1}{N_A}\sum_{a_i \in I} w\big(k - a_i\big), \qquad p_{AB}(k) = \frac{1}{N_A}\sum_{\substack{a_i \in I_A \\ b_i \in I_B}} w\big(k - a_i\big)\, w\big(k - b_i\big)$$

where $w$ is a properly-selected smooth, non-negative, symmetric, zero mean, and integrate to one function (Parzen window), $N_A$ denotes the number of randomly-chosen points $a_i$ , $b_i$ (usually several hundred) from images $I_A$ and $I_B$.

The computational complexity of the probability distribution estimator used in the paper by Helferty et al. [4] is on the order of $N$x$M$, where $N$ denotes the number of rows, and $M$ – the number of columns in the image. For typical images with 256 rows and 256 columns this results in checking the values of 65536 points. The estimator used by Viola and Wells [24] requires only about 200 randomly-selected image points which are used for calculation the value of function $w$.

Another advantage of the application of estimators based on Parzen window is due to the existence of an analytical expression of first (gradient) and second derivative (Hessian) of mutual information. Values of this derivative are required during the optimization process and, if they cannot be expressed analytically, they need to be approximated numerically. However, numerical approximation not only greatly increases the number of transformations and calculations of the similarity measure during registration but can lead to a lack of stability of optimization and therefore the whole registration process.

The efficiency of this method has been checked through registration of two images from video recordings of bronchofiberoscopy procedures. For test purposes, one image selected from this record was rotated and scaled, and the values of its intensity were changed to their opposites. The process of registration as a function of the iteration number is shown in Figure 3, while changes in values of the similarity measure, scale and rotation angle are presented on accompanying diagrams (Figure 4). It should be underlined that the number of iterations sufficient for accurate registration was really low. A further decrease of computational complexity may be achieved by the use of multi-resolution image registering algorithms [28].

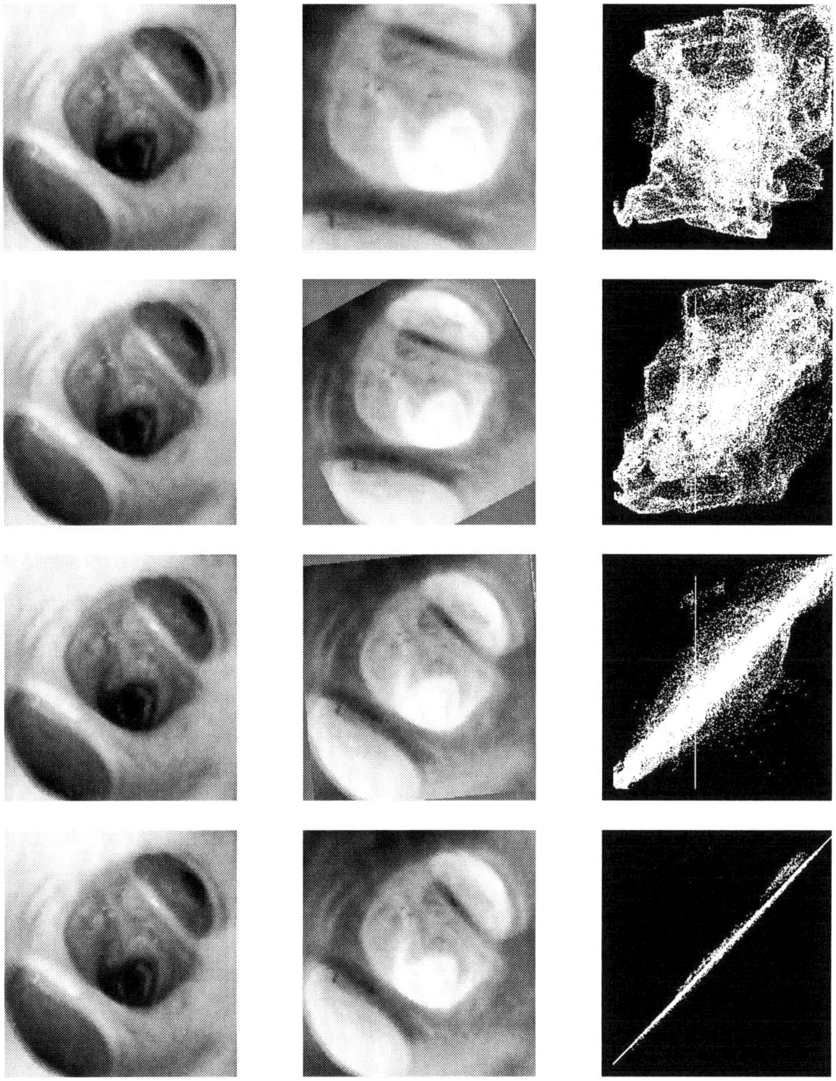

**Fig. 3.** A sequence of images as obtained during the registration process. Left column – reference image, middle column – image undergoing registration, right column – joint histogram. The rows correspond to iterations no.: 0, 3, 7 and 14 of the optimizer

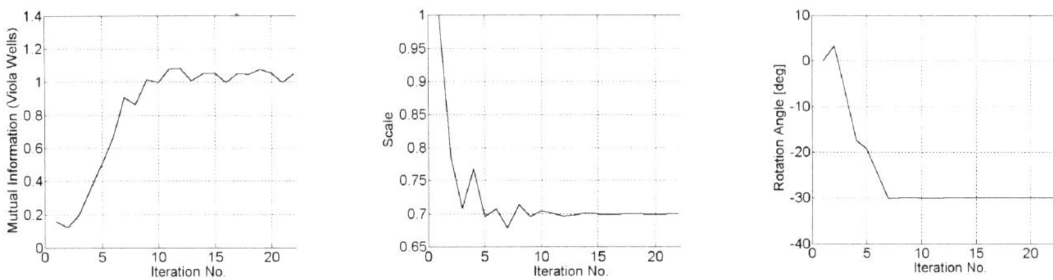


**Fig. 4.** The sequence of metric values, rotation angles and scales after each iteration of the optimizer

## References


[1] S.B. Solomon, P. White, C.M. Wiener, J.B. Orens, K.P. Wang, "Three-dimensional CT-Guided Bronchoscopy With a Real-Time Electromagnetic Position Sensor: A Comparison of Two Image Registration Methods", *Chest* vol. 118, pp. 1783-1787, 2000

[2] I. Bricault, G. Ferretti, P. Cinquin,. "Registration of real and CT-derived virtual bronchoscopic images to assist transbronchial biopsy", *IEEE Transactions on Medical Imaging* vol. 17, pp. 703-714, 1998

[3] K.Mori, Y.Suenaga, J.Toriwaki, et al., "Tracking of camera motion of real endoscope by using the Virtual Endoscope System", *Proc. of CARS2000*, pp. 85-90, 2000

[4] J.P. Helferty, W.E. Higgins, "Technique for registering 3D virtual CT images to endoscopic video", *IEEE Int. Conf. on Image Processing* 2001, pp.893-896, Oct. 7-10 2001

[5] K. Mori, J. Hasegawa, J. Toriwaki, et al., "Automated extraction and visualization of bronchus from 3-D CT images of Lung", In N.Ayache, (ed.) Computer Vision, Virtual reality and Robotics in Medicine, *Lecture Notes in Computer Science*, Springer-Verlag, Berlin Heidelberg New York, vol. 905, pp. 542-548, 1995

[6] K. Mori, J. Hasegawa, Y. Suenaga, J. Toriwaki, "Automated Anatomical Labeling of the Bronchial Branch and Its Application to the Virtual Bronchoscopy System", *IEEE Transactions on Medical Imaging*, vol. 19, pp. 103-114, 2000.

[7] A.P. Kiraly, W.E. Higgins, G. McLennan, E.A. Hoffman, J.M. Reinhardt, "Three-dimensional Human Airway Segmentation Methods for Clinical Virtual Bronchoscopy", *Radiology*, vol. 9, pp. 1153-1168, 2002.

[8] J.P. Helferty, Ch. Zhang, G. McLennan, W.E. Higgins, "Videoendoscopic Distortion Correction and Its Application to Virtual Guidance Endoscopy", *IEEE Transactions on Medical Imaging*, vol. 20, pp. 605-617, 2001.

[9] R. Shahidi, M.R. Bax, C.R. Maurer, et al, "Implementation, Calibration and Accuracy Testing of Image-Enhanced Endoscopy System", *IEEE Transactions on Medical Imaging*, vol. 21, pp. 1524-1535, 2002.

[10] K. Ramaswamy, W.E. Higgins, "Interactive Dynamic Navigation for Virtual Endoscopy", *Computers in Biology and Medicine*, vol. 29, pp. 303-331, 1999.

[11] M.L. Brady, K. Ramaswamy, R. Srinivasan, W.E. Higgins , "Dynamic Template-Based Method for 3D Virtual-Endoscopic Exploration", *Optical Engineering*, vol. 38, pp. 2162, 1999.

[12] K. Mori, D. Deguchi, J. Hasegawa, et al., "A Method for Tracking the Camera Motion of Real Endoscope by Epipolar Geometry Analysis and Virtual Endoscopy System", *Medical Image Analysis*, vol. 6, pp. 321-336 2002

[13] J.P. Helferty, W.E. Higgins, "Combined Endoscopic Video Tracking and Virtual 3D CT Registration for Surgical Guidance", *IEEE Int. Conf. Image Processing,* pp. II-961-964, 2002.

[14] B.K. Horn, R.J. Weldon. Jr. "Direct methods for recovering motion", *International Journal of Computer Vision*, vol. 2, pp. 51-76, 1988

[15] C. Studholme, D.L.G. Hill, D.J. Hawkes, "An overlap invariant entropy measure of 3D medical image alignment", *Pattern Recognition* vol. 32, pp. 71-86, 1999.

[16] W.E. Higgins, J.P. Helferty, D.R. Padfield, "Integrated Bronchoscopic Video Tracking and 3D CT Registration for Virtual Bronchoscopy", *SPIE Medical Imaging 2003: Physiology and Function–Methods, Systems, and Applications,* SPIE Proc., A. Clough and A. Amini, eds. vol. 5031, pp. 80-89, 2003.

[17] H. Lester, S.R. Arridge, "A survey of hierarchical non-linear medical image registration", *Pattern Recognition* vol. 32, pp. 129 –149, 1999.

[18] D.L.G. Hill, P.G. Batchelor, M. Holden, D.J. Hawkes, "Topical review, Medical image registration", *Physics in Medicine and Biology* vol. 46, pp. R1–R45, 2001.

[19] M.A. Audette, F.P. Ferrie, T.M. Peters, "An Algorithmic Overview of Surface Registration Techniques for Medical Imaging", *Medical image Analysis* vol. 4, pp. 201–217, 2000.

[20] B. Zitova, J. Flusser, "Image registration methods: a survey", *Image and Vision Computing* vol. 21, pp. 977–1000, 2003.

[21] J.P.W. Pluim, J. B. A. Maintz, M.A. Viergever, "Mutual information based registration of medical images: a survey", *IEEE Transactions on Medical Imaging*, vol. 22, pp. 986-1004, 2003

[22] J. Tsao, Interpolation Artifacts in Multimodality Image Registration Based on Maximization of Mutual Information, *IEEE Transactions on Medical Imaging*, vol. 22, pp.854-864, 2003

[23] R.P. Woods, S.R. Cherry, J.C. Mazziotta, "Rapid automated algorithm for aligning and reslicing PET images", *Journal of Computer Assisted Tomography* vol. 16, pp. 620-633, 1992.

[24] P. Viola, W.M. Wells III, "Alignment by maximization of mutual information", in International Conference on Computer Vision 1995 Eds.: E. Grimson, S. Shafer, A. Blake, K. Sugihara, *IEEE Computer Society Press*, Los Alamitos, CA., pp. 16-23, 1995.

[25] J.P.W. Pluim, J.B.A. Maintz, M.A. Viergever, "Image registration by maximization of combined mutual information and gradient information", *IEEE Transactions on Medical Imaging* vol.19, pp. 809-814, 2000.

[26] D. Rueckert, M.J. Clarkson, D.L.G. Hill, D.J. Hawkes, "Non-rigid registration using higher-order mutual information", *Proc. SPIE, Medical Imaging: Image Processing 2000, Ed K.M. Hanson*, vol. 3979 pp. 438- 447, 2000.

[27] J.A. Schnabel, D. Rueckert , et al, "A Generic Framework for Non-Rigid Registration Based on Non-Uniform Multi-Level Free-Form Deformations", *MICCAI 2001 Lecture Notes in Computer Science*, vol. 2208 pp. 573–581, 2001.

[28] F. Maes, D. Vandermeulen, P. Suetens, "Comparative evaluation of multiresolution optimization strategies for multimodality image registration by maximization of mutual information", *Medical Image Analysis* vol. 3, pp. 373-386, 1999.

*Transformation of Health Care with Information Technologies*
*M. Duplaga et al. (Eds.)*
*IOS Press, 2004*

# Segmentation of Human Brain MR Images Using Rule-Based Fuzzy Logic Inference

Marcin DENKOWSKI, Michał CHLEBIEJ, Paweł MIKOŁAJCZAK
*Laboratory of Information Technology, Institute of Physics,*
*Maria Curie Skłodowska University,*
*Pl. M. Curie-Skłodowskiej 1, 20-031 Lublin, Poland*
*e-mail: denmar@goblin.umcs.lublin.pl*

**Abstract.** The analysis of medical images for the purpose of computer-aided diagnosis and therapy planning includes the segmentation as a preliminary stage for the visualization or the quantification of such data. In this paper, we present a fuzzy segmentation system that is capable of segmenting magnetic resonance (MR) images of a human brain. The presented method consists of two main stages. The histogram analysis based on the S-function membership and Shannon's entropy function is the first step. In the final stage, pixel classification is performed using the rule-based fuzzy logic inference. After the segmentation is complete, attributes of different tissue classes may be determined (e.g., volumes), or the classes may be visualized as spatial objects. The implemented system provides many advanced 3D imaging tools, which enable visual exploration of segmented anatomical structures.

## Introduction

Image segmentation is a process of partitioning an image into a group of homogeneous regions according to characteristics such as the color and the texture. Threshold techniques, which make decisions based on local pixel information, are the simplest segmentation methods. The following equation describes the image that can be divided into $k+1$ homogenous regions:

$$g(k:x,y)=\begin{cases} k, & if \quad f(x,y)>T(k) \\ k-1, & T(k-1)<f(x,y)\le T(k) \\ \vdots & \\ 1, & T(0)<f(x,y)\le T(1) \\ 0, & otherwise \end{cases} \tag{1}$$

where $T(k)$ is the threshold level of the $k$-th region, $f$ is the intensity of the pixel in the $(x, y)$ position in the input image and $g$ is the output image. In this paper we present a numerical approach that enables us to find segmentation regions of human brain MR images. The main part of the proposed solution is implemented as a fuzzy rule-based inference algorithm [1] and a fuzzy-entropic algorithm based on S-function membership and Shannon's entropy function [2].

## 1. Methodology

Our segmentation algorithm consists of four main stages (see Figure 1). The first stage of our method is the preprocessing step. The main purpose of that stage is to reduce the background noise. The quality of the noise reduction is very significant for the accuracy of the whole segmentation process. At first, the standard "region growing" algorithm [3] eliminates the noisy background and the following binary opening operation [3] eliminates the remaining large noise clusters in the segmented background mask.

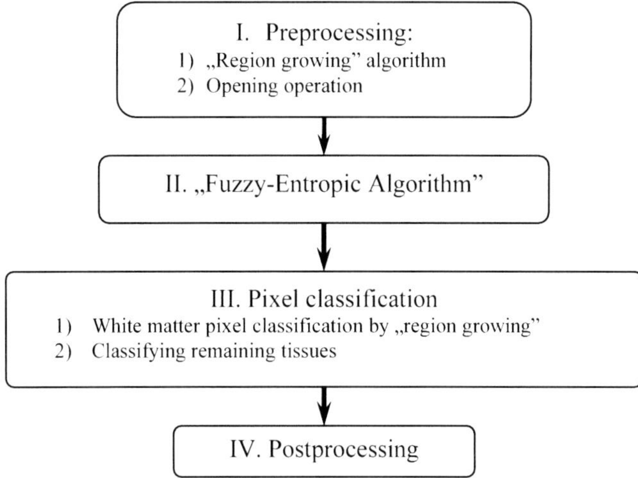


**Fig. 1.** The algorithm diagram

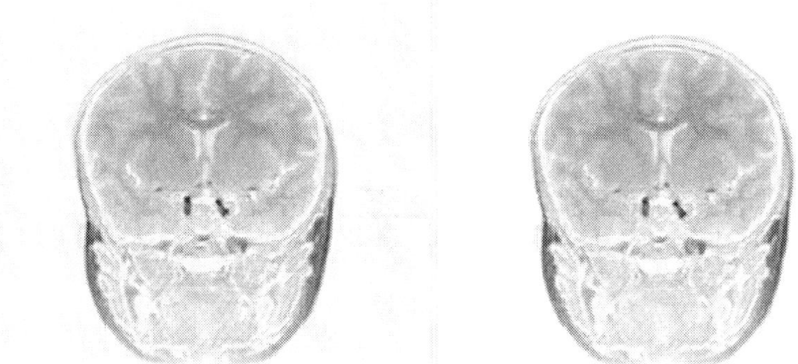

**Fig. 2.** The result of preprocessing – noisy image (left) and the same image following noise removal (right)

The second step is based on the "fuzzy entropic algorithm" [2]. From the point of view of a two-tone image, a gray-level image is fuzzy. We need to define a measure of fuzziness, which will enable us to find segmentation levels (boundary threshold values of a specified region) that would minimize fuzziness. The information theoretic entropy [4], which measures the mean value of the statistical uncertainty, is defined as follows:

$$H = -\sum_{i=1}^{n} p_i \log_2 p_i \qquad H[0,1] \tag{2}$$

$H$ is the average information supplied by a set of $i$ symbols whose probabilities are given by $p_1, p_2, p_3, \ldots, p_i, \ldots, p_n$ (respectively).

Fuzzy membership is regarded as a membership gradation of a set with some statistical uncertainty. This is equivalent to a situation where the image histogram does not display a smooth set of valleys between peaks.

In our approach, the standard *S*-function [1] has been selected for the purpose of membership gradation. Its generalized form is defined as follows:

$$\mu(x) = S(x,a,b,c) = \begin{cases} 0, & x \le a \\ k\left(\dfrac{x-a}{c-a}\right)^2, & a \le x \le b, k = \dfrac{c-a}{b-a} \\ 1-k\left(\dfrac{x-c}{c-a}\right)^2, & b \le x \le c, k = \dfrac{c-a}{c-a} \\ 1, & x \ge c \end{cases} \tag{3}$$

where $a$, $b$ and $c$ are the parameters which determine the shape of the S-function.

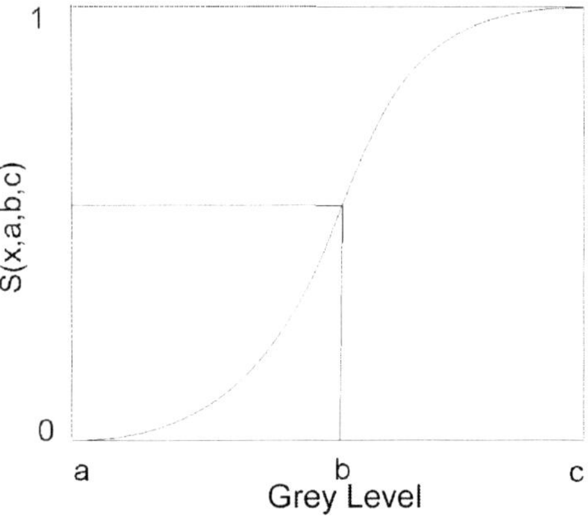


**Fig. 3.** Graph of the standard *S*-function, $b=a+c/2$, bandwidth $\Delta b=b-a=c-b$ and $k=2$

It is possible to apply Shannon's function (by substituting equation 2, 4 and taking $n=2$) to the membership function for a particular bandwidth:

$$S_n(x) = -\mu(x)\log_2\mu(x) - (1-\mu(x))\log_2(1-\mu(x)), \qquad 0 < x < n-1 \tag{4}$$

Now the fuzzy entropy measure is given by:

$$H_{fuzzy}(A) = \frac{1}{n\ln 2}\sum_{i=1}^{n} Sn(\mu_A(x_i)) \tag{5}$$

where $A$ is the fuzzy set of concern, containing $n$ members. To apply this equation to the image histogram $H$ with $n$ grey levels within the fuzzy region $g_i$ and width $h_i$ pixels in the $i$-th histogram bin, we use:

$$H_{fuzzy}(H) = \frac{1}{n\ln 2}\sum_{i=1}^{n} Sn(\mu_H(g_i))h_i \tag{6}$$

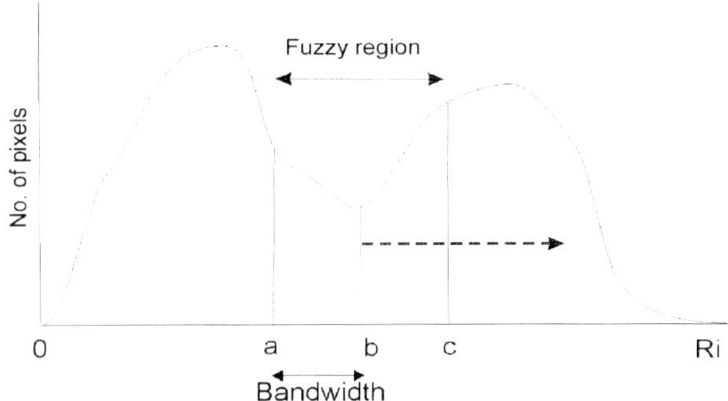


**Fig. 4.** Applying fuzzy region to the image histogram

The sample histogram and the bandwidth-dependent fuzzy entropy histogram are shown in Figure 5. To detect the fuzzy entropy valleys (local histogram minima) we need only to find where $e(k-1) < e(k) < e(k+1)$ for successive discretely-sampled values of fuzzy entropy $e(k)$ corresponding to each starting position of the bandwidth window.

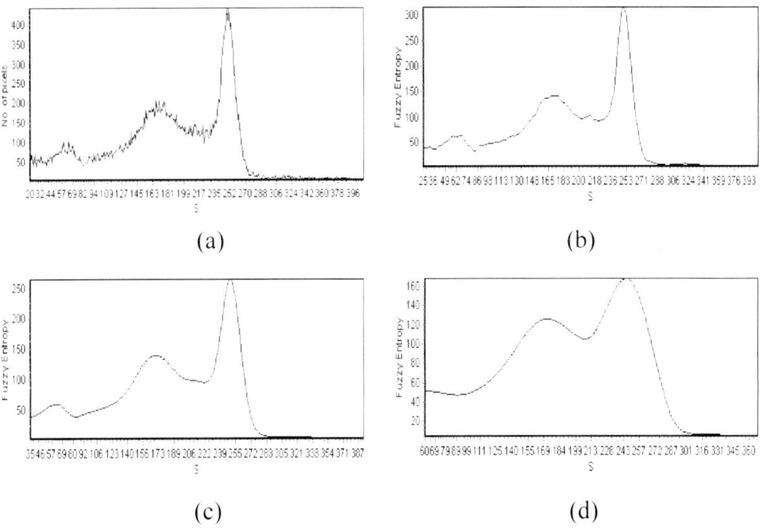


**Fig. 5.** The fuzzy entropy histogram of an MR slice for various bandwidths: the original histogram (a) and fuzzy histograms with bandwidth values of (respectively): $b=5$ (b), $b=15$ (c), $b=40$ (d)

The third stage of the presented algorithm is the pixel classification process. We use a fuzzy inference mechanism with IF-THEN rules.

IF-THEN rules for MRI T1 images:

IF *pixel* IS *bright* AND *Pixel* IS NOT *far* THEN *pixel* IS *white matter*

IF *pixel* IS *gray* AND *Pixel* IS NOT *far* THEN *pixel* IS *gray matter*

IF *pixel* IS *very bright* AND *Pixel* IS NOT *close* THEN *pixel* IS *CSF, muscle, fat*

IF *pixel* IS *dark* AND *Pixel* IS NOT *close* THEN *pixel* IS *bone*

MRI T2 images:

IF *pixel* IS *dark* AND *Pixel* IS NOT *far* THEN *pixel* IS *white matter*

IF *pixel* IS *gray* AND *Pixel* IS NOT *far* THEN *pixel* IS *gray matter*

IF *pixel* IS *very bright* AND *Pixel* IS NOT *close* THEN *pixel* IS *CSF*

IF *pixel* IS *dark* AND *Pixel* IS NOT *close* THEN *pixel* IS *bone, muscle*

Proton density:

IF *pixel* IS *gray* AND *Pixel* IS NOT *far* THEN *pixel* IS *white matter*

IF *pixel* IS *bright* AND *Pixel* IS NOT *far* THEN *pixel* IS *gray matter*

IF *pixel* IS *very bright* AND *Pixel* IS NOT *close* THEN *pixel* IS *CSF*

IF *pixel* IS *dark* AND *Pixel* IS NOT *close* THEN *pixel* IS *bone, muscle*

In the next step, we have to find the geometrical center of processed data set and for each pixel we have to create our own trapezoid membership function. The equations of this membership function are shown in (7) and its graph is presented in Figure 6 for a short, average and long distance from the center (respectively):

$$CLOSE: \begin{cases} r \in (0;\ 0.2r_m)\ F = 1 \\ r \in (0.2r_m;\ 0.4r_m)\ F = -\dfrac{5}{r_m}r + 2 \\ r > 0.4\ F = 0 \end{cases} \qquad FAR: \begin{cases} r \in (0;\ 0{,}75\,r_m)\ F = 0 \\ r \in (0{,}75\,r_m;\ 0{,}9r_m)\ F = \dfrac{5}{r_m}r - 1 \\ r > 0{,}9\ F = 1 \end{cases} \tag{7}$$

$$AVERAGE: \begin{cases} r \in (0;\ 0{,}2rm)\ F = 0 \\ r \in (0{,}2rm;\ 0{,}4r_m)\ F = \dfrac{5}{r_m}r - 1 \\ r \in (0{,}4r_m;\ 0{,}75\,r_m)\ F = 1 \\ r \in (0{,}75\,r_m;\ 0{,}9r_m)\ F = -\dfrac{5}{r_m}r + 4 \\ r > 0{,}9r_m\ F = 0 \end{cases}$$

where :

$r$ – the distance of the current pixel from the center of the dataset

$r_m$ – the maximum distance from the center of the dataset

$F$ – the fuzzy membership function

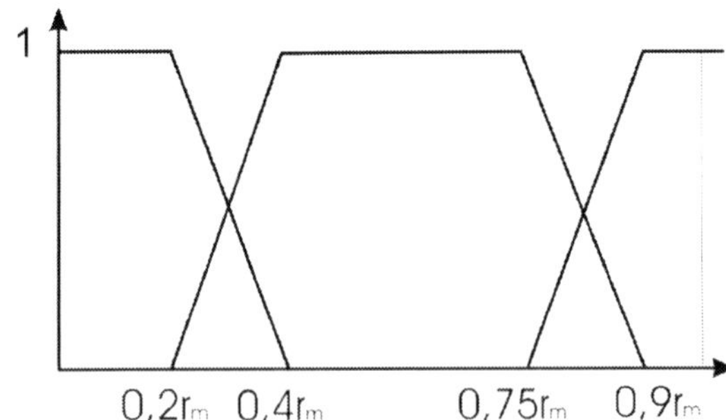


**Fig. 6.** The fuzzy membership function of the pixel distance from the geometrical center of the dataset

We have decided to choose the $G$ function [1] as the membership function for the pixel. This membership function is generated automatically on the basis of data obtained from the fuzzy-entropic stage. The typical $G$ membership function can be given as:

$$f(i)_N = \exp\left(\frac{-(i-c_N)^2}{2\sigma_N^2}\right) \tag{8}$$

where

$$c_N = \frac{V_N + V_{N+1}}{2} \text{ for } N \neq 0 \wedge N \neq N_{max}$$
$$c_N = 0 \text{ for } N = 0 \qquad \text{, and} \qquad \sigma_N^2 = \frac{-(V_N - c_N)^2}{2\ln(0.5)}$$
$$c_N = i_{max} \text{ for } N = N_{max}$$

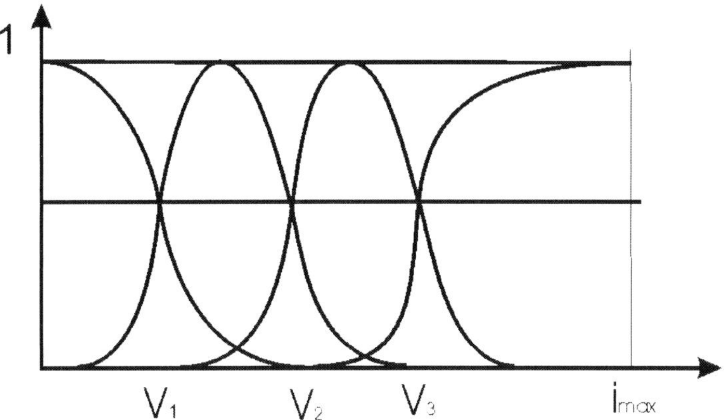


**Fig. 7.** The fuzzy membership function of pixel intensity

The inference process is of Takagi-Sugeno type [5], where the AND operator is defined as a minimum operator [5]. The defuzzyfication process is executed by the maximum height method [5].

This stage is divided into two phases. The first one involves the classification of the brain white matter. Only the first pixel classified as white matter by the inference mechanism is found iteratively from the geometrical center. This pixel is a seed for the 3D region growing algorithm, with the fuzzy inference as a homogeneity criterion.

After the white matter tissue is classified, the second phase classifies all remaining pixels, excluding the background. In this phase image pixels are examined sequentially, with fuzzy inference as the decision criterion.

In the pixel classification process we have to apply a low pass filter with the 3x3x3 mask to prevent classifying false single pixels:

$$\begin{bmatrix} 1 & 1 & 1 \\ 1 & 1 & 1 \\ 1 & 1 & 1 \end{bmatrix} \begin{bmatrix} 1 & 1 & 1 \\ 1 & 4 & 1 \\ 1 & 1 & 1 \end{bmatrix} \begin{bmatrix} 1 & 1 & 1 \\ 1 & 1 & 1 \\ 1 & 1 & 1 \end{bmatrix}$$
$$norm = 30$$

The last stage of the presented algorithm is the postprocessing step. Each pixel which remains unclassified is assigned to the class to which most of its neighbors belong. In that case, we also apply the 3x3x3 filtering mask.

## 2. Results

We have tested the method presented in this paper to segment the MRI data sets of a human head. The required computational time of the segmentation process for the test data set (256x256x128) was less then two minutes. The results of our fuzzy rule-based segmentation algorithm are presented in Figures 8 and 9. The separated segmented anatomical structures are illustrated in Figure 9. Selected images present good separation between air, bone, fat, soft tissues (such as skin and muscle), the cerebro-spinal fluid (CSF), grey matter (GM) and white matter (WM). Our system also enables three-dimensional visualization of datasets. It provides the ability to explore the spatial relationships of the anatomical structures (see Figure 10).

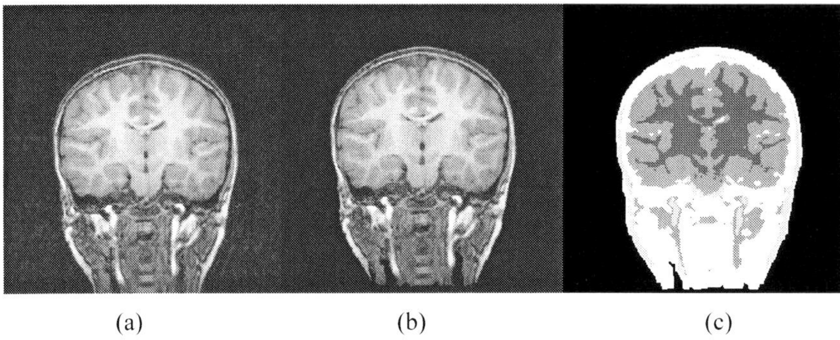

(a) (b) (c)

**Fig. 8.** Segmentation results of the MR human head: the original image (a), the image after background noise removal (b), the result of the segmentation process (c)

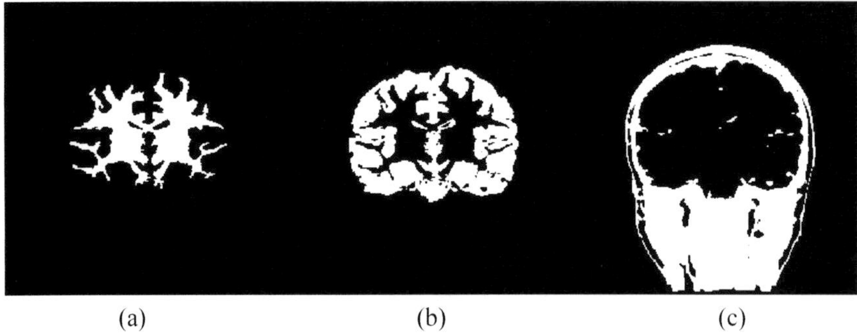

(a) (b) (c)

**Fig. 9.** Segmented tissue scan: the white matter (WM) (a); grey matter (GM) (b); skin, fat, CSF (c)

The acquired segmented images were compared to the expert's mask [7] for two similarity measures: difference between the number of pixels in our class and the expert's class (9) and pixels covering the measure in both data sets (10). The mask segmented by the expert contained only white matter and grey matter tissue. Because of this, we were only able to compare two structures.

$$r_{NP} = \left| \frac{N_{pat} - N}{N_{pat}} \right| \tag{9}$$

where

$r_{NP}$ – difference between the number of pixels in our class and the expert's class

$N$ – the number of pixels in the compared class in our image

$N_{pat}$ – the number of pixels in the compared class in the expert's image

$$r_{cover} = \left| \frac{N_{cover}}{N_{pat}} \right| \tag{10}$$

where

$r_{cover}$ – pixels covering measure

$N_{cover}$ – the number of covering pixels in the compared class in our image

$N_{pat}$ – the number of pixels in the compared class in the expert's image

**Table 1.** Results of comparison between our segmented image and the image segmented by experts

| Criterion | Results | |
|---|---|---|
| | White matter | Grey matter |
| $r_{NP}$ | 0,12 | 0,13 |
| $r_{cover}$ | 0,85 | 0,91 |

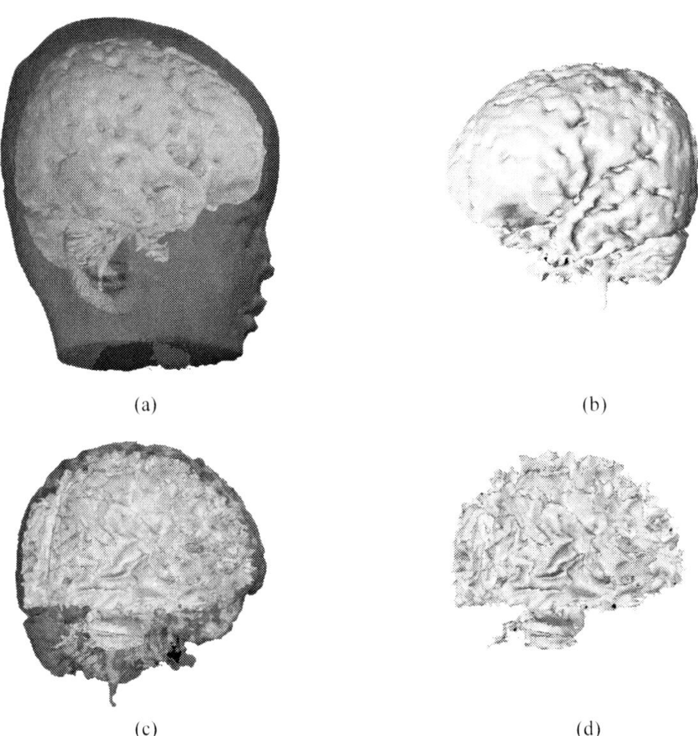

**Fig. 10.** Three-dimensional visualization of segmented anatomical structures: grey matter with semi-transparent skin (a), grey matter alone (b), white matter with semi-transparent grey matter (c), white matter alone (d)

## 3. Conclusions and Future Work

We have examined the idea of using the fuzzy rule-based inference system and the fuzzy entropy system as basics for the human head MR image segmentation algorithm. We used the fuzzy logic inference as a decision criterion for assigning pixels of the MR image to specified classes. Both of these methods are computationally fast, which is important in real-time systems.

**Acknowledgments.** We are very grateful to the National Library of Medicine [6, 7] for the permission to work with and publish the Visible-Human-Male datasets.

## References

[1] Zadeh L.A., Fuzzy Sets and their Applications to Cognitive and Decision Process, pp. 1-39, Academic Press, London, 1975

[2] Parallel entropic auto-thresholding, M. Fleury, L. Hayat, A.F. Clark, Image and Vision Computing, vol. 14, April, 1995

[3] Gonzalez R.C, Woods R.E., Digital image processing, Addison-Wesley Publishing Company, Inc., 1992

[4] Shannon C.E., A Mathematical Theory of Communication, The Bell System Technical Journal, vol. 27, pp. 379-423, 623-656, July, October, 1948.

[5] Łachwa A. Rozmyty świat zbiorów, liczb, relacji, faktów, reguł i decyzji, Wydawnictwo EXIT, Warszawa, 2001

[6] Spitzer V., Ackerman M.J., Scherzinger A.L., Whitlock D., The Visible Human male: A technical report, Journal of the American Medical Informatics Association, Vol. 3, pp. 118-130, 1996.

[7] National Library of Medicine, URL: *http://www.nlm.nih.gov/nlmhome.html*

# Developing Multimedia Software and Virtual Reality Worlds and their Use in Rehabilitation and Psychology

Cecília SIK LÁNYI[1], Viktória LAKY[1], Ádám TILINGER[1], Ilona PATAKY[2], Lajos SIMON[3], Bernadett KISS[4], Viktória SIMON[3], Júlianna SZABÓ[1], Attila PÁLL[1]
[1]*Colour and Multimedia Laboratory, University of Veszprém, Egyetem u. 10. H-8200 Veszprém, Hungary*
*e-mail: lanyi@almos.vein.hu*
[2]*National Centre of Brain Vein Diseases, Budapest, Hungary*
*e-mail: pataky@opni.hu*
[3]*Semmelweis Medical University in Budapest, Hungary*
*e-mail: simon@psych.sote.hu*
[4]*VerAnim, Budapest, Hungary*
*e-mail: bkiss@prim.hu*

**Abstract.** The multimedia and virtual reality projects performed at our laboratory during the last ten years can be grouped into the following groups: 1) tutorial and entertainment programs for handicapped children, 2) rehabilitation programs for stroke patients and patients with phobias. We have developed multimedia software for handicapped children with various impairments: partial vision, hearing difficulties, locomotive difficulties, mental retardation, dyslexia etc.

In the present paper we show the advantages of using multimedia software to develop mental skills in handicapped people and deal with the special needs of handicapped children. For the rehabilitation of stroke patients we have developed a computer-controlled method, which enables – contrary to methods used internationally – not only the establishment of a diagnosis, but also measurement of therapy effectiveness: 1) it enables us to produce a database of patients, which contains not only their personal data but also test results, their drawings and audio recordings, 2) it is in itself an intensive therapeutic test and contains tutorial programs. We are currently collecting test results.

We have also developed some virtual worlds for treating phobias: a virtual balcony and a ten-story building with an external glass elevator as well as an internal glass elevator in the virtual Atrium Hyatt hotel. We have developed a virtual environment for treating claustrophobia too: a closed lift and a room where the walls can move. For specific phobias (fear of travelling) we have modelled the underground railway system in Budapest. For autistic children, we have developed virtual shopping software too.

In this paper we present the advantages of virtual reality in the investigation, evaluation and treatment of perception, behaviour and neuropsychological disorders.

## Introduction

The term "multimedia" means literally "involving more than one medium", but it is used in three different and complementary senses: first to describe the channels through which information is delivered, including paper printouts, television, radio, telephone, CD-ROM and the Internet; second to describe the content as a mixture of still and moving images, text, graphics and sound; and third to describe the style of interaction through which the user may explore the content, taking advantage of the hierarchies and associations within the material via links connecting a variety of database resources. In this sense, multimedia is the meeting ground of technology, design and human factors [9].

Nowadays virtual reality (VR) is becoming very popular. It is an artificial world, which is created in a computer environment, where the user tries to fully enact a particular role in this unreal world. Virtual Environment (VE) technology has undergone a transition over the past few years that has taken it out of the realm of expensive toys and changed it into a functional technology. Recently, the considerable potential of VEs has been recognized in the field of mental healthcare and used in scientific studies. This paper summarizes the application of VR and presents the VR education and research performed at the University of Veszprém.

There are numerous definitions of virtual reality. one of these is the definition of Prof. Riva: virtual reality is multimodal interaction with dynamic and responsive computer-generated or so-called synthetic environments. [14] Its goal is to induce in the user the same feeling (or a similar feeling) as in the real world, thus it should produce the same effects as in vivo experience. Another definition is Prof. Rizzo's definition: VR is a way for humans to visualize, manipulate, and interact with computers and extremely complex data in a more natural-like fashion [15].

The virtual environment (VE) is a three-dimensional data set describing an environment based on real-world or abstract objects and data. The terms: virtual environment and virtual reality are usually used synonymously. However, some authors reserve the VE definition for describing the artificial environment that the user interacts with [19].

The concept has originally been used to label immersive virtual reality. This is an environment that corresponds as closely as possible to the real world. At present, the borders between both concepts are blurring, as e.g. it is common to also include in this definition three-dimensional worlds displayed on a graphic display or stereo projector, where the user can orient himself with the help of a mouse. There are also virtual realities that mix virtual objects with real environments (i.e. augmented/mixed realities).

Augmented reality involves the use of transparent glasses on which a computer displays data so that the viewer can view the data superimposed on real-world scenes [19].

When using VR, people often experience a feeling of actually being in the computer-generated environment, a feeling described as "presence" (illusion of being part of a virtual environment). The more immersive a VE experience is, the greater the sense of being part of it [19]. Presence can more explicitly be defined as a mediated experience that appears very much like a non-mediated one [2]. When a user experiences a high level of presence, it is even possible for the user to develop fear in response to simulated anxiety-provoking stimuli. Experiments have for instance shown that one can provoke in virtual reality the fear of heights [13]. This makes it possible for VR to be used in the treatment of phobia, where patients have to be exposed to the stimuli they fear. VR has already been shown to be effective in the treatment of the fear of heights, fear of flying, arachnophobia, claustrophobia and agoraphobia, as well as the fear of being in places from which escape might be difficult or embarrassing [16]. VE cannot and should not be viewed as a replacement for medical treatment [14].

## 1. The Application and Assets

Before we start developing multimedia software or virtual worlds we have to take into consideration for whom and in what order we will write it: we have to know the future users.

### *1.1 The Application of Multimedia*

Groups of multimedia applications are presented below [5]:

| **Application goal** | **Application types** |
|---|---|
| entertainment | computer games, video games |
| training | language education software, education, training and continuation courses, sales training, product training, simulation |
| promotion | point of Information (POI), product promos, demonstrations |
| sale | sales catalogue, Point of Sale (POS), travel promos, real advice |
| communication | videoconferencing, applications using sounds and video, Internet applications (e.g. World Wide Web) |
| information | civic and civil information systems |
| publication | image and video publications on CD-ROM and networking |
| documentation | online and offline documentation, online and offline help systems, user guides |

### *1.2 The Application of VR*

There are numerous applications of VR, for example:

- medicine – surgical training,
- NASA Space Program – Hubble repair procedures,
- military – terrain and battlefield simulation,
- training – manufacturing, firefighting,
- education – virtual science,
- entertainment – Disney Quest,
- mental health-phobias, pain, PTSD,
- physical, speech & occupational therapy,
- neuropsychology – assessment and rehabilitation of cognitive & functional behaviour, [15]
- micro- and nanotechnology,
- aerospace engineering,
- defense – air force avionics training, close range weaponry simulation, naval submarine qualification,
- heritage – heritage in the ceramics industry,
- database and scientific visualization. [19]

For us, the most important applications are those involving mental health (phobias), neuropsychology (rehabilitation of stroke patients), and education.

Education increasingly uses distributed virtual environments in training. Research currently concentrates on providing a theoretical basis for the use of simulation and virtual reality in individual and team training. These research efforts should address issues such as cognitive and perceptual processes, the conditions that promote transfer from simulated to real tasks, the use of feedback in training and the effects of spatial abilities [15].

### *1.3 The Multimedia Assets*

Computers attract children even more then picture books. Multimedia is a synergetic combination of audio, video, written text, pictures and animations. It is well suited for depicting situations, it can be interactive and it can develop skills. It is the task of the doctors, pedagogues and parents to use this possibility to train children by means of "games". The advantages of using multimedia software in develop skills are numerous:

- it is an audiovisual medium,
- it is interactive,
- the treatment or situation can be reproduced; the same condition can be repeated several times. This can help the treatment considerably,
- the display presentation can be configured. The size, form, contrast, color, size of line width, etc. of the objects and the background can be selected to better suit the needs of a particular patient,
- multimedia systems have an effect on more then one organ, and can thus be more effective,
- it can aid creativity,
- it works like a game: the child does not perceive the exercise as a chore, he/she likes it,
- the child feels success,
- motivating audio feedback can be used,
- multimedia can be used both in individual and small-group therapies,
- parents can also use it with success,
- most importantly, the child can become interested in the exercises for long periods of time. This is not an easy task, but multimedia presentations are very effective in this respect too,
- through multimedia programs one can introduce „games" that will increase the skills of the child.

### *1.4 What are the Special Needs of the Handicapped Children that have to be Considered when Developing Multimedia Software?*

In some cases amblyopic patients see only coloured patches. It is very important for them that single objects should be well separated from each other. For this, the objects have to be clearly demarcated. This demarcation can be achieved in several ways: One way is to increase the conspicuousness of the contour lines of the objects by increasing their contrast as well as the color contrast and the line width of the contour line. It is important to also introduce vivid contrast between the object and the background. This can be achieved by selecting appropriate coloration and structure of surfaces. Colors have significant importance in developing vision. (Figure 2)

Children with hearing impairments often have poor vocabulary, so in this case we have to use more pictures and short sentences.

For children with motion impairments we used a moving rectangle for navigation. In this case the child's task was only to hit a switch if the rectangle was over the selected part of the display. (Figures 1, 4 and 5)

We thus had to write short sentences, reduce complexity and use more illustrations for children with mental deficiencies.

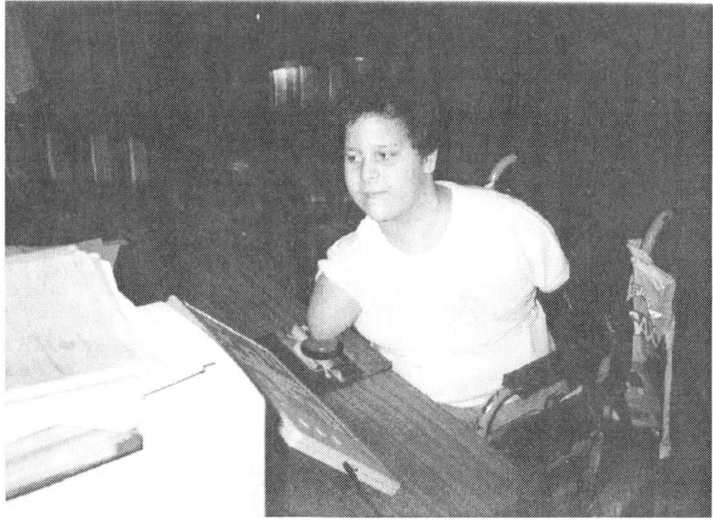

**Fig. 1.** A child with locomotive difficulties using our software

### *1.5 The VR Assets*

Virtual reality can help in three areas of mental hygiene and psychology: in the scientific investigation of perception and the study of processes, in neuropsychological studies and in cognitive rehabilitation (rehabilitation via cognition). Such a method can be applied to rehabilitate people who have suffered brain damage or neurological defects. (Alzheimer patients, cerebral haemorrhage, patients with Parkinson disease, etc.), who have learning or evolutionary problems (hiperactivity, autism, attention deficit, mental retardation, etc.) Virtual reality also has application in the investigation, evaluation and therapy of perception, behavioral and neuropsychological studies, such as:

- ecological validity,
- stimulus control and consistency,
- possibility of the delivery of repetitive and hierarchical stimuli,
- cueing stimuli for "errorless learning",
- real-time performance feedback,
- self-guided exploration and independent practice,
- stimulus and response modification contingent on the user's impairments,
- complete naturalistic performance record,
- production of a safe testing and training environment which minimizes risks due to errors,
- gradual, systematic exposure,
- distraction,
- gaming factors to enhance motivation,
- low-cost functional environments that can be duplicated and distributed [15].

## 2. Teaching, Research and Development

Multimedia and virtual reality courses have been offered to information technology students since 1998. These courses consist of two lecture hours and three hours of practice per week. In the practice classes, students learn the use of the Macromedia Director, Flash, Maya and VRML. They have to prepare some software, objects and virtual environments for the research work going on at the Laboratory. More then 32 software pieces have been developed for rehabilitation during the past ten years at our laboratory. [23] This software is used not only in Hungary but abroad as well. The following chapters present some examples.

### *2.1 Multimedia Software*

In 1999 and 2000 we created two programs to gain experience in developing aids for children with vision problems, and in 2001 we created a program for small children too [21]. These programs provide a multitude of visual stimuli; they increase the capabilities for observing and distinguishing shapes, they help see forms and generalize what is seen. Our programs teach amblyopic children to recognize objects in different colours and of different size, also on different backgrounds in a playful form, keeping their attention fixed.

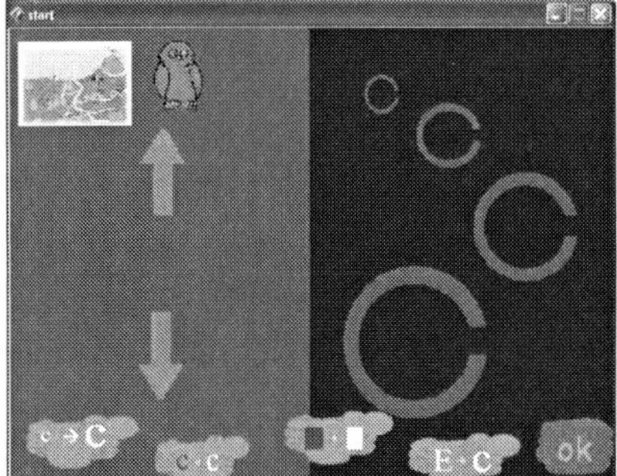


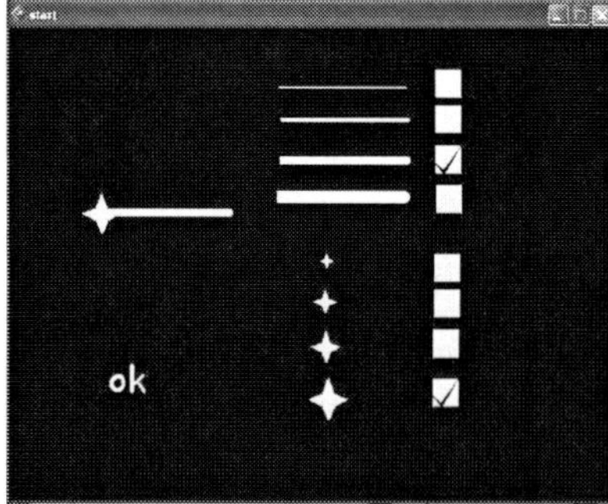


**Fig. 2.** The user can choose the color of objects and backgrounds, as well as the thickness of lines

Another program was developed for deaf children. [11] These children don't know the names of the surrounding objects, because they have never heard them. They must learn them through very hard work. Figure 3 shows the vocabulary sub-menu. It contains 14 sections, covering the most important words of our everyday life. The following sections are present: animals, parts of the human body, seasons, fruits, the house, domestic animals, verbs, school, traffic, at the doctor, closing, sports, flowers and vegetables.

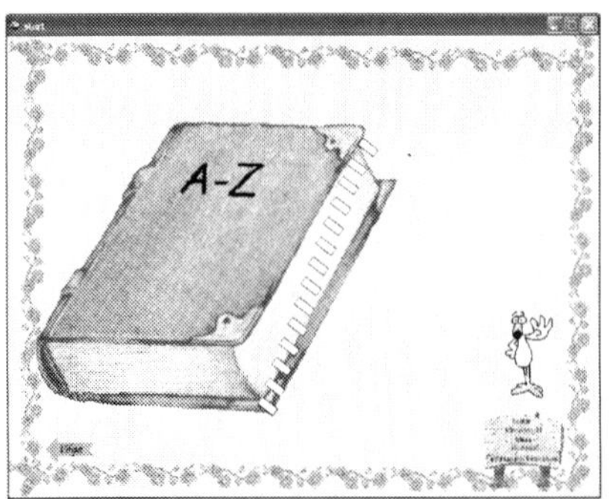


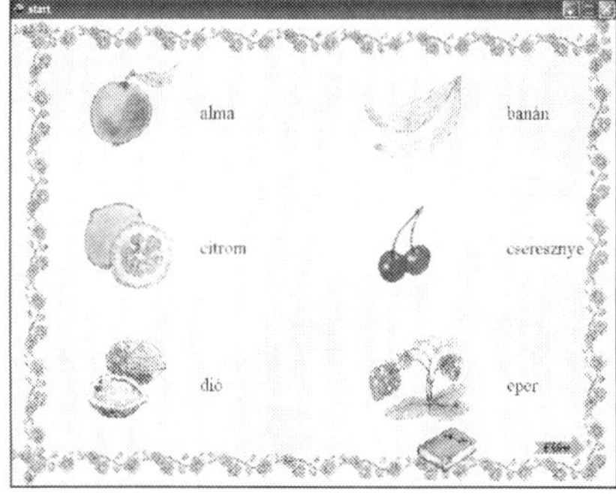


**Fig. 3.** The vocabulary sub-menu for deaf children

We have developed a test [20] and a memory game for disabled children, overcoming problems related to difficulties in movement. In our computer-based implementation we tried to adapt the test to the children's world. The pedagogical investigation part of the program is based entirely on the idea of the S.O.N. (Snijders – Oomen) test. It is a non-verbal intelligence test. The program contains several tasks the child will perceive as a playing opportunity. This test has no time limit. The first part deals with memory pictures: (Figure 4) In the lower part of the monitor screen are 5 hidden pictures, while the upper part contains 12 hidden pictures. In this task only one picture can be seen at a time. Subsequently, all top pictures are revealed. The child must locate matching pictures. The child can move the cursor with the mouse to select the picture, or, if it is handicapped and cannot use the mouse, there is the following possibility: Slowly, one picture after another is surrounded by a blue frame, as seen here in picture 3. When the picture the child would like to select is framed, he or she just has to hit the keyboard, or a special button, (Figure 1) to select the picture. This enables even severely handicapped children to complete the test. If the child gives a correct answer, the child gets a reward from a fairy (Figure 4) (such feed-back is important to motivate the child to perform well).

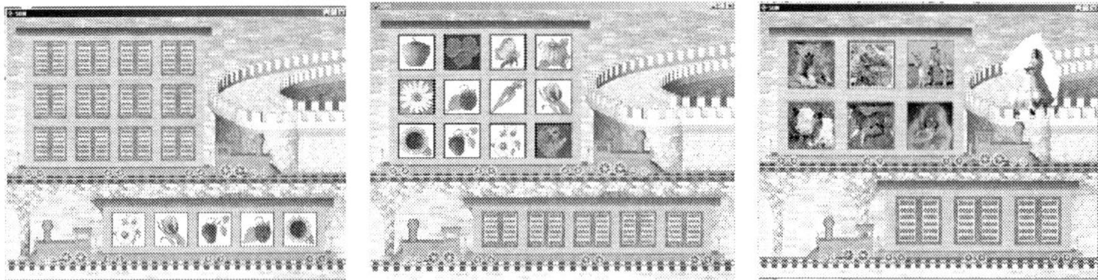

**Fig. 4.** Test for disabled children based on the S.O.N. test

In the memory test it is important to locate e.g. a picture similar to another one, match the number of points to a mathematical number, match lines to figures, match capital letters to other capital letters, small letters to other small letters, the first character of a word to a picture, the second character of a word to a picture, the third character of a word to a picture, etc. [4]. In this part of the program we have redesigned the conventional form tables into a computerised form. The animated (or jumping) number and the animated character in the $4^{th}$ row are the favourite memory toys of the children (Figure 5).

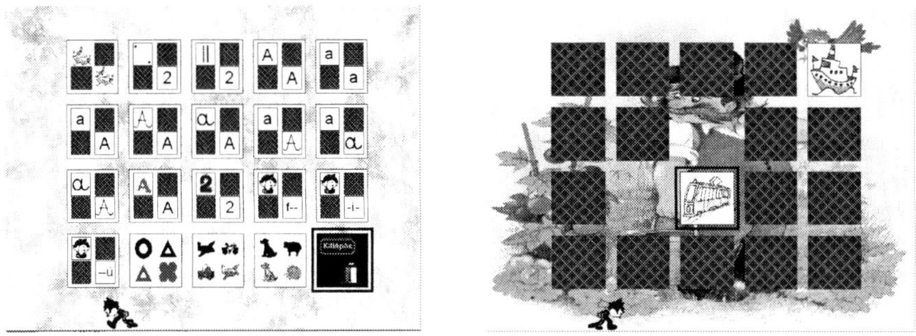

**Fig. 5.** The memory toy

As a next project, we have developed a computer-controlled method, which enables – contrary to methods used internationally – not only the establishment of a diagnosis, but also a measurement of the effectiveness of the therapy [18]:

- It can produce a database of patients that contains not only their personal data but also the results of the tests, their drawings and audio recordings.
- It is an intensive therapeutic test, supplemented by tutorial programs. It contains 22 tasks. Figure 6 shows some task types.

Materials and Methods: our approach uses syndrome analysis, thus it is more than a mere collection of computerized tests. It is built in such a form that it uses the solution provided by the patient to show the following task. As it does so, it shows the efficiency numerically. It also enables diagnostic and therapeutic programs according to the individual needs and, at the same time, it supplies exact results and comparative data. This means that we can investigate the cognitive and behavioral deficits while allowing other, intact functions to be expressed.

The system contains tasks that relate to perception, memory, attention, writing, reading, counting, etc. By this technique the patient controls the course through its procedures; he or she rehabilitates along his or her own path, i.e. becomes involved in the process and thus one can hope that the rehabilitation pace can increase in that way. A new aspect is that by using modern technical support within the described system, one can change the difficulty of the task by altering colors, changing the local or global intensity, adding noise, etc.

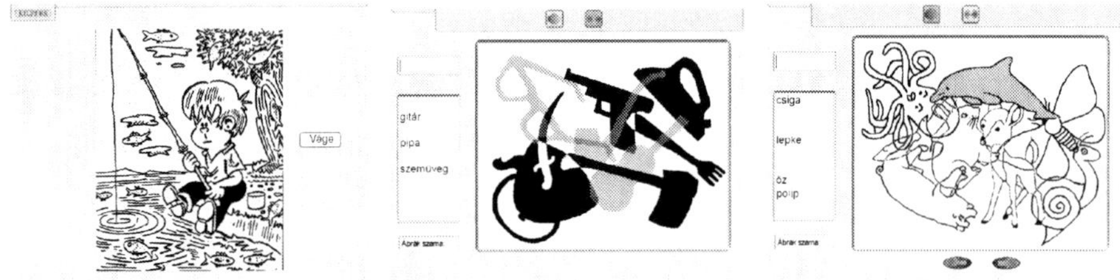


**Fig. 6.** The rehabilitation software for stroke patients provides only the necessary help

Three software pieces have been prepared for helping children with dyslexia. Figure 7 shows some tasks from the newest system. [10] The first is a drawing test, the second is a matching test and the third test involves locating opposites.

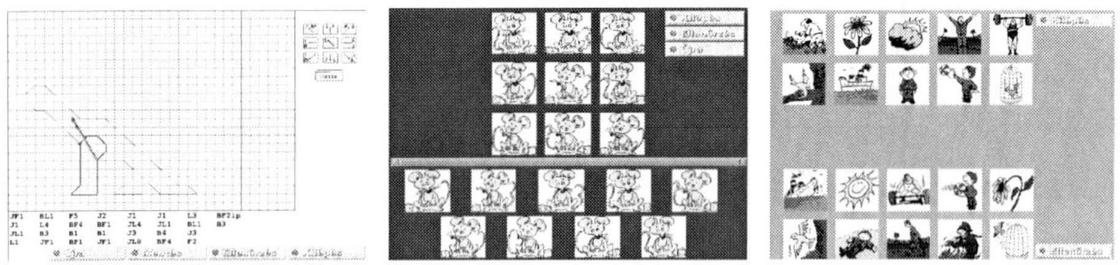

**Fig. 7.** Some tasks from the dyslexia software package

## 2.2 *Virtual Reality Worlds*

Some people suffer from various phobias and while most can surmount them by simple self-suggestion, for others this form of fear could significantly impact their lifestyle. A phobia is a type of anxiety disorder. Phobias can be divided into three categories: social phobia, agoraphobia and specific phobias. Social phobia is the fear of being judged in social or performance situations. Agoraphobia is the fear of public places and open spaces. Specific phobias are fears of a specific object or situation, such as airplanes, spiders or heights. [24] The aim of our work at the University of Veszprém and SOTE (Semmelweis Medical University in Budapest) was creating virtual environments, which could be used in treating phobias. Of course we are unable to deal with all the existing phobias, however we have created virtual worlds for treating agoraphobia (fear of wide, open spaces), acrophobia (fear of height) and a specific phobia (fear of travelling). Our investigation is the first of its kind in Hungary.

The first environment is a simple balcony of a two-story house. It has a large tiled floor and a low fence all around it. In the initial scene we can see the tops of some trees and some houses (Figure 8). After starting the animation the viewpoint takes the users closer and closer to the fence and makes them look down onto the garden (Figure 8) [7]

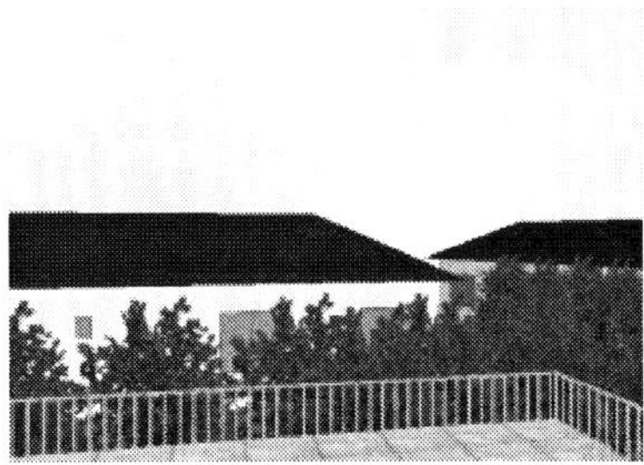

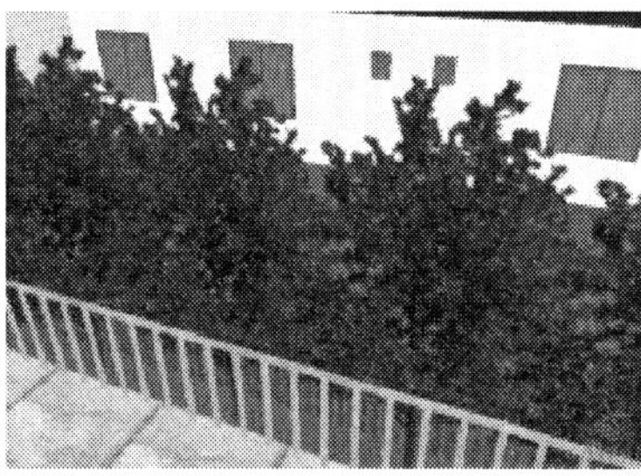

**Fig. 8.** Virtual balcony: the initial scene and looking down

The external glass elevator environment shows a ten-story building with an external glass elevator. At the beginning, the elevator is on the ground floor (Figure 9). Then the elevator starts moving up and finally the user can view the area from the top of the building. These VE simulations were created with the help of VRML.

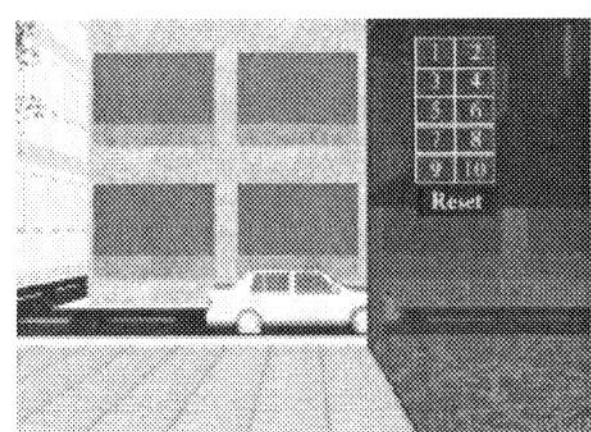


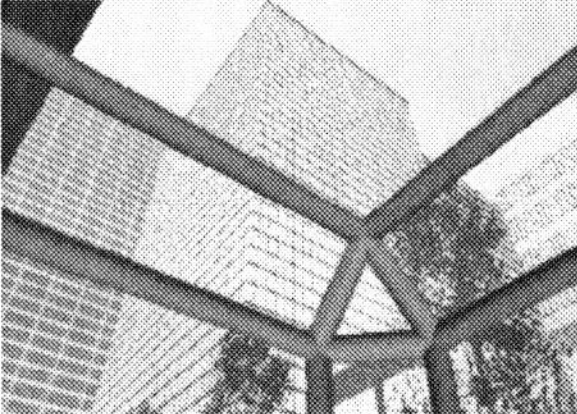

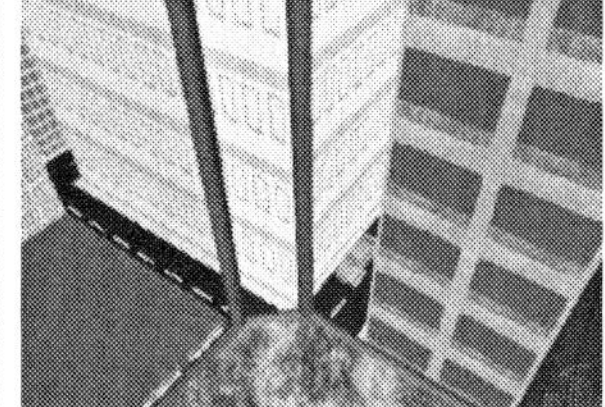

**Fig. 9.** The city from the ground floor, looking up from the 2nd floor and looking down from the 8th floor

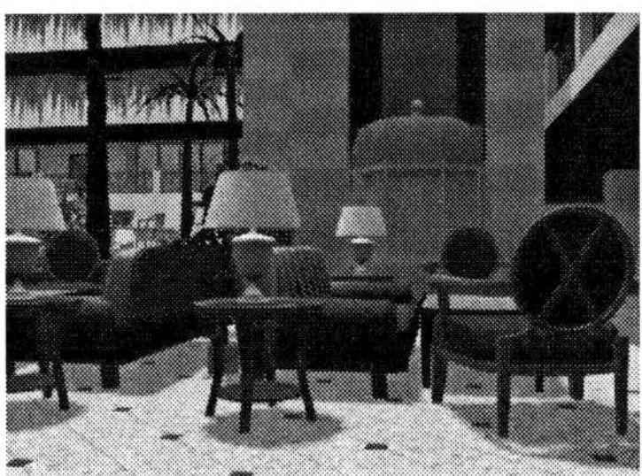

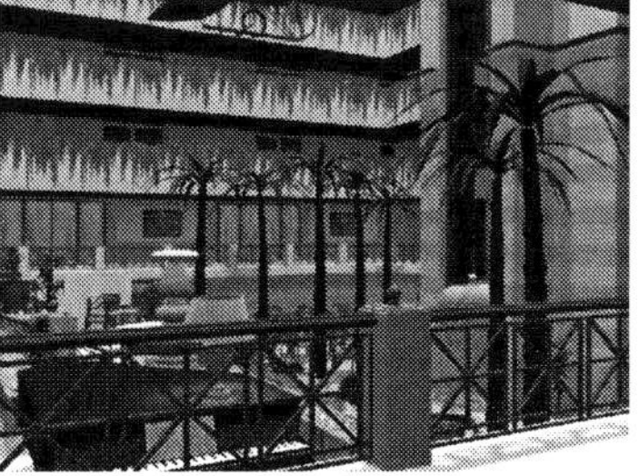

**Fig. 10.** Entering the virtual Atrium Hyatt Hotel and the view from the first floor

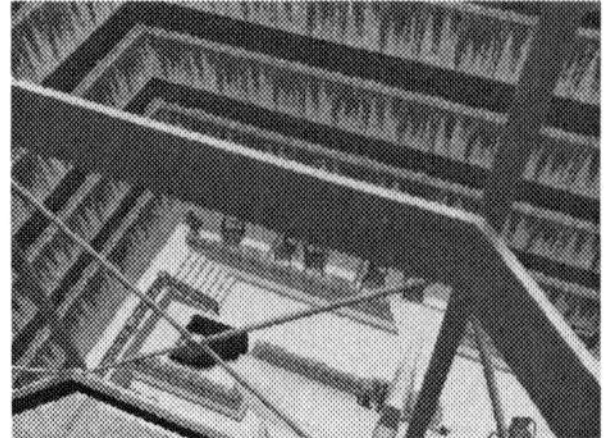
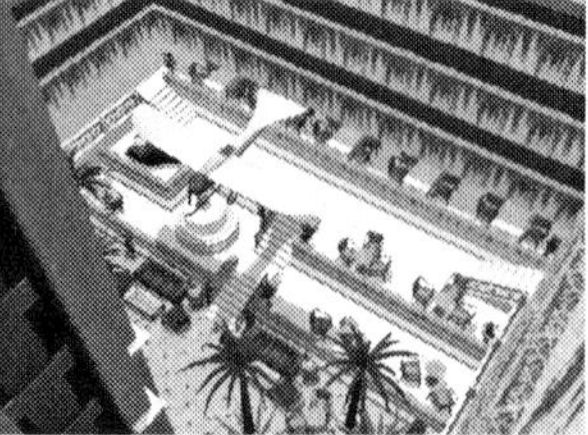

**Fig. 11.** Views from the glass elevator and from the 8th floor

The internal glass elevator is very similar to the external one, but there are some differences. The main difference is that we have developed this virtual environment by using the Maya program. The main reason for using another development method is to compare the environments being developed. First, we made a real video recording in the Atrium Hyatt Hotel in Budapest. The model of the internal glass elevator has been created on the base of real pictures of these video recordings. We would like to compare not only the developing environments (VRML and Maya) but also virtual worlds (Figures 10 and 11) with real video recordings in treating phobias [6].

For specific phobias (fear of travelling) we have modelled the underground transit system in Budapest (Figures 12 and 13) [12].

We have also developed a VE for treating claustrophobia: a closed lift and a room where the walls can be moved [8]. We are both locating and creating the appropriate hardware configuration for testing with the help of the SOTE psychological institute and some students, who suffer from light phobias. Thus far, we haven't tested environments for individuals, who suffer from complex phobias.

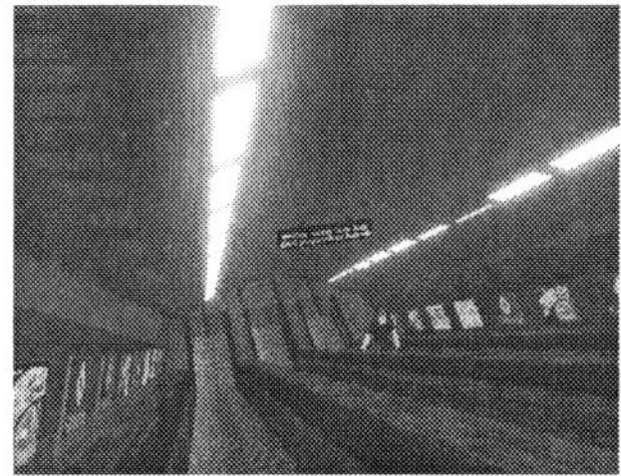
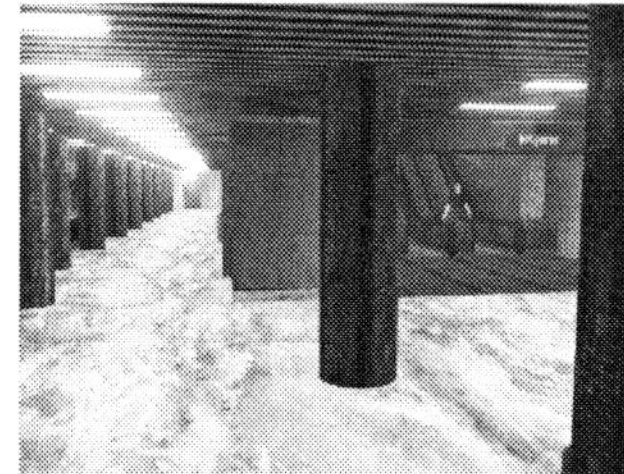

**Fig. 12.** The escalator and the underground waiting hall

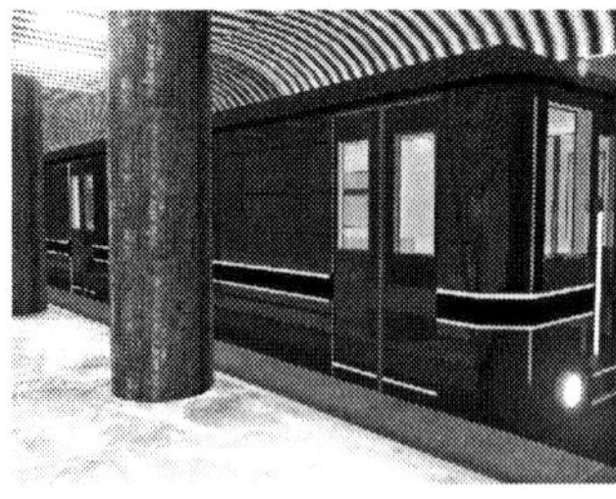
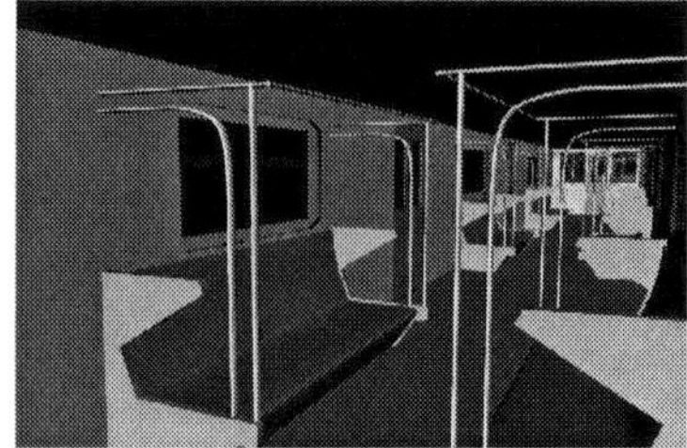

**Fig. 13.** The underground cars, outside and inside

For the education of autistic children, we have developed virtual shopping software (Figure 14). This educational software was developed using the Dark Basic programming language. We are testing the virtual shopping scenario in a special school for mentally-disabled children in Veszprém [17].

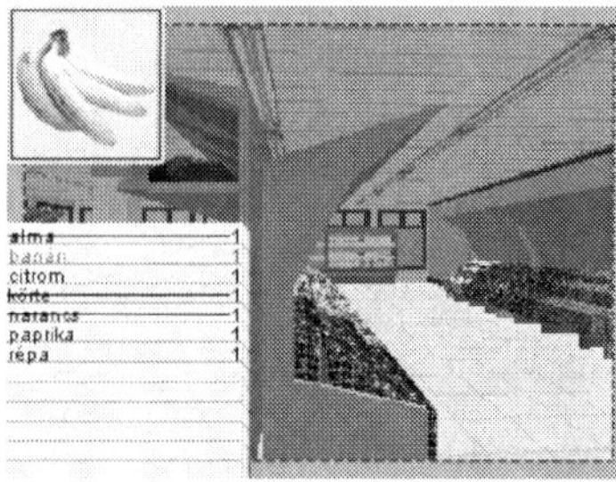


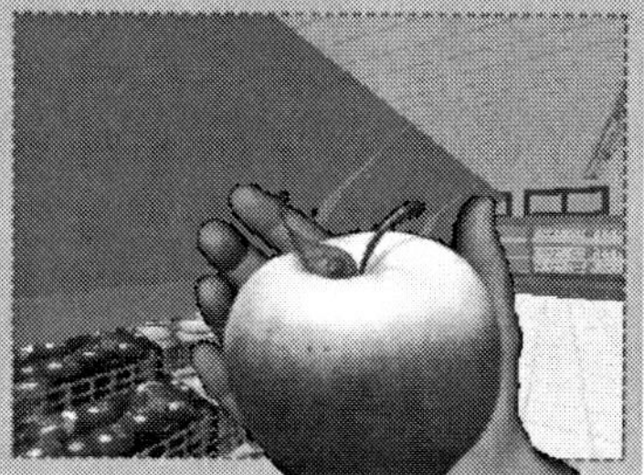

**Fig. 14.** Virtual shopping

## 3. Integrated Portable VR System

The applications presented above are currently being imported into a high performance portable virtual reality platform, called the Virtual Human Interface (VHI) [22]. The VHI was specifically developed to place the users in a closed-loop VE in which they would face a variety of challenges to help them to overcome their respective disorders in a fast and effective manner. To support this functionality, the VHI system not only presents complex, photo-realistic stimuli to its users but also measures reactions as part of the interaction process. A unique feature of the VHI is its ability to create and animate high-fidelity digital humans capable of expressing subtle facial expressions and nonverbal signals or body language. (Figure 16) Our goal is to integrate all previous applications into the VHI environment and use it as a foundation for future research [1], [3].

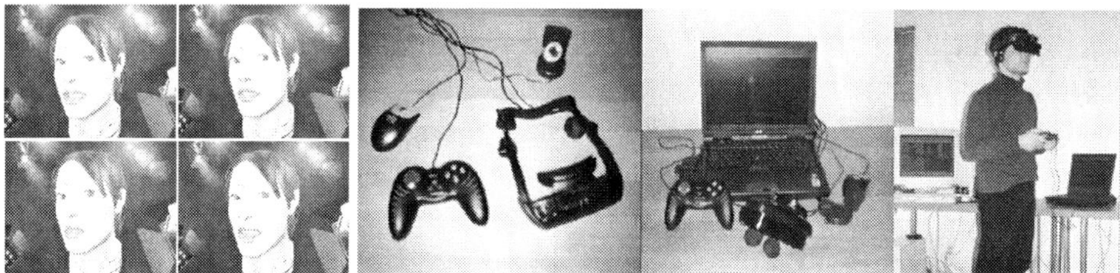

**Fig. 15.** Digital Face and the VR System

## 4. Future Plans

Our next plan is to develop VEs for rehabilitation of stroke patients (virtual home and everyday tasks). Another project involves developing a virtual class for young children, who exhibit fear of speaking and answering the teacher's questions in public. We intend to test this virtual class both in schools for healthy children and in schools for mentally challenged children. We are also developing a project which utilizes a collection of questionnaires asking children to select avatars from computer games they like the most. On the basis of these answers, we can develop new avatars and make recommendations for VE designers. This should help designers choose among the various avatars depending on the age groups for which they develop their programs.

## References


[1] Csukly, G., Simon, L., Benedek B., Szijarto, G., Kiss, B., Takács, B.: *Evaluating Psychiatric Patients Using High Fidelity Animated 3D Faces*, CyberTherapy, January 2004, San Diego, California.

[2] Ditton, T., Lombard, M., At the Hearth of it all: *The concept of presence, Journal of Computer-Mediated Communication*, 3(2), September, 1997

[3] Kiss, B., Benedek, B., Szijarto, G., Csukly, G., Simon, L., Takács, B.: *The Virtual Patient: A Photo-real Virtual Human for VR-based Therapy* , Medicine Meets Virtual Reality, January 2004, Newport Beach, California.

[4] Kosztyán, Zs: *Computer software of Memory game for accumulated handicapped children*, Scientific Youth Club Work, University of Veszprém, 2000

[5] Klimsa, P.: Multimedia, Anwendungen, Tools und Techniken, Grundkurs Computerpraxis, RORORO Computer,1997

[6] Laky, V., Sik Lányi, C.: *Using virtual reality in psychology (Virtual words in treating agoraphobia and acrophobia)*, 7th European Conference for the Advancement of Assistive Technology in Europe, Dublin, 31 August – 3 September, 2003. pp. 628-632.

[7] Laky, V., Sik Lányi, C: *To develop Virtual Reality worlds for treating agoraphobia and acrophobia*, VRIC Virtual Reality International Conference, Laval, 13-18 Mai, 2003. pp. 127-133.

[8] Laky, V.,: *Virtual Reality in the Psychology*, MSC Thesis Work University of Veszprém, 2002

[9] MacDonald, L.W., *Colour Image Reproduction*, The Evolution from Print to Multimedia, SPIE/Europto Conf. On Imaging Sciences and Display Technologies, Berlin, Proc. SPIE, Vol. 2949, pp 246-251, 1996

[10] Mátrai, R., Kosztyán, Zs., Sik Lányi, C.,: *Expandable Multimedia Software For Children Suffering From Dyslexia*, 6th International Conference on Applied Informatics, Eger, Hungary, January 27 - 31, 2004

[11] Molnár, O.: *Multimedia in improvement of deaf children*, MSC Thesis Work University of Veszprém, 2002

[12] Posztós, N., Tóth, G.: *To develop wirtual worlds for treating fear of travelling*, Scientific Youth Club Work, University of Veszprém, 2003

[13] Regenbrecht, H.T., Schubert, T.W., Friedmann, F.,: *Measuring the Sence of Presence and its Relation to Fear of Heights in Virtual Environments*, International Journal of Human-Computer Interaction, 10(3), 1998, 233-249,

[14] Riva, G., Wiederhold, B.K., Molinari e.(Eds.): Virtual Environments in Clinical Psychology and Neuroscience, From Toy to Tool: The Development of Immersive Virtual Reality Environments for Psychotherapy of Specific Phobias, IOS Press Amsterdam, 1998

[15] Rizzo, A.S.: *Virtual Reality as an Assessment, Treatment and Research Tool for Psychological, Cognitive and Physical Disorders*, Tutorial on the Laval Virtual 5th Virtual Reality International Conference, Laval, 13-18 May 2003

[16] Schuemie, M.J., van der Mast C.A.P.G.: *Presence: Interacting VR? http://www.schuemie.net*

[17] Sik Lányi, C., Tilinger Á.: *Producing virtual worlds for the rehabilitation of disabled people (Simulating shopping for autistic children)*, 7th European Conference for the Advancement of Assistive Technology in Europe, Dublin, 31 August – 3 September, 2003. pp. 633-636.

[18] Sik Lányi, C., Szabo, J., Pall, A., Pataky, I.: *Development of a computer controlled cognitive diagnostics and rehabilitation method for the use on the Internet*, The 4th International Conference on Disability, Virtual Reality and Associated Technologies ICDVRAT 2002 , Veszprém, Sept. 18-20. 2002, pp. 149-154.

[19] Stanney, K.M.: *Handbook of Virtual Environments*, LEA, London, 2002

[20] Szabo, J., Pall, A., Csuti, P.,: *Multimedia capacity developer application for accumulated handicapped children*, Scientific Youth Club Work, University of Veszprém, 2000

[21] Szendrő, S.: *Multimedia program for low vision children*, MSC Thesis Work University of Veszprém, 2002

[22] Takács, B., Kiss, B.: *The Virtual Human Interface: A Photo-realistic Digital Human*, in IEEE Computer Graphics and Applications Special Issue on Perceptual Multimodal Interfaces, September-October 2003.

[23] The Colour and Multimedia Laboratory, *http://www.knt.vein.hu*

[24] The Virtual Reality Medical Center, *http://www.vrphobia.com*

[25] Wiederhold, B.K., Davis, R., Wiederhold, M.D.: *The effect of immersiveness on psychology*, In Riva, G., Wiederhold, M.D. (Eds.) Virtual environments in clinical psychology and neuroscience. Amsterdam: IOS Press 1998

*Transformation of Health Care with Information Technologies*
*M. Duplaga et al. (Eds.)*
*IOS Press, 2004*



# Methods of Bronchial Tree Reconstruction and Camera Distortion Corrections for Virtual Endoscopic Environments

Mirosław SOCHA[1], Mariusz DUPLAGA[2], Paweł TURCZA[3]
[1] *AGH University of Science and Technology, al. Mickiewicza 30, 30-059 Kraków, Poland*
*e-mail: mireksocha@op.pl*
[2] *Jagiellonian University Medical College, Skawińska Str. 8, 31-066 Kraków, Poland,*
*e-mail: mmduplag@cyf-kr.edu.pl*
[3] *Department of Instrumentation and Measurement,*
*AGH University of Science and Technology*
*al. Mickiewicza 30, 30-059 Kraków, Poland,*
*e-mail: turcza@agh.edu.pl*

**Abstract:** The use of three-dimensional visualization of anatomical structures in diagnostics and medical training is growing. The main components of virtual respiratory tract environments include reconstruction and simulation algorithms as well as correction methods of endoscope camera distortions in the case of virtually-enhanced navigation systems. Reconstruction methods rely usually on initial computer tomography (CT) image segmentation to trace contours of the tracheobronchial tree, which in turn are used in the visualization process. The main segmentation methods, including relatively simple approaches such as adaptive region-growing algorithms and more complex methods, e.g. hybrid algorithms based on region growing and mathematical morphology methods, are described in this paper.

The errors and difficulties in the process of tracheobronchial tree reconstruction depend on the occurrence of distortions during CT image acquisition. They are usually related to the inability to exactly fulfil the sampling theorem's conditions. Other forms of distortions and noise such as additive white Gaussian noise, may also appear. The impact of these distortions on the segmentation and reconstruction may be diminished through the application of appropriately selected image prefiltering, which is also demonstrated in this paper. Methods of surface rendering (ray-casting, ray-tracing techniques) and volume rendering will be shown, with special focus on aspects of hardware and software implementations. Finally, methods of camera distortions correction and simulation are presented. The mathematical camera models, the scope of their applications and types of distortions were have also been indicated.

## Introduction

Three-dimensional visualization is widely used in medicine, mainly due to the rapid growth of computing power and teleinformatic infrastructures available in healthcare institutions. The use of computer technologies for advanced visualization of data obtained during diagnostic procedures has become commonplace in many fields. Virtual bronchoscopy is one of the examples of the presentation of computer tomography data. It may be used as an accessory noninvasive method, broadening pulmonary diagnostics, as a tool supporting real bronchofiberoscopic procedures or as an element of a training environment.

The software tools delivered with modern CT equipment enable generation of virtual images of trachea and bronchial tree from the data obtained during standard examination. The diagnostic value of virtual endoscopy is still limited and requires further validation, but with new generations of equipment and software tools, new options become available. Standard bronchofiberoscopy is clearly a method of choice in pulmonary diagnostics. However, virtual bronschoscopy may be an important, additional tool under some conditions, especially when the planning of surgical procedures is involved.

Even if the scope of diagnostic applications of virtual bronchoscopy is limited, this method is perceived as a promising supporting tool for procedures performed in the course of standard bronchofiberoscopy. Systems based on virtual bronchoscopy visualization may enhance the sensitivity of sampling approaches carried out during bronchofiberoscopy, e.g. tranbronchial needle aspiration or transbronchial lung biopsy. The presentation of CT data in the form of virtual bronchoscopy allows for overcoming the anatomical barrier of the bronchial wall and presentation of the structures surrounding the bronchial tree. The specific application of the virtual bronchoscopy technique is a development of navigation systems, supporting endoscopy of the respiratory tract. Such systems explore the algorithms of registration of images obtained in virtual bronchoscopy and cropped from an endoscopic camera.

The use of virtual reality systems depicting the structure of the bronchial tree brings real opportunity for improvement of training methodologies in interventional medicine. The main benefit of such training systems is related to the improved preparation of health professionals undergoing such training to performing real-life procedures. It is usually expected that training systems offer interactivity and imaging environments resembling real-life conditions. Furthermore, the use of available visualization techniques, e.g. volume rendering, offers additional attractive options such as seeing through walls of the respiratory tract during procedures.

The potential use of advanced data presentation techniques like virtual bronchoscopy is quite wide, but their implementation in specific applications requires addressing various types of problems. The adoption of virtual bronchoscopy in practical diagnostics or training systems, particularly in navigation systems, is associated with several types of operations. They include data preparation, data segmentation, visualization of the trachea and the bronchial tree and adjustment for distortions occurring in the optical system of the bronchofiberoscope. Data preparation should result in the improvement of CT data quality. It relies on such techniques as filtering or data interpolation. Data segmentation is performed for extraction of tracheobronchial tree surfaces from all the available data and narrowing the range of data for processing. The stage of visualization of the tracheobronchial tree leads to a digital image representing airways. Adjustment for distortions occurring in the optical system of the endoscope may follow two opposite directions. The distortions can be simulated in a training system to establish a realistic environment, resembling real endoscopy. However, in navigation systems aimed at support of real-life bronchofiberoscopic procedures, the distortions should be corrected in order to ensure maximum accuracy.

This paper addresses all the mentioned issues and explores the opportunities related to the development of interactive virtual environments for diagnostics and training purposes.

## 1. Preprocessing of Computer Tomography Data

### *1.1 Deformations of CT Data*

Input data for virtual bronchoscopy is obtained in the course of computer tomography (CT). CT is an indirect imaging method which means that cross-sections of the human body are generated as a result of mathematical processing of data obtained during many series of X-ray exposition of the same region of the body, but performed at changing angles [8]. Physical parameters of images like resolution or accuracy of reconstruction depend mainly on the characteristics of CT equipment.

The most frequent deformations and limitations of CT data include:

- *reconstruction artefacts*, which depend on the use of mathematical analysis of projections. Ethical reasons (lowering the dose of radiation) force us to limit the total number of projections. The reconstruction algorithm is thus fed little data and this results in distortions seen on images, e.g. shadow-like effects (shown in Fig. 1).

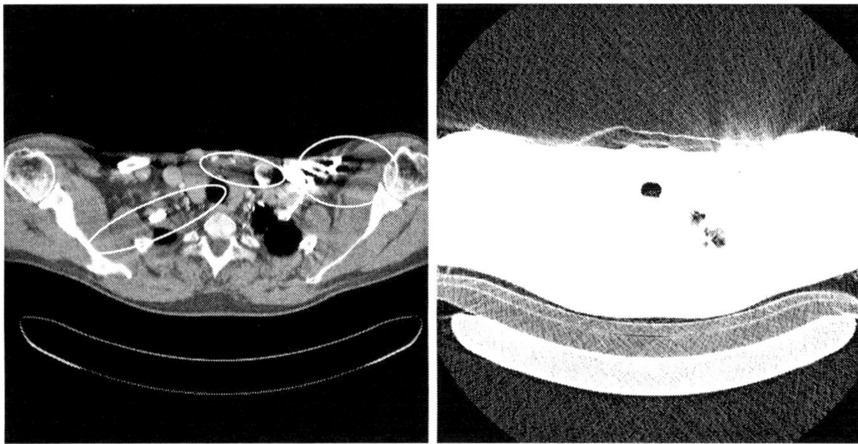

**Fig. 1.** Examples of distortions occurring in computer tomography. Reconstruction artefacts (left); noise and shadow effects (right)

- *noise*, is intrinsic phenomenon of data acquisition and processing.
- *insufficient resolution*, depending on the method of reconstruction and resolution of the X-ray detector available in the CT device. Usually, the resolution of one slide depicting a cross-section of the whole thorax is 512x512 pixels. The part occupied by the lumen of the bronchial tree is relatively small in relation to the whole chest scan and intensity values of those pixels result from averaging the densities of air, soft tissues of the wall, cartilages and other structures. Insufficient resolution leads to violation of sampling theory conditions which, in turn, results in the impossibility of unambiguous determination of bronchial tree surface.
- *distortions* related to breathing and patient movements result in the effect of discontinuity of anatomical structures in successive scans.

There are many methods for improving digital data quality. One of them is median filtering which enables removal of data points differing considerably from the values of neighbouring points. The main advantage of a median filter is avoiding the inclusion of new values and preserving edges which are not blurred. The next technique of CT data improvement is smoothing by low-pass filtering. Unfortunately, such filtration leads to blurring of image details which is in some cases unacceptable.

Data interpolation may be used for artificial increase of resolution, without augmentation of information carried by the data. Higher-order interpolation is particularly useful for additional slides creation.

### *1.2 Data Segmentation*

The main objective of the segmentation process is selection of data related to the specific anatomical structure from data contained in the image of the whole chest. Segmentation performed for virtual bronchoscopy should envisage the bronchial tree only. Any decrease of the processed data volume results in acceleration of visualization. Distinguishing chosen structures makes it possible to mark them with different colours during the visualization process. In this way, the visualization of chest structures may present the walls of the bronchial tree in one colour and the neighbouring lymph nodes in another.

The simplest segmentation method is region-growing. Starting the segmentation requires supplying the process with coordinates of the first seed point located within the extracted object and with values of minimum and maximum density. The algorithm checks 26 nearest neighbouring points for every seed point and determines if the criteria of inclusion are fulfilled for the specified density interval. If the criterion is fulfilled for the selected pixel, it is included in the segment and becomes a new seed point. The algorithm terminates when no new seed points are available. It works smoothly when the density of the structure is different from the density of surrounding tissues and the accurate density interval is known. Unfortunately, this method frequently fails when applied to bronchial tree segmentation because of discontinuity of data in lower anatomical parts of this structure. As a result, lung fragments are added to the bronchial tree.

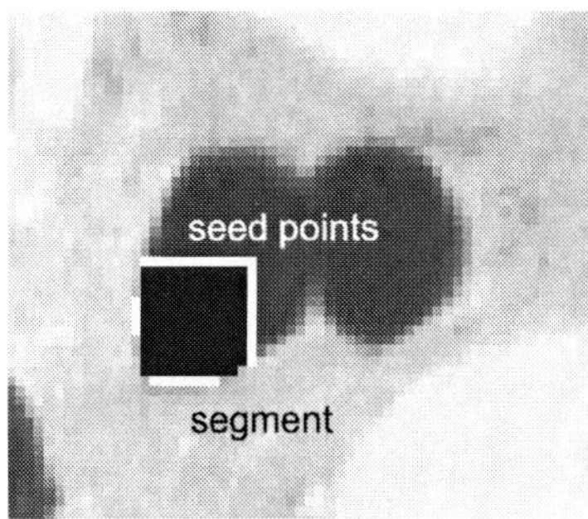


**Fig. 2.** Two-dimensional segmentation

This problem is solved with application of modified region-growing algorithms, e.g. adaptive region-growing or hybrid methods [9], [3], [13]. The adaptive method is characterized by the modification of the density interval after adjustment for volume and values of included pixels. Hybrid methods combine the adaptive region-growing algorithm with methods relying on mathematical morphology and statistical analysis (probability distribution of collected data).

Segmentation errors are usually associated with insufficient resolution of CT data, overwide intervals between successive scans (discontinuity of structures), artefacts related to CT scan reconstruction or shifts of anatomical structures caused by patient's movements. The data selected during the segmentation process are used for visualization.

## 2. Data Visualization

The basic form of visualizing CT data is a series of scans presented as two-dimensional images showing consecutive cross-sections of the body. Such a series is available as a film processed after a CT examination. CT data carry information about radiation absorption which can vary in a very wide range (the number of possible values for 12-bit data representation is 4096). The lowest values are characteristic for structures containing air and the highest – for bones. To deal with the problem of the wide range of possible data, a selected data interval is calibrated according to a grey scale. This interval is characterized by a central value, level and data range called the window width. Such an approach enables preparation of films depicting soft tissues and denser structures in the same grey scale, from one data package. The grey scale may be substituted with a colour scale and in some situations this modification enhances the legibility of data. Colour scans may be browsed only on monitors, as the preparation of colour films would not be cost-effective. Such a method of data presentation requires considerable experience and imagination from physicians using advanced imaging methods in their practices.

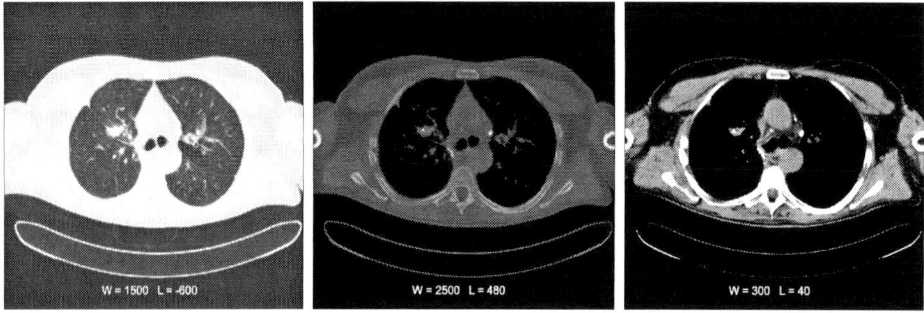


**Fig. 3.** Traditional method of CT data presentation (W – window width, L – level)

Three-dimensional reconstructions of the bronchial tree enhance CT data viewing options. The relatively limited use of three-dimensional visualization is related to the available technical resources. Data obtained during a CT examination of the chest, yielding 360 scans, 512x512 pixels each, takes up about 200 MB of disk space. Processing of such volume of data in real time would require not only a very high bandwidth of CPU and memory buses but also extremely fast CPUs, although modern-day PC systems can indeed cope with such volumes of data.

Nowadays, graphic cards also allow for the most demanding processing associated with three-dimensional visualization on PC systems. Specialized hardware acceleration enables development of fully interactive virtual environments available in operating rooms. The main three-dimensional visualization techniques include ray-tracing, surface rendering and volume rendering.

### *2.1 Ray Tracing*

Ray tracing is a visualization method, which generates images through the simulation of the light rays' routes in the real world. Light rays are generated by the source and they illuminate the observed scene. As most of rays do not reach the observer, the backward tracing method is applied. The rays are generated from the centre of the camera through the centre of the pixel towards the scene to check if they hit any object in the scene. The operation is repeated for every pixel of the image. Every time when a ray hits some object, the colour of the object surface at the intersection point is calculated. This calculation requires information about the amount of light coming from all light sources in the scene, the viewing angle and assigned optical properties. Information about light amounts can be easily collected by sending rays from this point to each light source. The concept of ray-tracing is depicted in Figure 4.

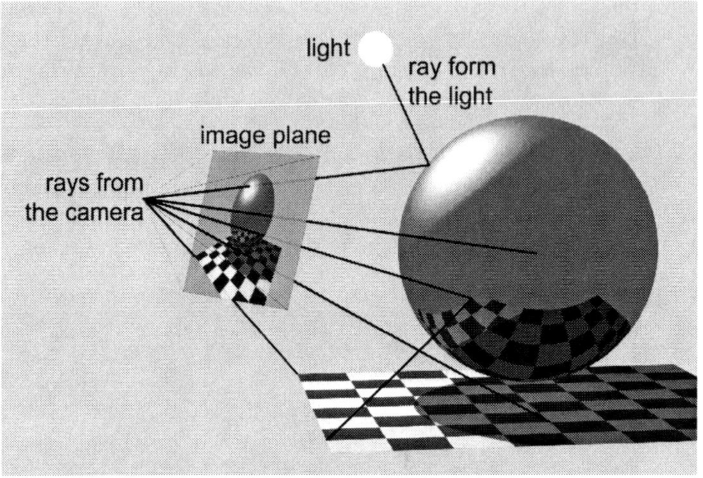


**Fig. 4.** A diagram showing the concept behind the ray-tracing technique

Secondary rays led from the intersection point are also helpful for determination if the chosen point remains in the shadow. If the object reflects rays (mirror surface) or is translucent, new rays are led from the intersection point in order to find the ultimate colour of the surface. This method yields high-quality images, but is very slow. Ray tracing methods are usually applied for objects which can be described by mathematical formulas. The existence of mathematical descriptions allows for algebraic determination of intersection points of rays and the object.

The segmentation methods described in previous chapter do not produce such surfaces. The information resulting from this procedure indicates if a specific voxel belongs to the tracheobronchial tree or not. On the basis of this information, the surface has to be generated during the ray tracing process. For each ray passing through the voxels, a local approximation of the surface according to the values of neighbouring voxels is generated. If the ray intersects the surface representing a desired value of density, the colour of the intersection point is determined as described above.

The efficiency of this method is the main restraint limiting its use in interactive applications. Each change of position or direction of the camera view requires total recalculation of the image. Efficiency may be improved with multiprocessor systems, but such solutions are more expensive and the obtained results are not very spectacular.

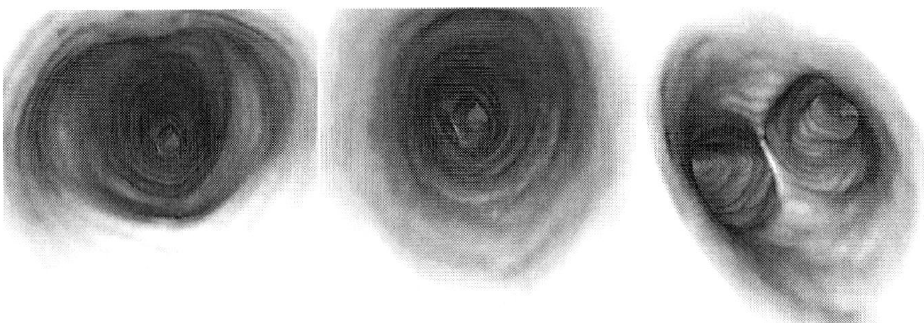

**Fig. 5.** An image of virtual bronchoscopy obtained with the ray-tracing technique

Examples of images produced with the ray tracing method implemented in VolVis [20] software are shown in Figure 5. The time of generation of one image with a 2GHz PC and 1GB of RAM was about 3s, which appears to prevent the application of this method in interactive solutions. The ray tracing method may be perceived as a starting point for more efficient methods addressed below.

## 2.2 *Surface Rendering*

Surface rendering yields images of high quality through the presentation of the surface of three-dimensional structures. This method includes two stages: generation of a three-dimensional surface from CT data and an essential visualization process relying on the image generation on the basis of prepared surfaces.

Visualization is preceded by segmentation. Subsequently, segments are transformed into a grid of triangles forming a continuous surface. This grid of triangles is found through the so-called marching cube technique [11]. It encompasses the determination of a surface fulfilling specified criteria for each eight adjacent points, then searching for values of normal vectors for apices of triangles forming this surface and finally, conformation of the surface in adjacent cubes in order to achieve a continuous surface.

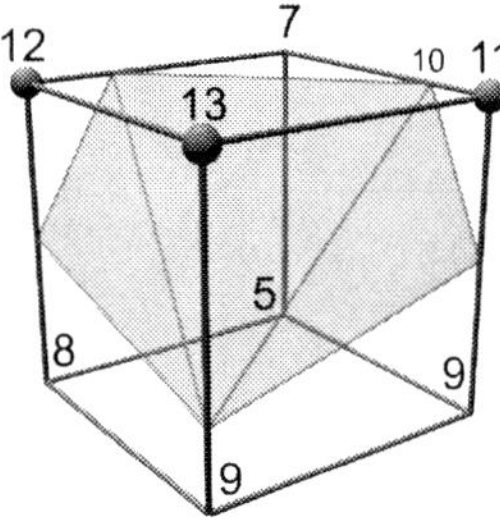


**Fig. 6.** Marching cube

The process of searching for the aforementioned grid of triangles is presented in Figure 6. The apices of the cube represent data after segmentation. Filled circles designate apices located above the surface, which is being defined, while apices without circles are situated below. As one can see, the apices of triangles are located along the edges of the cube. Their coordinates are determined with linear interpolation.

The surface of the tracheobronchial tree produced by the marching cube technique is defined by a list of triangle apex coordinates and corresponding normal vectors. Such a defined surface can already be visualized by any graphic card. However, in order to increase its visualization quality, a colour interpolation algorithm proposed by Phong [16] has to be applied. The colour interpolation process requires calculation of normal vectors at each triangle apex. The number of triangles necessary for the visualization of the bronchial tree surface may exceed one million.

Currently-available graphic cards are characterized by an immense capability for three-dimensional data processing [19]. Commonly-used cards enable hardware-based implementation of such tasks as relocation, rotation and scaling of triangles, lighting of points, texturing of several images on objects (texture mapping) and other operations, with a speed of 300 million triangles per second, and a rendering power of 4000 million pixels per second. Such performance makes it possible to develop fully interactive systems generating images with frame rates of up to 30 per second.

The efficiency of the visualization process may be increased considerably by initial determination of three-dimensional surface representing the chosen level of tissue density. Rapid improvements in graphic card performance over the last few years assure appropriate hardware support for visualization techniques.

### *2.3 Volume Rendering*

Volume rendering enables direct data visualization without creating intermediate surfaces consisting of triangles. Additionally, this method provides the option of "seeing inside" and "seeing through". The volume rendering technique is the extension of the ray tracing method. Rays sent by each pixel of the image pass through volumetric data for determination of the pixel value from all data points located along the ray route. Each ray is not stopped on a specific level, but it intersects all data for the purposes of collecting information. Through appropriate assignment of colours and transparency for specific tissues, images providing much more information than in the case of methods described above, may be produced. Examples of images generated with the VolView [21] software are presented in Figure 7.

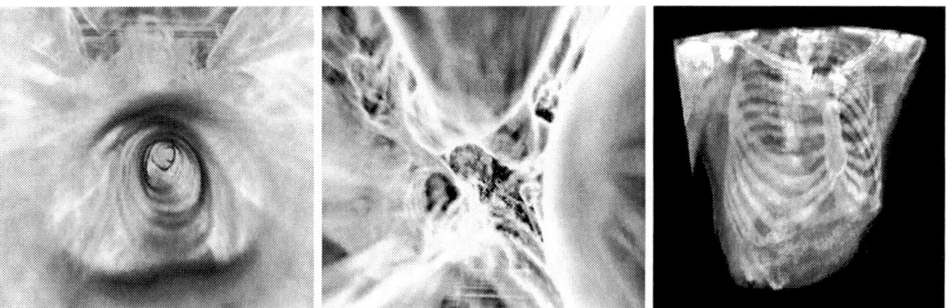

**Fig. 7.** Images produced with the volume rendering technique

Numerous algorithms accelerating the process of volumetric visualization [10], [5], [12], [16] and performance of graphic cards [2], [4], [1], [14], [18], [17] are available. Modern graphic cards are also characterized by performance sufficient for building interactive systems. Additionally, there are special cards, enabling hardware-based generation of entire volumetric images [15], but they are not commonly used, due to their high prices.

## 3. Correction Methods of Camera-Based Distortions

Images distortions related to camera characteristics are inevitable. They are associated with the presence of lenses in the optical system of the camera. In wide-angle systems, such as bronchofiberoscopes, lenses are the source of distortions manifesting themselves by bending straight lines [7]. Images from virtual bronchoscopy are devoid of these deformations, so in training systems which are supposed to depict real-life situation such distortions should be included. The inclusion of distortions in virtual training systems considerably increases the authenticity of images. Furthermore, systems developed for the support of bronchofiberoscopy based on registration of real camera images and views from virtual bronchoscopy, require correction of distortions occurring in images acquired by the camera or simulation of distortions in virtual images. Such a strategy assures improved performance of image registration algorithms and diminishes the occurring errors.

The model of a wide-angle camera consists of a linear and a non-linear part. The linear part carries out the transformation of points viewed from the scene to the coordinates of the camera. It is based on the pinhole camera model. The non-linear part is responsible for distortions related to the optical path of the camera. Distortions are usually modelled by two components: radial distortion, which determines the shift of the image pixel along the line going through the centre of the image and the actual position of the pixel, and the tangential distortion component, related to pixel dislocation around a circle [7], [6], [16].

$$q_i = FMTp_i = \begin{bmatrix} w_i u_i \\ w_i v_i \\ w_i \end{bmatrix} = \begin{bmatrix} x \\ y \\ 1 \end{bmatrix} = \begin{bmatrix} f & 0 & 0 \\ 0 & f & 0 \\ 0 & 0 & 1 \end{bmatrix} \cdot \begin{bmatrix} m_{11} & m_{12} & m_{13} \\ m_{21} & m_{22} & m_{23} \\ m_{31} & m_{32} & m_{33} \end{bmatrix} \cdot \begin{bmatrix} 1 & 0 & 0 & -x_0 \\ 0 & 1 & 0 & -y_0 \\ 0 & 0 & 1 & -z_0 \end{bmatrix} \cdot \begin{bmatrix} X \\ Y \\ Z \end{bmatrix}$$

**Equation 1.** Pinhole camera model; $q_i$ – image point coordinate, F – focus length matrix, M – rotation matrix, T – translation matrix, pi – point in scene coordinate

$$\begin{bmatrix} x_{dist} \\ y_{dist} \end{bmatrix} = \left(1 + a \cdot r^2 + b \cdot r^4 + c \cdot r^6\right)\begin{bmatrix} x \\ y \end{bmatrix} + \begin{bmatrix} 2 \cdot d \cdot x \cdot y + e\left(r^2 + 2x^2\right) \\ d\left(r^2 + 2y^2\right) + 2 \cdot e \cdot x \cdot y \end{bmatrix}$$

**Equation 2.** Mathematical model of radial (parameters a, b and c) and tangential (parameters d and e) distortions; r denotes the distance from the pixel to the centre of the image

Camera calibration, that is the determination of all model coefficients, is performed in two phases. During the first phase, perspective transformation coefficients (linear part of the camera model) are calculated with the use of algebraic matrix equations from known dimensions of the calibration pattern and its images obtained with the calibrated camera. The second phase encompass calculation of coefficients of non-linear parts of the model that are responsible for distortions. Iterative methods taking into account the sum of mean square errors between real and model-derived characteristic points of the pattern are commonly used. Appropriate selection of the pattern size and a high number of test images enable an accurate determination of distortions.

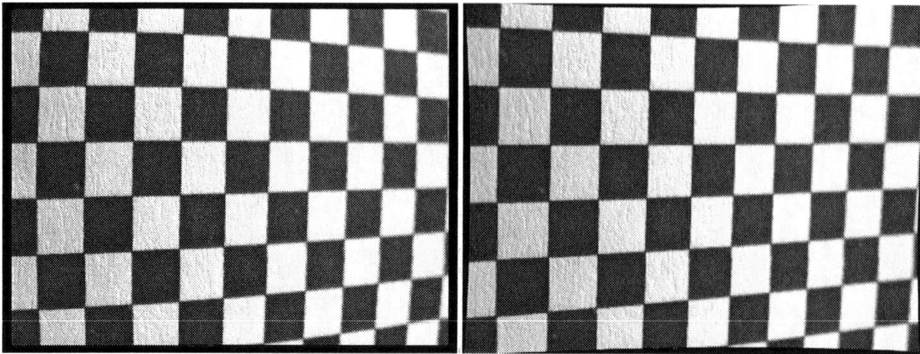

**Fig. 8.** Images showing correction of distortions related to the optical system

As one can observe in Figure 8 the image on the left-hand side is convex. The images obtained after correction are shown on the right-hand side – grid lines are straight.

## 4. Conclusion

The authors have focused on three main visualization techniques and their applicability to creating an interactive virtual endoscopic environment of the respiratory tract. It should be underlined that only those visualization techniques which explore the performance of hardware acceleration are suitable for development of interactive applications. Surface rendering techniques demonstrate good performance and produces images of reasonable quality. Furthermore, they can fully use the features of hardware acceleration, which considerably improves the efficiency of the system. Volume rendering simulated through three-dimensional textures may also be applied in interactive training systems.

The main factors influencing the quality of visualization include, apart from the visualization technique itself, distortions occurring in input data. Possible origins of these distortions were also evaluated in this paper. High-quality visualization requires data at an appropriate resolution, obtained in a short period. Decrease of the acquisition time is associated with lower data discontinuity effects. One should bear in mind that for the moment of data acquisition, the patient should hold his/her breath. High-quality data are obtained from modern CT equipment. The quality of data also has a considerable impact on the efficiency of the segmentation algorithm used in visualization techniques, e.g. in surface rendering. The simplest and fastest algorithms, like region-growing, fail in cases of data discontinuity or low data resolution. More advanced algorithms require longer periods for data preprocessing. An important element of the virtual diagnostic and training environments in medicine is the management of distortions related to the optical systems of endoscopes.

## References

[1] Berger Ch., Hadwiger M., Hauser H.: A Flexible Framework for Hardware-Accelerated High-Quality Volume Rendering. Technical Report: TR VRVis 2003 001, VRVis Zentrum für Virtual Reality und Visualisierung Forschungs-GmbH, 2003.

[2] Cabral B., Cam N., Foran J.: Accelerated volume rendering and tomographic reconstruction using texture mapping hardware. In Proc. Symp. Volume Visualization 1994. IEEE Computer Society Press, October 1994.

[3] Chang YL, Li X: Adaptive Image Region-Growing. IEEE Trans. Image Processing 1994; 3: 868-872.

[4] Cullip T.J., Newman U.: Accelerating volume reconstruction with 3d texture hardware. Technical Report: TR93-027, University of North Carolina, Department of Computer Science, Chapel Hill, NC, 1993.

[5] Hege H-C., Höllerer T., Stalling D.: Volume rendering – mathematicals models and algorithmic aspects. Technical report of Konrad-Zuse-Zentrum für Informationstechnik Berlin, TR 93-07, 1993.

[6] Heikkilä, O. Silvén: A four-step camera calibration procedure with Implicite Image correction. IEEE Computer Society Conference on Computer Vision and Pattern Recognition (CVPR'97) 1997, San Juan, Puerto Rico, pp. 1106-1112.

[7] Helferty J.P., Zhang C., McLennan G., Higgins W. E.: Videoendoscopic distortion correction and its application to virtual guidance of endoscopy. IEEE Trans Med Imag 2001; 20:605-617.

[8] Kak A.C., Slaney M.: Principles of Computerized Tomographic Imaging, Society of Industrial and Applied Mathematics, 2001.

[9] Kiraly, W.E. Higgins, G. McLennan, E.A. Hoffman, J.M. Reinhardt: Three-dimensional Human Airway Segmentation Methods for Clinical Virtual Bronchoskopy. Radiol 2002;9:1153-1168.

[10] Kwan-Liu Ma, Cohen M.F., Painter J.S.: Volume Sedes: A Volume Exploration Technique. The J Visual Computer Animation 1991;2: 135-140.

[11] Lorensen W.E., Cline H.E.: Marching cubes: a high resolution 3D surface construction algorithm. Comput Graph 1987; 21:163–169.

[12] Meissner M., Huang J., Bartz D., Mueller K., Crawfis R.: A Practical Evaluation of Popular Volume Rendering Algorithms. In: Proc. Volume Visualization and Graphics Symp2000:81–90.

[13] Mori K., J. Hasegawa, J. Toriwaki J., Anno H., Katada K.: Recognition of Bronchus In Three-Dimensional X-ray CT Images with Applications to Virtualized Bronchoscopy System. ICPR '96;3: 528-532.

[14] Pfister H., Kaufman A., Wessels F.: Towards a scalable architecture for real-time volume rendering. Proc Eurographics Workshop on Graphics Hardware 1995, Maastricht, The Netherlands, pp. 123-130.

[15] Pfister H., Hardenbergh J., Knittel J., Lauer H., Seler L.: The VolumePro real-time ray-casting system. In: SIGGRAPH, 1999: 251–260.

[16] Tsai R.Y.: An Efficient and Accurate Camera Calibration Technique for 3D Machine Vision. In: Proc IEEE Conf Computer Vision and Pattern Recognition 1986, Miami Beach, FL, pp. 364-374.

[17] Schulze J.P., Niemeier R., Lang U.: The Perspective Shear-Warp Algorithm In A Virtual Environment. IEEE Visualization, 2001: 207-213.

[18] Weiler M., Westermann R., Hansen C., Zimmermann K., Ertl T.: Level-Of-Detail Volume Rendering via 3D Textures. Proc. IEEE Volume Visualization 2000: 7 –13.

[19] *www.ati.com, www.nvidia.com*

[20] *www.cs.sunysb.edu/~volvis*

[21] *www.kitware.com*

# MEDIM – Software System for Content-Based Visual Retrieval Study in Databases with Medical Images

Liana STANESCU, Dumitru Dan BURDESCU, Anca ION
*University of Craiova, Faculty of Automation, Computers and Electronics*
*Lapus Str. Nr.5 Craiova, Romania*
*e-mails: {stanescu, soimu}@nt.comp-craiova.ro,*
*burdescu@topedge.com*

**Abstract.** This paper presents the MEDIM software system created for the study of a number of methods used in the content–based visual retrieval, based on color characteristics. The problems studied with the help of this system are content–based image query and extraction of color regions. The study of the implemented algorithms was conducted from the point of view of the retrieval quality and complexity, in different cases of transformation and quantization of color spaces, on a database with color medical images from the digestive apparatus sphere, collected with the help of an endoscope.

## Introduction

Content-based visual information retrieval has been one of the most active research areas in the field of computer vision over the last ten years. The availability of large amounts of visual and multimedia data, and the development of the Internet underline the need to create access methods that offer more than simple text-based queries based on matching exact database fields.

In the medical field, images, and especially digital images, are produced and used for diagnostics and therapy in large amounts. In some medical areas, hundreds or even thousands of images are produced daily. A large fraction of them are color images, like the images collected with an endoscope, so taking into consideration the color characteristic in the content-based visual retrieval process is of special importance.

Several access methods have thus been proposed, based on the content and also several scenarios of integrating medical images in the diagnosis process have been formulated. However, still very few systems can be integrated in the diagnosis process.

There are several important reasons that explain the need for supplementary methods in image retrieval. In the process of clinical decisionmaking, it may be very important to supply an image as a query and return all the images that are similar to it, together with the accompanying diagnoses. Also, it may be useful to query one or more regions of the image for a relevant diagnosis and to locate all images from the database that contain those regions of interest.

With the exception of the diagnosis process, the education and research activity can be improved by means of utilization of visual access methods. The inclusion of visual characteristics in medical studies is another interesting point of view in a large part of the medical domain. The visual characteristics allow not only the retrieval of patients' having the same disease, but also of cases where visual similarities exist, albeit the diagnoses differ.

The content-based visual query may be realized either at the level of the entire image, or limited to the color regions existing in images (content-based region query) [2]. In this article we present a software system, MEDIM, used for realizing two important tasks, namely:

- **content-based image retrieval study on a database with medical color images;** In this study five metrics were taken into consideration to evaluate the similarity of images, namely: the Euclidean distance, the intersection of histograms, the quadratic distance between color histograms, the quadratic distance between color sets and the Hamming distance between color sets. These five metrics are utilized in three cases of transformation and quantization of the color space: the images were transformed from the RGB format to the HSV format, afterwards they were quantized to 166 colors; the images in the RGB format were quantized to 64 colors, then transformed from the RGB format to CIE-LUV, and afterwards quantized to 512 colors. Three cases of color spaces were thus taken into consideration for viewing, in which the properties of the color spaces and the quantization degree affect the quality of the medical images retrieval with a large complexity factor (hues, which can have extensive medical significance). Two methods of color information presentation were used: color histograms and the color sets. These two modalities were taken into consideration for gauging the influence of the quality of the content–based visual process. The presented methods were studied from two points of view, namely: the retrieval quality (the ratio precision/recall) and the temporal algorithms complexity. The comparative study was effectuated on a collection of medical images from the digestive apparatus sphere. These images were collected with the help of an endoscope and they represent stomach and duodenum ulcer, ulcerous cancer, gastric cancer, hernia and esophagus varicose.

- **detection of color regions from medical images;** an automated algorithm for realizing this is very important. It is desired for such an algorithm to correctly extract the color regions significant for medical image diagnoses. We thus focused on a color set back-projection algorithm. This technique provides automated extraction of regions and representation of their color content. The algorithm performs a reduction of insignificant color information and evidences significant color regions, followed by the generation, in an automatic fashion, of regions which share a single color, two colors, of three colors (respectively). The color set back-projection algorithm was applied after the transformation of images from the RGB color space to the HSV color space and after the quantization of the HSV color space in two cases (166 colors and 328 colors). Two schemes of quantization of the HSV color space were used for making a comparison between the color regions detected in the two cases and for deciding upon the better solution.

## 1. MEDIM System Functions

The MEDIM software system was created as a part of the research process on content-based visual retrieval in databases with medical images, keeping in mind the most important factor in these images: color information [6]. The first problem presented involves content-based image retrieval. Because there does not exist a unanimously accepted solution on the appropriate color space to be used in content-based image queries, the study realized with the MEDIM system takes in consideration three solutions:

1. The transformation of the RGB color space to the HSV color space and quantization at 166 colors [2].

   The transformation from RGB to HSV is realized by means of the following equations [2]: given the triplet $v_c = (r, g, b)$ representing a color point in the RGB color space and also given $w_c = (h, s, v)$ – the color point transformed in the HSV color space, such that $w_c = T_c(v_c)$, for $r, g, b \in [0\ldots1]$, then $T_c$ generates the $h, s, v \in [0\ldots1]$ such that:

$$v=\max(r,g,b) \qquad s=\frac{v-\min(r,b,g)}{v}$$

$$r' = \frac{v-r}{v-\min(r,b,g)} \qquad g' = \frac{v-g}{v-\min(r,b,g)} \qquad b' = \frac{v-b}{v-\min(r,b,g)}$$

$$\begin{array}{l}
ßh=5+b' \text{ if } r = \max(r,g,b) \text{ and } g = \min(r,b,g) \\
ßh=1-g' \text{ if } r = \max(r,g,b) \text{ and } g \# \min(r,b,g) \\
ßh=1+r' \text{ if } g = \max(r,g,b) \text{ and } b = \min(r,b,g) \\
ßh=3-b' \text{ if } g = \max(r,g,b) \text{ and } b \# \min(r,b,g) \\
ßh=3+g' \text{ if } b = \max(r,g,b) \text{ and } r = \min(r,b,g) \\
ßh=5-r' \text{ otherwise}
\end{array} \qquad (1)$$

2. The use of the RGB color space quantized to 64 colors.

3. The transformation of the RGB color space to the CIE-LUV and the quantization to 512 colors.

   For example, pursuant to the recommendations of CCIR 601-1, the transformation from RGB to XYZ is given by [2]:

$$\begin{vmatrix} X \\ Y \\ Z \end{vmatrix} = \begin{vmatrix} 0.6069 & 0.1735 \\ 0.2989 & 0.5866 \\ 0.0000 & 0.0661 \end{vmatrix} \begin{vmatrix} 0.2003 \\ 0.1145 \\ 1.1162 \end{vmatrix} \begin{vmatrix} R \\ G \\ B \end{vmatrix} \qquad (2)$$

   The conversion from the XYZ space to LUV is the following:

$$\begin{array}{l}
L^{-} = 116\,(Y/Y_n)^{1/3} - 16 \text{ if } Y/Y_n>0.008856 \\
L^{-} = 903.3\,(Y/Y_n) \text{ if } Y/Y_n<=0.008856 \\
u^{-} = 13\,L^{-}\,(u' - u_n') \\
v^{-} = 13\,L^{-}\,(v' - v_n')
\end{array} \qquad (3)$$

   where

$$\begin{array}{l}
u' = 4X / (X + 15Y + 3Z) \\
v' = 9Y / (X + 15Y + 3Z) \\
u_n' = 4X_n / (X_n + 15Y_n + 3Z_n) \\
v_n' = 9Y_n / (X_n + 15Y_n + 3Z_n)
\end{array}$$

   Xn, Yn, Zn are the X, Y, Z values of the white color reference point. The color distance between two color stimuli points is computed as:

$$\Delta E^{-}_{uv} = [(\Delta L^{-})^2 + (\Delta u^{-})^2 + (\Delta v^{-})^2]^{1/2} \qquad (4)$$

The CIE color space represents in an equal manner the luminosity, the color and the hue, but it has the inherent disadvantage of requiring a nonlinear transformation.

The choice motive behind selecting these three methods is that HSV and CIE-LUV color spaces are uniform, complete, compact and natural [2]. The RGB color space is also considered, because of its widespread use, even though it does not possess the above mentioned properties.

Two modalities of color information are used in the presentation: color histograms and binary color sets [2]. Color histograms memorize the quantity from each color existing in the image, unlike the binary color set, which indicates only the presence of a color in a quantity that exceeds a threshold. The two modalities were used for assessing to what degree they influenced the quality of the content-based visual process.

The MEDIM system is used for performing a comparative study on the five metrics of image similarity, namely:

- the **intersection of the histograms** [2]:

$$d_{q,t} = 1 - \frac{\sum_{m=0}^{M-1} \min(h_q[m], h_t[m])}{\min(|h_q|, |h_t|)} \quad (5)$$

- the **Euclidean distance** [2]:

$$d_{q,t} = \sum_{m=0}^{M-1} (|h_q[m] - h_t[m]|)^2 \quad (6)$$

- the **Hamming distance between color sets** [2]:

$$d_{q,t} = \frac{|s_q - s_t|}{|s_q||s_t|} \quad (7)$$

- the **quadratic distance between histograms** [2]:

$$d_{q,t} = \sum_{m_0=0}^{M-1} \sum_{m_1=0}^{M-1} (h_q[m_0] - h_t[m_0]) a_{m0,m1} (h_q[m_1] - h_t[m_1]) \quad (8)$$

  where $A=[a_{i,j}]$, and $a_{i,j}$ represents the similarity between the elements with indices i and j (respectively)

- the **quadratic distance between the color sets** [2] :

$$d_{q,t} = \sum_{m_0=0}^{M-1} \sum_{m_1=0}^{M-1} (s_q[m_0] - s_t[m_0]) a_{m0,m1} (s_q[m_1] - s_t[m_1]) \quad (9)$$

These five metrics are computed in each of the three cases of transformation and quantization of the color space, following the way in which the quality of retrieval is affected by factors such as the color space and the degree of quantization.
The studies are conduced on medical images from the area of the digestive apparatus.

The presented methods are studied from two points of view, namely:

- the retrieval quality (the ratio precision / recall),
- the temporal complexity of the algorithms [1].

So, if we denote by A the set of relevant articles, by B the set of retrieved articles, then a, b, c, d are defined as follows:

a = relevant and retrieved articles
b = irrelevant and retrieved articles
c = non-retrieved and relevant articles
d = non-retrieved and irrelevant articles

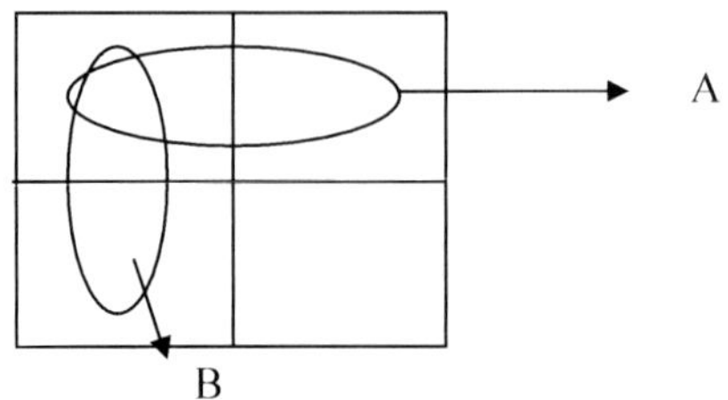


**Fig. 1.** A – the set of relevant articles; B – the set of retrieved articles

Then:

Recall = a / (a + c)
Precision = a / (a + b)

In practice, the two parameters (recall and precision) should be considered together. In this case, the better the recall, the lower be the precision. This happens due to the fact that in trying to retrieve all the relevant articles for a query, it may be possible to also retrieve irrelevant articles, which reduce precision. A system with a large value of the recall parameter, but with a lesser value of the precision parameter, will return a long list of retrieved articles, but most of them will be irrelevant. From another point of view, a system offering a large value of the precision parameter, but only a small value of the recall parameter indicates that a lot of relevant articles for the query would not be retrieved. We may thus conclude that a good retrieval system has to assure equilibrium between the two parameters.

The study realized with the help of the MEDIM, regarding the problem of content-based image query is complete. Many experiments have been performed, allowing the extraction of useful conclusions. Some such conclusions are presented in [5], resulting from conducting four types of queries based on images catalogued with the following diagnoses: stomach and duodenum ulcers, ulcerate cancers, hernias, esophagus varicose.

Another problem studied with the help of the MEDIM system is that of the detection and extraction of color regions. An automated algorithm here is absolutely necessary for calculating the absolute and relative spatial visual query.

The algorithm being studied and implemented is that of content-based visual retrieval systems realized at the Columbia University, namely the binary color set back-projection algorithm [2]. This algorithm, which can be executed in the preprocessing phase, detects regions sharing a single color and, afterwards, regions sharing two colors.

The extraction system for color regions consists of four steps [2]:

1. image transformation, quantization and filtering,
2. back-projection of binary color sets,
3. labeling of regions,
4. extraction of region features.

The algorithm implemented for this study is in fact a depth-first traversing algorithm, described in detail in [3]. Regions sharing a single color, two colors or many colors are memorized in a database, together with all the afferent information (the binary color set, surface, the minimum bounding rectangle coordinates, centroid coordinates, etc. [4])

J.R.Smith in [2] proposed a quantization of the HSV space, which should produce a compact set of 166 colors.

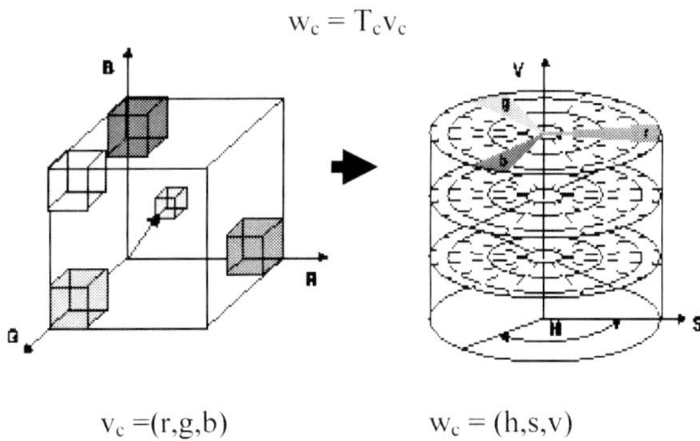


**Fig. 2.** Transformation $T_c$ from RGB to HSV

Because hues represent the most important color feature, a fine quantization is necessary here. In the circle that represents color information, the primary colors (red, green and blue) are separated by 120 degrees. A circular quantization with a 20-degree step sufficiently separates the colors, such that the primary colors, as well as yellow, magenta and cyan are each represented by three subdivisions. The saturation and the value are each quantized to three levels. This quantization produces 18 hues, 3 saturations, 3 values and 4 greys, therefore giving 166 distinct colors in the HSV color space. Nevertheless, studies effectuated in this case of quantization have shown that, for a large majority of medical images from the digestive apparatus sphere, it is not possible to detect color regions with the greatest significance for the diagnosis related to the image. In these conditions, we propose a finer quantization of the HSV color space at 328 colors. Taking into consideration the fact that the hues are of great importance for medical images, we have doubled their number, resulting in 36*3*3+4=328 colors in the HSV quantized color space.

## 2. User Interface

With the aim to fulfill the previously presented objectives, the MEDIM system offers a graphical interface for the user, implemented in the Visual Basic 6.0 development environment.

One of the most important windows of the MEDIM system is the preprocessing of images (Figure 3).

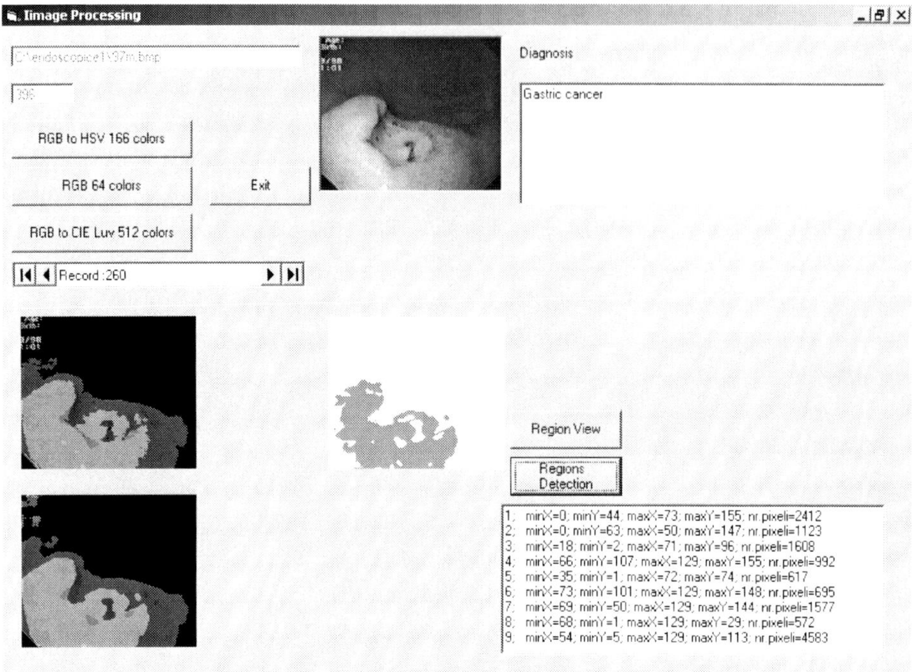


**Fig. 3.** The image preprocessing window

In this window, the user can activate the following operations: the selection of a certain image from the database, image transformation to the HSV color space, image quantization to 166 colors or 328 colors, execution of the color set back-projection algorithm with the aim of detecting color regions of the image.

The window also displays the image file names with the related diagnoses, the image quantized to 166 colors and to 328 colors respectively, as well as the filtered images for the two cases of quantization. In the bottom right corner the detected color regions in the two cases of quantization (166 colors and 328 colors) are displayed.

The image collection is thus prepared to be presented for different queries.

Another window of the MEDIM system is that which allows the study of the proposed objectives as part of the content-based image query (Figure 4). The window in Figure 4 allows the activation of the following operations:

- choosing an image query,
- setting relevant images for the current query,
- computing the five metrics in all the three cases of transformation and quantization of the color space.

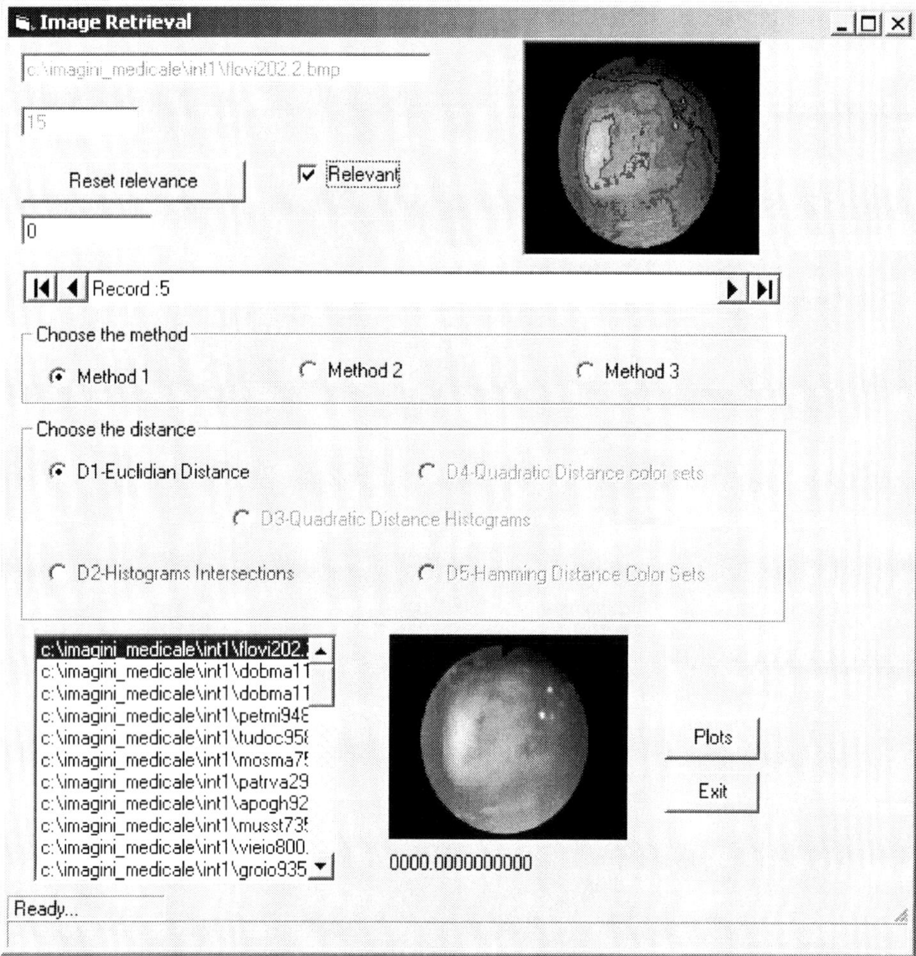


**Fig. 4.** Content-based image query

The visualization of the results obtained in the content-based image retrieval process can be performed in two ways.

The first form includes the displaying of the image file name, the image and the value of the computed distance for each distance and quantization method. The images appear in an ascending order, based on the distance computed for a certain quantization method (Figure 4).

The second modality includes the display of a complete set of graphics that allows the user to compare query results as a function of the method used or of distance. The graphical visualization allows for comparisons between distances, and also for comparisons between methods.

The comparison between distances includes the selection of a method for transformation and quantization and the construction of a graphics precision vs. recall chart for all computed distances (Figure 5).

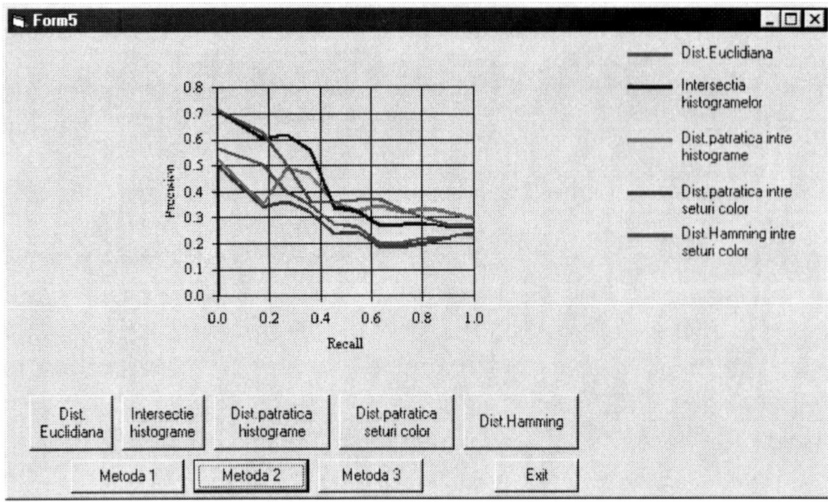


**Fig. 5.** Graphical visualization of the content-based image query

The comparison between methods includes the selection of one of the five distances computed and the construction of the graphic precision vs. recall chart for all three methods of transformation and quantization (Figure 6).

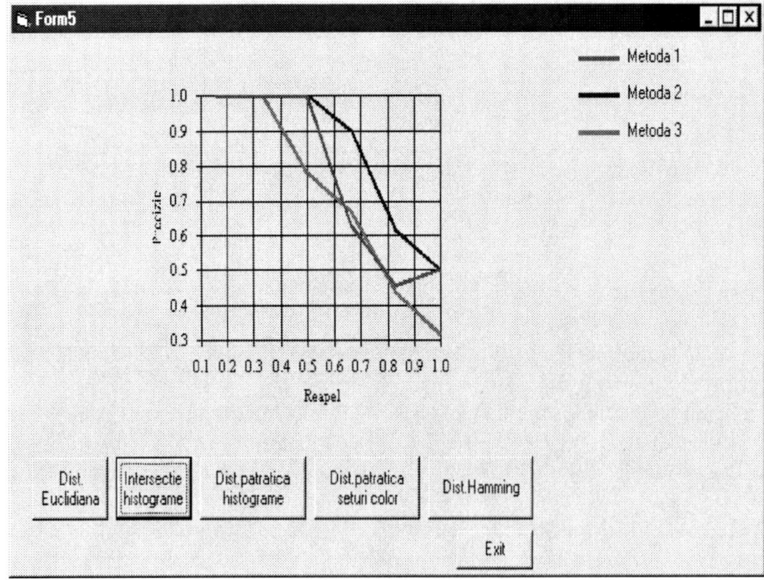


**Fig. 6.** Another graphical visualization of the content-based image query

In Figure 7 we presented some images retrieved in the case of quantization at 166 colors and using the histograms intersection.The first image is the query image.

These images originate from patients with a duodenum ulcer.

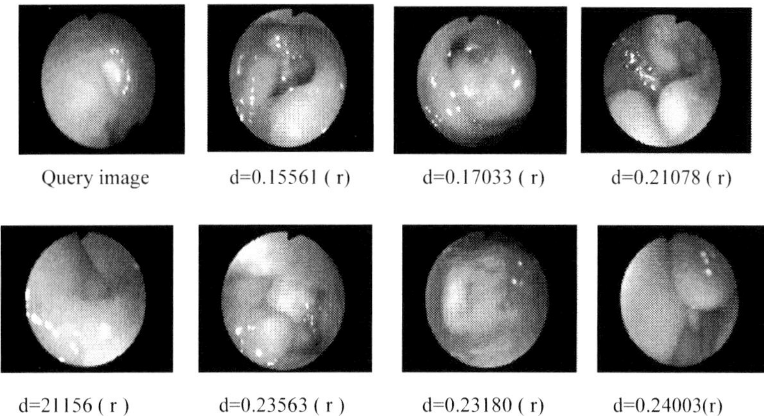


**Fig. 7.** The retrieved images using the histograms intersection in the case of quantization at 166 colors for the query image from the first position

The “r” symbol indicates that the image was found to be relevant, and the "nr" symbol labels the image as irrelevant.

The software system also presents another window that allows (for a selected image) the parallel visualization of the detected color regions using the color-set back projection algorithm – in the case of the HSV color space quantized at 166 and 328 colors respectively, as in Figure 8.

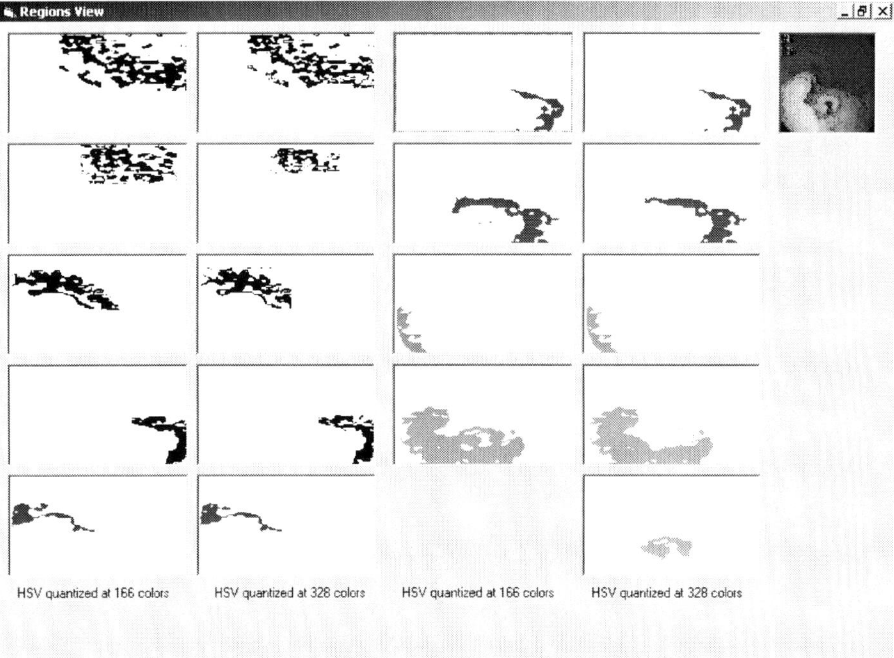


**Fig. 8.** A comparative study in the two cases of quantization at 166 colors and 328 colors respectively

## 3. Database Structure

The database which this software system is based on, contains a series of tables whose structure is presented here.

The Imtest table memorizes the image information and is organized in the following way:

- id (the unique identifier of an image),
- the path and the name of the image file,
- relevance (True when the image is relevant for the query that follows to be displayed); established through human evaluation,
- colorset1, colorset2, colorset3 (memorize the color sets with 166 positions, with 64 positions and with 512 positions respectively),
- d11, d12, d13, d14, d15 (memorize the computed values for the 5 distances in the case of the first method that includes a transformation from RGB to HSV and quantization at 166 colors),
- d21, d22, d23, d24, d25 (memorize the computed values for the 5 distances in the case of the second method that includes the quantization of the RGB space at 64 colors),
- d31, d32, d33, d34, d35 (memorize the computed values for the 5 distances in the case of the third method that includes the transformation from RGB to CIE-LUV and quantization at 512 colors),
- width (the image width),
- height (the image height),
- im_query (True when the image is chosen as a query image).

The **Color1** table memorizes the color histograms of the images from the Imtest table in the case of transformation from RGB to HSV and quantization at 166 colors:

- id_image (represents the image identifier for which we compute the histogram),
- id_color (represents the color number),
- hist (memorizes the color percent represented by id_color).

The **Color2** and **Color3** tables have the same structure as **Color1** and memorize the image histograms in the case of the RGB quantization at 64 colors, as well as the RGB transformation to CIE-LUV and quantization at 512 colors.

The storage of regions extracted with the color set back-projection algorithm, in the case of quantization at 166 colors, is done by the **RegiuniBP166** table that is in an 1:m relationship with the Imtest table. The **RegiuniBP166** table has the following structure:

- idregion (the unique identifier of the detected region),
- id_image (the foreign key),
- colorset (the color set of the region),
- minX,maxY (the coordinates of the upper left corner of the minimum bounding rectangle),
- maxX,minY (the coordinates of the bottom right corner of the minimum bounding rectangle),
- nr_pixels (represents the effective number of pixels corresponding to the considered color set, i.e. the surface of the region).

The storage of regions extracted with the color set back-projection algorithm, in the case of quantization at 328 colors, is done by the **RegiuniBP328** table, which is in an 1:m relationship with the Imtest table. The **RegiuniBP328** table has the same structure as the table **RegiuniBP166** presented above.

## 4. Conclusions

The MEDIM software system, presented in this paper, has been implemented for studying the algorithms used in content-based visual retrieval. Experiments were conducted on medical images from the digestive apparatus sphere, collected with the help of an endoscope.

The images in question originate from patients with gastric cancer, ulcer, hernia and esophagus varicose. Such a study is necessary because the algorithms, which are otherwise satisfactory in the case of a pure image collection, can lead to worse results in the case of medical images, whose complexity is usually higher.

For example, the color set back-projection algorithm applied in the case of the HSV color space quantized at 166 colors did not correctly detect the all color regions specific to the diagnosis. Quantization at 328 colors is shown to improve the results.

The MEDIM system can be used in the educational process, for example the presentation conducted by a lecturer could be augmented by information derived from medical images. MEDIM can also take the role of a support tool in computer-aided medical diagnosis, since it proves its efficiency in the case of tests performed on a color medical image collection.

In order to improve execution speed, the C language was used for the implementation of algorithms and the user interface bases on the Visual Basic 6.0 development environment.

## References

[1] Burdescu Dumitru, Algorithms Complexity Analysis, Editura Albastra Cluj-Napoca,1998

[2] Smith J.R,Integrated Spatial and Feature Image Systems: Retrieval, Compression and Analysis, Ph.D. thesis, Graduate School of Arts and Sciences, Columbia University, 1997

[3] Stanescu L., Cojocareanu C.,The Colour Set Back-Projection Method for Colour Image Retrieval, Sintes 10, Craiova,2000

[4] L.Stanescu, D.D.Burdescu, An Application for the Content-Based Visual Retrieval Study, Control Engineering and Applied Informatics Journal, vol. 5, no. 2, 2003, pag. 48-56, ISSN 1454-8658.

[5] L.Stanescu, D.D.Burdescu, A Study of Content-Based Retrieval From a Database with Medical Images, The 1st International Conference on Medical Informatics & Engineering MEDINF 2003. October 9-11 2003 Craiova

# Telelearning Standards and their Application in Medical Education

Mariusz DUPLAGA[1], Krzysztof JUSZKIEWICZ[2], Mikolaj LESZCZUK[2]
[1] *Department of Medicine,*
*Jagiellonian University Medical College, Krakow, Poland*
[2] *Department of Telecommunications,*
*AGH University of Science and Technology, Krakow, Poland*

**Abstract.** Medial education, both on the graduate and postgraduate levels, has become a real challenge nowadays. The volume of information in medical sciences grows so rapidly that many health professionals experience essential problems in keeping track of the state of the art in this domain. e-learning offers important advantages to medical education continuation due to its universal availability and opportunity for implementation of flexible patterns of training. An important trace of medical education is developing practical skills.

Some examples of standardization efforts include: the CEN/ISSS Workshop on Learning Technology (WSLT), the Advanced Learning Infrastructure Consortium (ALIC), Education Network Australia (EdNA) and PROmoting Multimedia access to Education and Training in European Society (PROMETEUS). Sun Microsystems' support (Sun ONE, iPlanetTM ) for many of the above-mentioned standards is described as well.

Development of a medical digital video library with recordings of invasive procedures incorporating additional information and commentary may improve the efficiency of the training process in interventional medicine. A digital video library enabling access to videos of interventional procedures performed in the area of thoracic medicine may be a valuable element for developing practical skills. The library has been filled with video resources recorded at the Department of Interventional Pulmonology; it enhances training options for pulmonologists and thoracic surgeons. The main focus was put on demonstration of bronchofiberoscopic and videothoracoscopic procedures. The opportunity to browse video recordings of procedures performed in the specific field also considerably enhances the options for training in other medical specialties. In the era of growing health consumer awareness, patients are also perceived as the target audience for medical digital libraries.

As a case study of Computer-Based Training systems, the Medical Digital Video Library is presented

## Introduction

Medical education, both on the graduate and postgraduate levels, has become a real challenge nowadays. The volume of information in medical sciences grows so rapidly that many health professionals experience essential problems in keeping track of state-of-the-art in the domains. E-learning offers important advantages to medical education continuation due to its universal availability and opportunity for implementation of flexible patterns of training. An important trace of medical education is the development of practical skills.

## 1. Computer-Based Training Standards

### *1.1 AICC*

The Aviation Industry CBT (Computer-Based Training) Committee (AICC) [8] is an international association of technology-based training professionals. The AICC develops guidelines for aviation industry in the development, delivery and evaluation of CBT and related training technologies.

The AICC generates and distributes three different types of documents. The first type of documentation includes the AICC Guidelines and Recommendations (AGR). AGRs represent the official voice of the AICC with respect to a designated area. All AGRs have been formally voted upon and approved by the general voting membership of the AICC. The technical reports are the second type of documentation. Technical reports typically contain the technical details underlying an AGR. White papers and working documents are the third type of documentation. All the publications are available on the AICC website.

The areas of AICC interest include guidelines for courseware delivery stations, digital audio, operating/windowing systems, digital video and user interfaces, peripheral devices and interoperability with other CBT systems. The AICC has developed a free automated testing program for verifying conformance with file-based and web-based computer managed instruction Systems and CBT Courseware.

### *1.2 ADL*

The Advanced Distributed Learning (ADL) Initiative [9], sponsored by the Office of the Secretary of Defense (OSD), is a collaborative effort between government, industry and academia to establish a new distributed learning environment that permits the interoperability of learning tools and course content on a global scale. ADL's vision is to provide access to the highest quality education and training, tailored to individual needs, delivered in a cost-effective manner, anywhere and anytime.

The ADL Initiative is developing the concept and implementation of ADL specifications and guidelines such as the Sharable Content Object Reference Model (SCORM). The SCORM is a reference model that defines the interrelationship of course components, data models and protocols so that learning content objects are shareable across systems that conform with the same model. The SCORM contains a collection of specifications adapted from global specification bodies and consortia to provide a comprehensive suite of e-learning capabilities, enabling interoperability, accessibility and reusability of Web-based learning content.

The SCORM applies current technology developments to a specific content model by producing recommendations for consistent implementations by the vendor community. It is built upon the work of the AICC, IMS, IEEE, ARIADNE and others to create one unified "reference model" of interrelated technical specifications and guidelines designed to meet DoD's high-level requirements for Web-based learning content. The SCORM includes aspects that affect learning management systems and content authoring tool vendors, instructional designers and content developers, training providers and others (Figure 1).

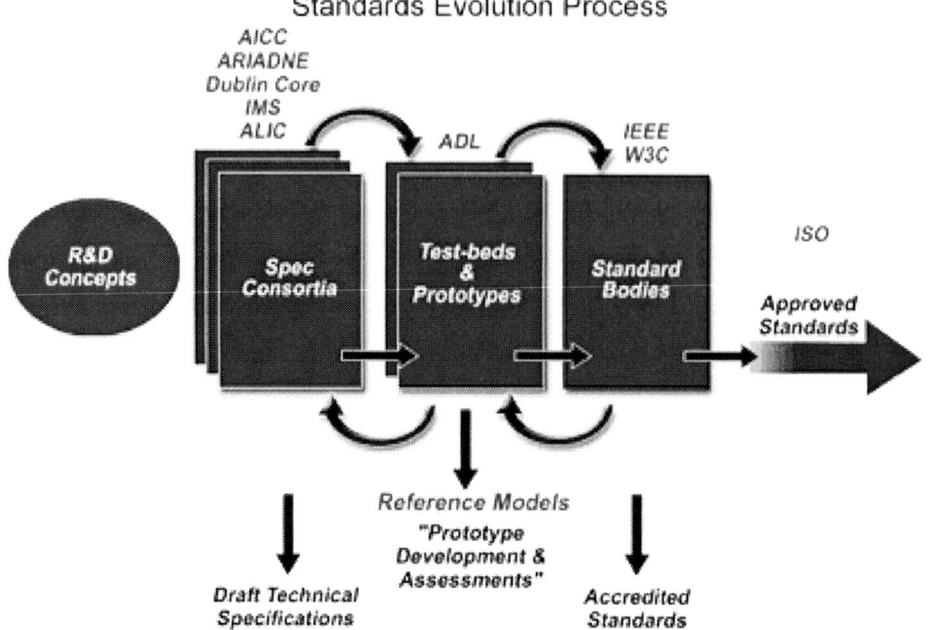


**Fig. 1.** Standards creation path [9]

### 1.3 IMS

In 1997, IMS [10] came into existence as a project within the National Learning Infrastructure Initiative of EDUCAUSE. While IMS commenced with focus on higher education, the specifications published to date as well as ongoing projects address requirements in a wide range of learning contexts, including K-12 schools and both corporate and government training.

The scope for IMS specifications, broadly defined as "distributed learning" includes both online and offline settings, taking place synchronously (in real time) or asynchronously. This means that the learning contexts benefiting from IMS specifications include Internet-specific environments (such as Web-based course management systems) as well as learning situations that involve offline electronic resources (such as a learner accessing learning resources on a CD-ROM). The learners may be in a traditional educational environment (school classroom, university), in a corporate or government training setting, or at home. For example, the IMS Learning Resources Metadata Specification benefits the learner looking for information with a metadata-aware search tool, both when the search is for Web-based resources and when searching through a CD-ROM or DVD-ROM encyclopedia on a home PC. Content developers who have implemented the IMS Learning Resources Metadata Specification will have made it much easier for people performing the search to find the resources they want, since metadata allows users to be much more specific in their search terms.

Specifications used to describe, discover and exchange content, content interaction and tracking, as well as application system interoperability include the Simple Sequencing Specification, the Content Packaging Specification, the Learning Resource Metadata Specification and the Learning Design Specification.

### *1.4 ARIADNE*

The ARIADNE Foundation [11] was created to exploit and further develop the results of the ARIADNE and ARIADNE II European projects, which created tools and methodologies for producing, managing and reusing computer-based pedagogical elements and telematics-supported training curricula. The main goals are the following:

- foster cooperation between educational bodies through the set-up and exploitation of a truly European Knowledge Pool,
- maintain social and citizenship aspects dominating education, combat the evolution towards making it a mere marketable item,
- uphold and protect multilinguality and the use of national/regional languages in education,
- define by international consensus which aspects of ICT-based formation should be standardized and what should be left local.

Since December 1997, ARIADNE has been involved in standardization activities performed under the auspices of the IEEE LTSC Committee. In this context, ARIADNE has agreed to collaborate with the US-funded Educause IMS Project, in view of reaching (as quickly as possible) an educational metadata set that would be widely acceptable. This collaborative work has produced various successive IEEE Working Documents that draw largely on ARIADNE's inputs. Version 2.2 and then version 3.4 of this document have been adopted by the IMS Project for its own use (IMS is now working to synchronize its metadata with LOM 6.1).

ARIADNE is also active in the standardization activities initiated by the European Commission, taking place under the auspices of CEN/LTWS (Learning Technologies Workshop). Work in this forum is now (amongst other subjects) concentrating on the "localization" of the mainly English language results obtained so far by the IEEE.

ARIADNE has recently established cooperation with the ADL Initiative US Project, whose SCORM specification relies on LOM metadata.

### *1.5 LTSC*

The IEEE Learning Technology Standards Committee (LTSC) [12] is chartered by the IEEE Computer Society Standards Activity Board to develop accredited technical standards, recommended practices, and guides for learning technology.

The LTSC coordinates formally and informally with other organizations that produce specifications and standards for similar purposes. Standards development is done in working groups via a combination of face-to-face meetings, teleconferences, and exchanges on discussion groups. The LTSC is governed by a Sponsor Executive Committee (SEC) consisting of working group chairs and elected officers. The main working areas include: the Architecture and Reference Model (LTSA), the Digital Rights Expression Language (DREL), Computer-Managed Instruction (CMI), Learning Object Metadata (LOM) and Competency Definitions (RCD).

### *1.6 CEN/ISSS Workshop on Learning Technology (WSLT)*

One of the European organizations developing e-learning standards is CEN (Committee European de Normalization, European Committee for Standardization). Its ISSS division (Information Society Standardization System) develops industry standards, mostly aimed at the promotion of European companies. The effect of their work on the area of e-Learning is the Workshop on Learning Technology [1]. Membership in this workshop is only by invitation.

The areas the WSLT is working on, are as follows:

- internationalization of the Learning Object Metadata,
- standardized educational copyright,
- quality assurance process standards (similar to ISO 9000),
- educational modeling language (EML),
- a repository of taxonomies (standardized codes) for European learning.

### *1.7 Advanced Learning Infrastructure Consortium (ALIC)*

ALIC is a Japanese consortium (composed of public and private organizations), which promotes the adoption e-learning in Japan. ALIC is supported by industry, academia and government bodies, and it participates in international meetings. ALIC is managed as a part of IPA (the Information Technology Promotion Agency, a special certification authority of the Ministry of Economy, Trade and Industry) business [2].

ALIC's objectives are:

- to reasonably and effectively provide a learning environment which enables anyone to learn anytime and anywhere, according to the goals, pace, interests and understanding of individuals and groups,
- to foster people of expertise,
- to achieve global competitiveness,
- to build an active society.

### *1.8 Education Network Australia (EdNA)*

The Australian consortium EdNA [3] is a collaborative framework involving all Australian training and education authorities focused on maximizing the benefits of the Internet to their stakeholders. EdNA Online is the 'portal' or 'gateway' to information and creation of a range of technical standards. AICTEC (the Australian ICT in Education Committee) is the guiding committee of EdNA.

As an information service, EdNA Online provides two key functions:

- a directory on education and training in Australia,
- a database of Web-based resources useful for teaching and learning.

### *1.9 PROmoting Multimedia access to Education and Training in European Society (PROMETEUS)*

In March 1999, an open initiative called PROMETEUS was introduced. The initiative is sponsored by the European Commission with the aim of building a common approach to the production and provision of e-learning techniques and content in Europe. It operates via a Memorandum of Understanding (MoU) signed by all members, sponsors and expert communities [5].

The objectives of the PROMETEUS signatories, as laid out in the MoU, are:

- to improve the effectiveness of cooperation between education and training authorities and establishments, users of learning technologies, service and content providers and producers within the European Community including the Commission of the European Communities (the European Commission),
- to foster the development of common European and international standards for digital

multimedia learning content and services,
- to give a global dimension to their cooperation, and to conduct open and effective dialogues on issues relating to learning technologies policy with policymakers in other regions of the world, while upholding Europe's cultural interests and specificities,
- to consider that the way to achieve these goals is by following certain common guidelines organizing their future cooperation,
- to consider that these guidelines should be based upon an analysis of the needs expressed by users of the information and communication technologies (ICT) in the education and training sector.

### *1.10 The Sun ONE Architecture and the iPlanet™ Products*

Sun Microsystems supports many of the above mentioned learning standards. The Sun ONE architecture and the iPlanet™ product suite are well-suited to supporting demands of e-learning in education, composed of tools and content from multiple vendors working together through e-learning interoperability standards. Sun platforms and technology allow the education community to pick and choose the best tools and content without being locked into any particular product or environment (in truth – except those provided by Sun) [6] [7].

Sun's e-learning standards are aimed at:
- utilization of open standards and techniques in order to ensure operability across heterogeneous platforms, systems and environments,
- leverage on existing systems while affording services-on-demand flexibility,
- accommodation of short and long-term software architecture needs,
- impact on immediate business challenges with proven, scalable products,
- limiting software integration costs by operating out-of-the-box with other Sun ONE products,
- cooperation with network infrastructure companies that understands mission-critical product and support needs.

## 2. The Opportunities Related to Telelearning in Medical Education

Health professionals remain under continuous pressure for presenting high-quality up-to-date competencies concordant with evidence-based medicine guidelines. This pressure comes from the empowered consumers well aware of their health status needs. Furthermore, the relative shortage of health professionals all over the world pushes those professionals to take on additional responsibilities and services. The domain of medical sciences and practice is particularly extensive and still growing. In most countries, physicians are supposed to undertake educational and training activities in order to achieve an annual credit points threshold. Such activities are time-consuming and therefore telelearning is perceived as an efficient tool to ensure appropriate training opportunities for health professional. In this context, their extensive integration with tasks performed in the workplace seems to be a reasonable option. Harun has proposed a classification of telelearning activities including just-in-time continuing of medical education (information enhancing consecutive patients management), formal distant learning (online courses enabling certification by accredited organizations), modular distance learning (condensed modules maintaining the level of competencies and skills) and, finally, personalized continuing medical education, designating information and skills chosen according to individual needs and interests of health professionals [13].

The track of continued professional education in medicine depends strongly on individual preferences as well as on the variety of tasks performed and career steps faced by the physician. As the continuation of medical education and training is a highly individualized process, distance learning is an efficient tool to reach the personal objectives related to professional formation. E-learning strategies enable us to overcome the challenges of postgraduate medical training, including different patterns of study, availability and learning needs of health professionals [14]. The key benefits related to the use of the e-learning approach encompass time flexibility, cost savings, self-paced and "just-for-me" learning opportunities and unlimited use of learning resources.

The impact of information technology on medical education is clearly appreciated by organizations responsible for medical education on various levels. The results of a survey published in 2000 by the Association of American Medical Colleges indicated that 45 of 130 schools require students to have their own computers upon admission to medical schools, and others offer round-the-clock computer facilities to students [15]. Furthermore, the Internet is commonly perceived as a platform for self-directed medical learning and research. Finally, many faculties develop software used in their courses and computers are used to teach EBM strategy and to search through literature.

The World Federation for Medical Education Standing Advisory Committee issued a set of guidelines on use of IT tools in this area [16]. Its recommendations include development of online learning materials, provision of access to computer technologies in medical education, integration of computer science into curricula, planning the migration from conventional learning methods and assuring advice on production of electronic learning materials.

It also seems that e-learning may be an attractive strategy for the development of training programs in interventional and surgical domains of medicine [17]. Multimedia contents delivery improves e-learning results as multi-sensory environment accelerates information retention. The use of multimedia materials may also accelerate the process of practical skills development. Furthermore, advanced visualization techniques allow for creation of virtual environments resembling real-life conditions. Browsing digital video resources with recordings of interventional procedures prepares physicians for situations which may occur during their training. Medical digital video libraries may also be used as a basis for a problem-based learning approach during specialization courses.

## 3. Case Study (Medical Digital Video Library)

The development of a medical digital video library with recordings of invasive procedures incorporating additional information and commentaries may improve the efficiency of the training process in the interventional domains of medicine. The digital video library, enabling access to videos of interventional procedures performed in the range of thoracic medicine, may be a valuable element of developing practical skills. The library has been filled with video resources recorded at the Department of Interventional Pulmonology, enhancing training options for pulmonologists and thoracic surgeons. The main focus was put on demonstration of bronchofiberoscopic and videothoracoscopic procedures. The opportunity to browse video recordings of procedures performed in the specific field considerably enhances the options for training in other medical specialities. In an era of growing health consumer awareness, patients are also perceived as the target audience for medical digital libraries (Figure 2).

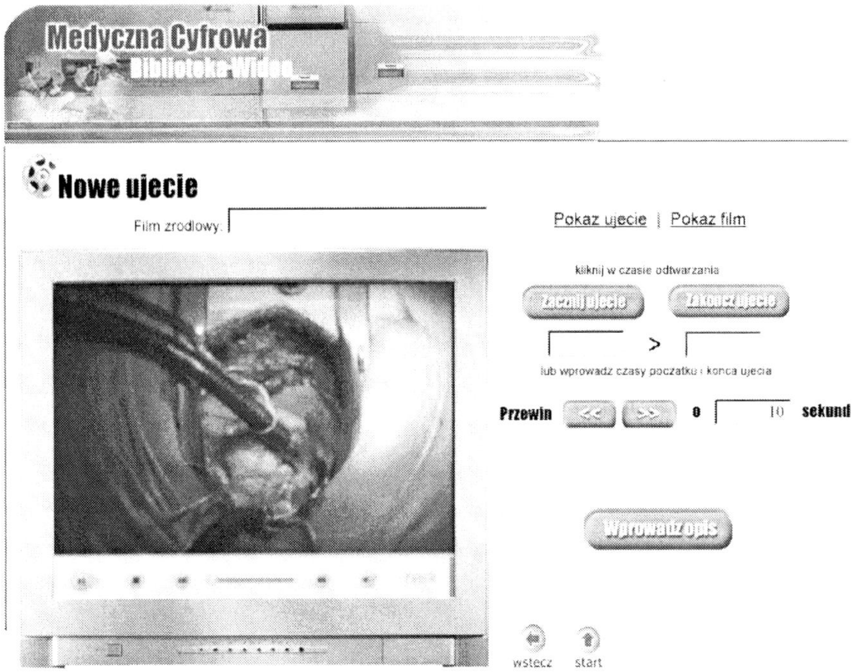


**Fig. 2.** Medical Digital Video Library

Digitized recordings are stored on hard disks to be described by the library administrator. The first information consists of dimensions and duration, which is extracted automatically and added to the database. The second step is creating human-readable descriptions, such as titles, authors, keywords and other medical-specific explanations, by leading doctors for final presentation. Subsequently, the prepared films are processed by specialists.

Doctors isolate the most interesting scenes by specifying theirs beginning and ending timestamps. The scenes can be viewed separately or can be joined in separate sequences, with their own descriptions.

Each material prepared for viewing, has some description fields, such as title, author and other medical-specific information. Each of them can serve as a key for a search. The end user can obtain access to materials prepared earlier, using any user interface. The most popular and easiest way to implement this functionality is through a Web browser. This eliminates the necessity of installing any software on the end user's computer, other than an operating system with a plugin-enabled browser.

## 4. Conclusions

Nowadays, many e-learning standards are emerging, some of them are described in this paper. The most advanced standard is the SCORM model, created by the ADL consortium. It consolidates the results of efforts by various bodies and it is accepted by the ISO standardization organization as a key model for e-learning standards. A simplified model was presented in the MDVL case study. The digital library is also used as a diagnostic medical tool and will be further developed to better match local needs.

## References


[1] "CEN Learning Technologies Workshop" *http://www.cenorm.be/*
[2] "About ALIC", *http://www.alic.gr.jp/eng/index.htm*
[3] "Welcome to EdNA Online", *http://www.edna.edu.au/*
[4] "Welcome to AICTEC", *http://www.aictec.edu.au/*
[5] "PROMETEUS", *http://www.prometeus.org/*
[6] Sun Microsystems, "e-Learning Applications Infrastructure", *http://www.sun.com/products-n-solutions/edu/whitepapers/pdf/eLearning_Application_Infrastructure_wp.pdf*
[7] Sun Microsystems, "e-Learning Interoperability Standards", *http://www.sun.com/products-n-solutions/edu/elearning/eLearning_Interoperability_Standards_wp.pdf*
[8] "AICC", *http://www.aicc.org/*
[9] "ADL", *http://www.adlnet.org/*
[10] "IMS", *http://www.imsproject.org/*
[11] "ARIADNE", *http://www.ariadne-eu.org/*
[12] "IEEE LTSC", *http://ltsc.ieee.org/*,
[13] Harun M.H.: Integrating e-Learning into the workplace. Internet and Higher Education 2002; 4: 301-310,
[14] Grant J.: The Flexible Use of Distance Learning in a Professional Context: the Medical Experience. In: Distance Education Futures, ed. Ted Nunan, 1993, pp.309-329,
[15] Anderson M.B.: A guide to the 130 reports in this Snapshot supplement to Academic Medicine. Acad Med 2000; 75: 0-b,
[16] Winding O. and WFME Standing Advisory Committee. Guidelines for Using Information and Communication Technology in Medical Education. *http://www.sund.ku.dk/wfme/Activities/WFME%20Guidelines%20Info%20and%20Communic%20Tech.htm*
[17] El-Khalili N.H., Brodlie K.W.: Surgical training on the web. Future Generation Comp Sys 2000; 17: 147-158

# 5. PRO-ACCESS – Lessons Learned

# Beyond Wishful Thinking; Medical Community Presence on the Web and Challenges of Pervasive Healthcare

Ioana MOISIL, Boldur E. BARBAT
*Lucian Blaga University of Sibiu, Hermann Oberth Faculty of Engineering, Sibiu, Romania*
*e-mail: ioana.moisil@ulbsibiu.ro*

**Abstract.** Romanian healthcare is facing a number of challenges, from the growing general costs, through requests for better services, inadequate territorial coverage, medical errors and a growing incidence of chronic diseases, to the burden of debt toward the pharmaceutical industry. For the last 14 years decision factors have been searching for the magic formula in restructuring the healthcare sector. Eventually, the government has come to appreciate the benefits of IT solutions. Our paper presents recent advances in wireless technologies and their impact on healthcare, in parallel with the results of a study aimed to acknowledge the presence of the medical community on Romanian WWW and to evaluate the degree of accessibility for the general population. We have documented Web sites promoting health services, discussion forums for patients, online medical advice, medical image teleprocessing, health education, health research and documentation, pharmaceutical products, e-procurement, health portals, medical links, hospitals and other health units present on the Web. Initial results have shown that if the current trend in price decreases for mobile communications continues and if the government is able to provide funding for the communication infrastructure needed for pervasive healthcare systems together with the appropriate regulations and standards, this can be a long-term viable solution of the healthcare crisis.

## Introduction

The brave new world of telecommunications that we are witnessing is a very challenging one. It seems that we have voted for a wireless world and more and more people everywhere are benefiting from and even enjoying the possibilities of communicating in a world without wires.

Wireless technology, with all kinds of intelligent mobile devices, wearable networks, handheld devices, remote micro-cameras sending images from inside the human body to the physician's computer or picturing the environment, are now present in all corners of the world and tend to become ubiquitous and pervasive.

*Ubiquitous* is the property of being present in different places, *everywhere, at the same time*, emphasizing the disappearance of distance between any two points in space. *Pervasive computing* is a concept with a heavier meaning, for it assumes the property being not only omnipresent but also having an insidious character, being able to override all barriers and cross borders.

## 1. Pervasive Healthcare

Healthcare all over the world is facing difficulties. Managers and professionals have to face limited financial and human resources, the exponential grows of the information to be captured, populations with a great degree of mobility and with a higher life expectancy, new diseases, health and environmental hazards and health-related terrorism. And all this in the context of a world economy that also seems to be ill.

It has been proved that IT applications, when well designed, developed and implemented, can dramatically reduce health costs and improve the quality of health services. There are strong hopes that wireless/mobile technology integrated with existing middleware information systems will be a solution for the healthcare crisis. The main argument in favor of this approach is that information delivery is critical to all healthcare aspects and if we manage to have good information delivered "anytime, anywhere, to the right person" we will be able to cope with the scarce resources and ensure an increase in the quality of health services.

Supposing that we have the ideal technical and organizational infrastructure for pervasive healthcare, we will now briefly examine the benefits of using this new technological paradigm.

- *Wireless handheld devices* will reduce the access time to the electronic health record (EHR), to clinical guidelines, medical textbooks, drug information and patient health insurance data. Various healthcare providers can easily exchange information about the patient, about new treatments and drugs; handheld devices can upload information on history and insurance status to the healthcare provider's databases; laboratory results can also be browsed and a patient with a mobile device can stay updated on the health status of the whole family, receive health alerts and information about vaccination periods or health hazards – all these resulting in reducing the risks of medical errors and saving time both for the patient and for the health professional .
- *Wireless Local Area Networks (LANs) and Personal Area Networks (PANs)* will route biomedical and environmental data collected from sensors on the patient's body and from her/his environment directly to the main computer system that will process this data and a multi-agent application, that will evaluate risk. In this way interventions, if needed, are made in due time, advice is delivered in real time and the amount of false alarms is reduced. This will ensure true real-time physiological monitoring. The patient and the physician can both obtain information concerning prescriptions, drug choices, drug interactions and dosages. The level of patient compliance is also easier to check. Patients in post-operative care can be easily monitored and even discharged from the hospital if they are placed under electronic surveillance.
- *Location tracking technology* can be used for intelligent management of emergencies and disasters, for supervising elderly patients and patients who are restricted to a certain area; it can direct people to a nearby healthcare facility and last but not least, locate potential donors for blood transfusion and organ transplants.
- *Lifestyle management* can be easier both for the individual who, given a handheld device, will have all the needed information and advice for her/his diet, and for the health authorities trying to combat obesity, smoking etc.
- The use of *wireless PDAs* can dramatically save time in the process of collecting and recording health-related data.
- Wireless handheld devices can be used to enable direct charge at the point of care and thus for better monitoring of billing for health services.

## 2. Side Effects

We have briefly explored the most important applications of pervasive technology in healthcare. However, we must not neglect that healthcare also has other links to technology.

Wireless technology is a source of radio frequency (RF) radiation that can interact with other devices used in healthcare, producing failures of life support equipment such as ventilators, dialysis machines, and defibrillators, on one side, and on the other side, it can directly interact with people.

It is worth mentioning that wireless technology, in order to obtain connectivity, includes a large range of tools, devices and equipment that act in different segments of the electromagnetic spectrum (figure 1). We can mention wireless LAN, infrared and other line-of-sight devices, wireless Web applications using protocols such as WAP (Wireless Application Protocol) and WML (Wireless Markup Language) to communicate via cellular phone channels, and data synchronizing techniques for mobile, intermittently-wired devices such as PDAs.

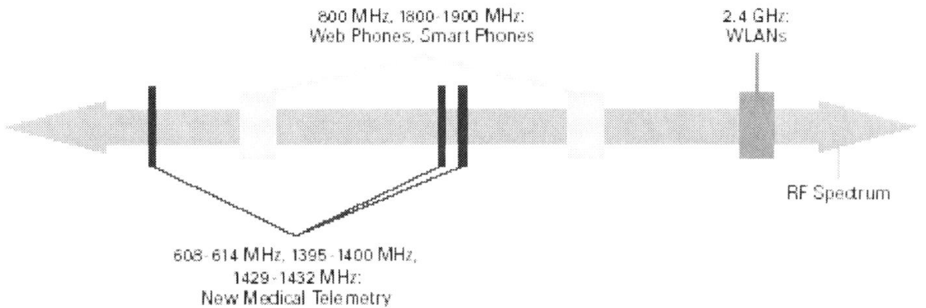


**Fig. 1.** RF spectrum utilization (from the FCG report on Wireless & Mobile Technologies in Healthcare)

Research on the effects of electromagnetic fields interference is gaining momentum, however a sound verdict still cannot be issued. For example, several studies have been published documenting that digital mobile phones can exceed the immunity level of 7V/m recommended by FDA for medical equipment and cause interference and alarm conditions [14, 15, 16]. Some studies recommend maintaining a separation distance of at least six inches between pacemakers and wireless phones, but also observe that pacemakers revert to normal operation when an interfering phone is turned off [17].

A reverse situation appears when considering the effect of wireless technology on human beings who interact with it: providers of healthcare services and clients or any other individual. It has been emphasizes that because many wireless phones operate at 300 MHz and 6 GHz at power levels <1.6W/kg, being in their proximity can induce non-thermal biological effects that eventually end up becoming risk factors for brain cancer, lymphomas and leukemia [26, 27].

Last but not least, social and economic effects of pervasive healthcare, from network privacy violation and misuse of individual data and information to corporate abuse must not be neglected.

## 3. Presence of Physicians on the Web

A recent marketing study has shown, among other conclusions, that *one of every three Romanians owns a mobile phone*. Following this study, our government has concluded that the Romanian Communications and Information Technology market is an example for Europe, a model for the way in which the acquis communitaire has been implemented. It is, no doubt, a very active market, exhibiting spectacular evolution. If we look, for instance, at the trends in mobile telephony we notice that the number of subscribers has risen continuously, from 2.6 million in 2000 to approximately 7 million at this moment. As regards information technology, Romania has recorded increased turnovers and profits between three and five times the European average" [16]. Another interesting conclusion was that citizens are willing to interact online with the authorities of the public administration.

Keeping these results in mind we have tried to document physician on-line connectivity as well as physicians' use and expectations with regard to computers. In this context we have analyzed the possibility and the benefits of introducing pervasive healthcare systems, taking into account that more than seven million citizens own mobile phones and, if they want and can interact online with public administration, they can also communicate with healthcare providers.

We have not take into account advanced medical clinics, transplant clinics and heart surgery units, where telemedicine applications and intensive use of computers is almost natural.

The study has been carried out in the district of Sibiu (online and offline questionnaires), involving 125 physicians (about 20% of the total number, excluding specialists in stomatology) and, in parallel, by evaluating Web accesses (over 400 medical Romanian sites) and health portals. Sibiu is a medium-sized town, with about 140,000 inhabitants and about 500 physicians offering health services.

92% of physicians taking part in the study are using the Internet at least several times per week, which means an increase of more than 100% from 1995. 46% are using the Internet daily. Communicating via e-mail shows spectacular growth with 97% of the subjects using e-mail to correspond with their colleagues and friends. On the other side, correspondence with patients is at a very low level, i.e. 6%. This can be explained by the fact that, when sending e-mail and navigating the Web, physicians are using their own computers and connections and not the ones provided by the health unit. Also, only 10% of the population own computers and less than 10% have Internet connections. The costs imposed by the national telecom for cable links are still relatively high.

In browsing the Web, priority is on the search for general information (weather forecasts, currency exchange rates, etc.) rather then medical news and literature, entertainment, music or games. An important barrier in accessing Web documents is the predominance of the English language. In spite of this inconvenience, foreign sites are much more frequently visited than domestic ones.

32% of the subjects are using more than one computer and connection to the Internet and 50% of those frequent Internet cafes.

Concerning medical sites, only 101 from a total of over 400 are registered with *www.statistica.ro*. Information on these sites is neither organized nor structured, so searching is a real burden.

Recently, academic medical libraries at the foremost universities in the country have started discussions on creating a national digital library for medicine.

76% of those interviewed are aware of wireless technology and had at least once used a PDA or a handheld device. 67% are confused about the meaning of telemedicine and consider that it only involves teleconsultation and e-learning. All physicians graduating in the last five years have followed a program of continuing education in medical information technologies. Also, postdoctoral studies in medicine are possible only if the candidate completes a course on medical IT.

Physicians over 45 years old consider that a drawback in ICT literacy was effected by restricting the number of medical competencies (as imposed by the EU), therefore making it impossible to have such programs on e-health.

Only 23% of the subjects knew about the e-health initiative in connection with other "e-..." developments.

To the question "where to you think *e* is coming from?", 93% answered "from *electronic*", only 2% – "from *enabling and electronic*" and 5% did not know.

74% of those interviewed think that wireless technology has a bright future even in Romania, especially in the private sector. 23% are worried about the sides effects of pervasive healthcare, considering viruses and hackers more dangerous than radiation.

## 4. Challenges

In spite of their growing popularity, pervasive technologies are extremely challenging. First of all, there is a need for serious, continuous funding in order to create and maintain the infrastructure. This means that governmental bodies must be persuaded by the long-term benefits of pervasive healthcare in order to release the money. We must also note that existing technologies do not interoperate well, that there is a need for standards, regulations and laws accepted at a global level. It has also been demonstrated [1] that users of mobile phones and of the Internet are often not the same kinds of persons. Mobile users and Internet users have different profiles, hence broadband services for mobile users should be different from broadband services for Internet users. Also, we need to consider both faces of the coin: access to and practical use of mobile technologies and the Internet are not one and the same.

The pervasive healthcare paradigm involves a wide variety of actors: healthcare providers, patients playing the role of clients, drug providers, insurers, industries, communications operators etc. and any potential solution has to include all these actors. Clients will need to change their behavior and take an active part in the play, providing greater feedback and accepting the new technology. This last aspect is very important in countries from Central and Eastern Europe where there are justified susceptibilities towards being supervised by a mobile eye or tracked by network or satellite positioning systems. If we have accepted to implant a chip in the ear of a horse, this is because we may sell it one day, but to implant a chip in our own ear is quite different.

Perhaps the most challenging aspect is the need to ensure privacy and security and to protect the whole wireless world from terrorism of all kinds, for potential damage resulting from a malfunction or a system crash grows together with the sophistication of the technology.

## 5. Conclusions

Pervasive technology, like any new technology, will probably "invade" the market and eventually also the healthcare sector. Concerning Romania, we do not foresee a problem with acquiring the technology or training the actors, but we will have a very important infrastructure problem. And when we say "infrastructure" we do not mean wireless communications, but a good and safe privacy and security policy, a sound modality to make the system run *à la longue*, to integrate providers, clients and insurers and to offer them the common goal of better healthcare.

## References

[1] A social ecology of wireless technology by Critical Friends of Technology, First Monday, volume 8, number 8 (August 2003)

[2] *http://inventors.about.com/library/inventors/blpager.htm.*

[3] *http://www.californiahealthline.org/.*

[4] Wearable device for monitoring multiple physiological signals as part of a Personal Area Network (PAN). E. Jovanov, D. Raskovic, J. Price, J. Chapman, A. Moore, and A. Krishnamurthy, 2001. "Patient monitoring using personal area networks of wireless intelligent sensors," *Biomedical Sciences Instrumentation,* volume 37, pp. 373-378.

[5] "New frequencies for medical telemetry. FCC's plan is final — now what?" *Health Devices,* volume 29, number 9 (September 2000), pp. 335-337.

[6] K.J. Clifford, K.H. Joyner, D.B. Stroud, M. Wood, B. Ward, and C.H. Fernandez, 1994. "Mobile telephones interfere with medical electrical equipment", *Australasian Physical & Engineering Sciences in Medicine,* volume 17, number 1 (March), pp. 23-27.

[7] J. Hamilton, 1996. "Electromagnetic interference can cause hospital devices to malfunction, McGill group warns", *Canadian Medical Association Journal,* volume 154, number 3 (1 February), pp. 373-375.

[8] W. Irnich and R. Tobisch, 1998. "[Effect of mobile phone on life-saving and life-sustaining systems]", *Biomedizinische Technik* (Berlin), volume 43, number 6 (June), pp. 164-173.

[9] R.E. Schlegel, F.H. Grant, S. Raman, and D. Reynolds, 1998. "Electromagnetic compatibility study of the in-vitro interaction of wireless phones with cardiac pacemakers", *Biomedical Instrumentation & Technology,* volume 32, number 6 (November-December), pp. 645-655.

[10] J.M. Lyznicki, R.D. Altman, and M.A. Williams, 2001. "Council on Scientific Affairs. Report of the American Medical Association (AMA) Council on Scientific Affairs and AMA recommendations to medical professional staff on the use of wireless radio-frequency equipment in hospitals", *Biomedical Instrumentation & Technology,* volume 35, number 3, pp. 189-195.

[11] K.S. Tan and I. Hinberg, 2000. "Effects of a wireless local area network (LAN) system, a telemetry system, and electrosurgical devices on medical devices in a hospital environment", *Biomedical Instrumentation & Technology,* volume 34, number 2, pp. 115-118.

[12] P. Gilligan, S. Somerville, and J.T. Ennis, 2000. "GSM cell phones can interfere with ionizing radiation dose monitoring equipment", *British Journal of Radiology,* volume 73, number 873 (September), pp. 994-998.

[13] E. Hanada, K. Takano, Y. Antoku, K. Matsumura, Y. Watanabe, and Y. Nose, 2002. "A practical procedure to prevent electromagnetic interference with electronic medical equipment", *Journal of Medical Systems,* volume 26, number 1 (February), pp. 61-65.

[14] R.W. Morgan, M.A. Kelsh, K. Zhao, K.A. Exuzides, S. Heringer, and W. Negrete, 2000. "Radiofrequency exposure and mortality from cancer of the brain and lymphatic/hematopoietic systems", *Epidemiology,* volume 11, number 2 (March), pp. 118-127.

[15] M.A. Stuchly, 1998. "Biomedical concerns in wireless communications", *Critical Reviews in Biomedical Engineering,* volume 26, numbers 1-2, pp. 117-151.

[16] *http://www.mct.ro*

[17] *http://www.ms.ro*

# Implementing the HL7v3 Standard in Croatian Primary Healthcare Domain

Miroslav KONČAR
*Ericsson Nikola Tesla d.d.*
*Krapinska 45, P.O.Box 93, HR-10002 Zagreb, Croatia*
*e-mail: miroslav.koncar@ericsson.com*

**Abstract.** The mission of HL7 Inc. is to provide standards for the exchange, management and integration of data that supports clinical patient care and the management, delivery and evaluation of healthcare services. The scope of this work includes the specifications of flexible, cost-effective approaches, standards, guidelines, methodologies, and related services for interoperability between healthcare information systems. In the field of medical information technologies, HL7 provides the world's most advanced information standards.

Versions 1 and 2 of the HL7 standard have on the one hand solved many issues, but on the other demonstrated the size and complexity of the health information sharing problem. As the solution, a complete new methodology has been adopted, which is being encompassed in version 3 recommendations. This approach standardizes the Reference Information Model (RIM), which is the source of all domain models and message structures. Message design is now defined in detail, enabling interoperability between loosely-coupled systems that are designed by different vendors and deployed in various environments.

At the start of the Primary Healthcare Information System project, we have decided to go directly to HL7v3. Implementing the HL7v3 standard in healthcare applications represents a challenging task. By using standardized refinement and localization methods we were able to define information models for Croatian primary healthcare domain. The scope of our work includes clinical, financial and administrative data management, where in some cases we were compelled to introduce new HL7v3-compliant models. All of the HL7v3 transactions are digitally signed, using the W3C XML Digital Signature standard.

## Introduction

HL7 is one of the many Standards Developing Organization (SDO) working in the field of medical information technologies. It is a non-profit organization with a headquarters in the United States and a number of licensed affiliates in different countries around the world. HL7 was founded in 1987, with the mission "to provide standards for the exchange, management and integration of data that support clinical patient care and the management, delivery and evaluation of healthcare services. Specifically, to create flexible, cost-effective approaches, standards, guidelines, methodologies, and related services for interoperability between healthcare information systems" [1]. Following that mission, HL7 produces standards in the field of medical IT, with the domain of interest including administrative, clinical and financial transactions and data exchange. "Level Seven" in HL7 definition refers to the highest level of the International Standardization Organization (ISO) [2] communications model for Open Systems Interconnection (OSI), called the application level. The application level addresses definition of data to be exchanged, the timing of the interchange, and the communication of certain errors to the application. The seventh level supports such functions as security checks, participant identification, availability checks, exchange mechanism negotiations and, most importantly, data exchange structuring [1].

Since 1987 the influence of the HL7 standards and recommendations has crossed the borders of the United States, and today they represents the world's leading standard efforts in the field of medical IT. It is also worth mentioning that HL7 standards are accepted by the ANSI (American National Standard Institute) organization [3]. Furthermore, the organization is working in close collaboration with other recognized SDOs like ISO and CEN (European Committee for Standardization) [4] that serves as the basis for providing interoperability mechanisms and support for other medical information standards. Given all that, HL7 is envisioned as being the unavoidable part of next-generation medical information systems, application solutions and advanced medical diagnostic devices.

The work on Version 3 of HL7 standard started in 1996, and the first official release is expected to be announced somewhere in 2004. HL7v3 represents one of the most advanced information standards for the highest level of communication protocols. It is based on well-defined formal mechanisms that employ advanced information modeling techniques like UML (Unified Modeling Language) and the Unified Process. HL7v3 artifacts such as message information models, storyboards and interaction diagrams are mostly based on the scenarios and trigger events encountered in the US healthcare domain. In order for HL7v3 to be implemented in specialized environments, the standard introduces guidelines for creating local profiles that formally define how the standard would be implemented in a particular setting. However, the localization process is by no means easy; on the one hand, one has to be fully familiar with the healthcare business processes, legal regulations and scenarios encountered in a particular domain, and on the other hand it is imperative to use the formal mechanisms, guidelines and artifacts that are required by the standard.

This paper discusses the challenges and efforts inherent in working with the HL7v3 implementation. The target domain of interest includes primary healthcare in the Republic of Croatia, which is part of the e-Government initiative officially led by the Croatian government. The current scope of work includes primary healthcare domain transition from paper-based to paperless business environments. The paper is organized as follows: Section 1 introduces the main characteristics and issues involving HL7 Version 2 standard; Section 2 provides the basic concepts and the rationale for HL7 Version 3 standard; Section 3 introduces localization methods and mechanisms, and our experience with the HL7v3 standard implementation; Section 4 elaborates the usage of digital signatures in HL7 messages; Section 5 discusses the issues involving the HL7v3 standard conformance testing; and, finally, Section 6 provides final remarks and our future plans and actions.

## 1. Main Features and Issues of the HL7v2.x Standard

The HL7v2.x standard defines the concept of a message as an atomic unit of data that is transferred between systems. The message is comprised of a group of segments in a defined sequence, and every segment is composed using a set of message fields. Both message segments and data fields can be defined as required and optional, and can be reused in different messages (see example in Figure 1). Message construction rules allow Technical Committees to define locally-used messages and segments when needed. Certain data fields are furthermore allowed to use locally-defined tables and sets of values. As it is defined on the application level of the communication stack, the standard does not enforce application architectures, design and business rules, or a specific transport mechanism on lower layers of communication (it assumes that error-free transmission, support for unlimited message length, and character conversion are guaranteed). At the moment, the latest officially released HL7 standard refers to version 2.5 (approved as an ANSI standard June 26, 2003) [1].

Currently there are different HL7v2.x implementations deployed in various environments and countries around the world. While these implementations have by all means solved many requirements and issues, they have also demonstrated a great deal of complexity stated in the mission. As it is recognized by the HL7 community, there are some very fundamental issues and barriers in HL7v2 specifications, making it practically impossible to completely follow the goals. The process of building HL7v2.x messages is entirely *ad hoc*, and there is no formal methodology followed by the standards artifacts. Most of the data fields are optional, and there are no application responsibility requirements that would be enforced by the standard and respected in certain scenarios and real-life trigger events [5]. While this provides a great deal of flexibility, it also makes it impossible to have reliable conformance tests of any vendor's implementation and also forces implementers to spend more time analyzing and planning their interfaces to ensure that both parties are using the same optional features. Basically, when creating an HL7v2.x message for a particular setting, the Technical Committee edits word processing documents directly. The metadata is not available in a structured form, which makes it extremely hard to provide any kind of interoperability outside controlled working environments.

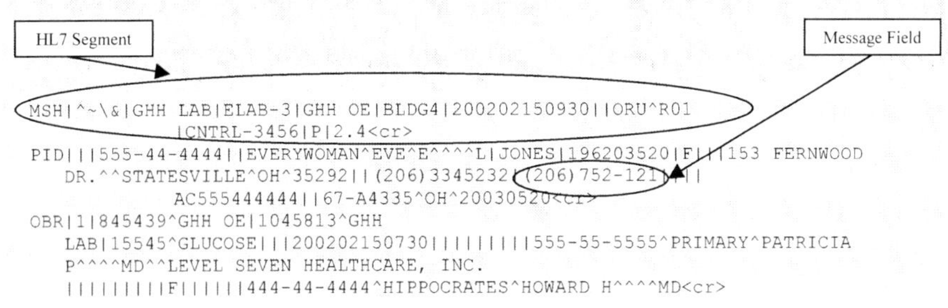


**Fig. 1.** HL7v2.x Message Example (source HL7v3 Ballot)

## 2. The Key Concepts of HL7v3 Methodology

Version 3 addresses the issues detected in HL7v2.x by using a well-defined methodology based on a Reference Information Model (RIM), which serves as the source of all derived models defined in the standard. The RIM represents the essential part of the HL7v3 development methodology, as it provides an explicit representation of the semantic and lexical connections that exist between the information contained in HL7 messages. The process of message building is explicitly documented and supported by training classes and computerized tools, and as such represents a part of the standard that needs to be respected by the Technical Committees working on different aspects of standard definition and implementation [6].

The HL7v3 specification starts at the business level, where Technical Committees are using Use Case modeling and the Storyboarding mechanism that depict sequences of events encountered in specific healthcare environments (Figure 2). Every event represents a recognizable, meaningful moment in the sequence, and provides the illustration of key actors involved in the event and their interactions with other playing entities included in the sequence. A single interaction is defined in the standard with one real-life Trigger Event, one sending and one receiving Application Role, and Message Types that the message exchange is based on (see Figure 3).

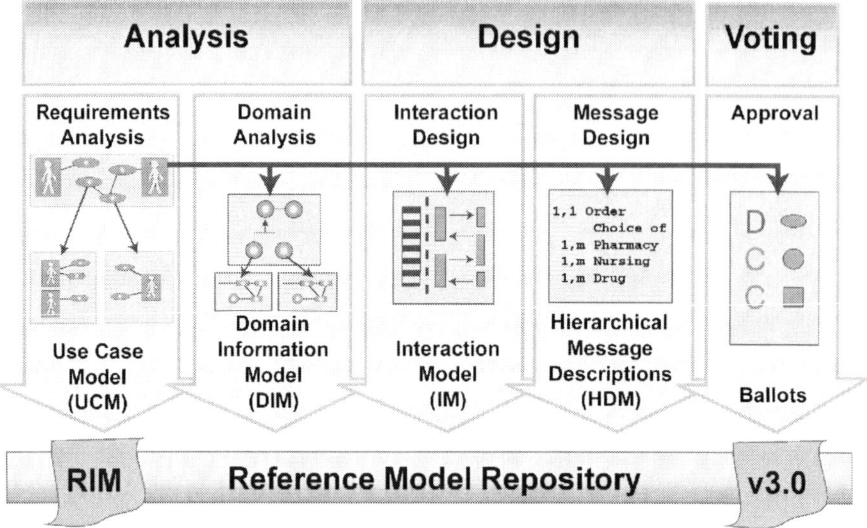


**Fig. 2.** HL7v3 Methodology

One of the most important quality features in HL7v3 is the concept of Application Roles, which serves as the basis for application conformance testing and claims. An Application Role is an abstraction that expresses a portion of the messaging behavior of an information system. It embodies the responsibilities of the applications that claim to conform to it. In essence, every Application Role is bound to two sets of interactions; one where it acts as the sender, and another where it acts as the receiver. Furthermore, for the interactions it receives, the application role is given additional post-receipt responsibilities.

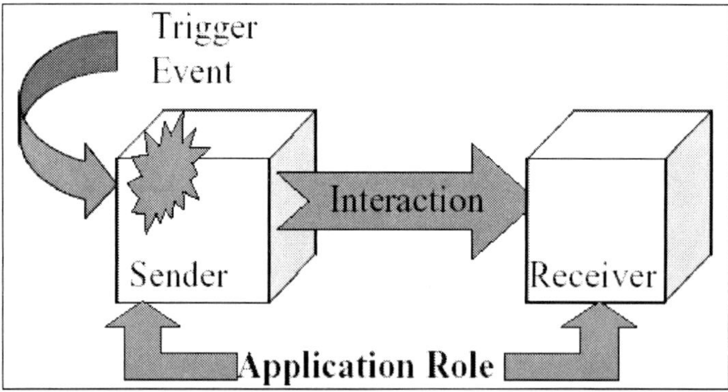


**Fig. 3.** HL7v3 Storyboard Interaction Diagram and Trigger Event Ilustration (source: HL7v3 ballot4 package)

In making a conformance claim, a system developer identifies the application roles to which he/she wishes to claim conformance. For these application roles, the HL7v3 specification will state directly the trigger events the system shall recognize, messages that the system shall send in response to trigger events or other messages, and the data content for these messages. The specification also states the messages that a system conforming to the Application Role shall receive and process [7].

### 2.1 HL7v3 Information Models

In Version 3 of the HL7 standard the RIM is a static information model for health and healthcare information as viewed within the scope of HL7 standards development activities. It is the combined consensus view of information from the perspective of the HL7 working groups and the HL7 international affiliates. The RIM is the ultimate source from which all HL7v3 protocol specification standards draw their information-related content [7].

RIM is an UML-based information model that is comprised of six "backbone" classes:

- ***Act*** represents the actions that are executed and must be documented as healthcare is managed and provided,
- ***Participation*** expresses the context for an act in terms such as who has performed it, for whom it has been done, where it has been done, etc.,
- ***Entity*** represents the physical things and beings that are of interest to, and take part in healthcare,
- ***Role*** establishes the roles that entities play as they participate in healthcare acts,
- ***ActRelationship*** represents the binding of one act to another, such as the relationship between an order for an observation and the observation event as it occurs,
- ***RoleLink*** represents relationships between individual that is defined with the four base classes.

RIM contains round 70 classes that are the basis of all other information models developed by the Technical Committees[8]. In that manner, every single information model or a healthcare event is modeled using these six types of classes. Furthermore, by using the cloning mechanism, the information content is preserved throughout the refinement process up to the lowest levels of standard, represented by HL7 message types. Based on the RIM, the following information models are derived:

- ***Domain Message Information Model (DMIM)*** is used to express the information content for the work of a specific Technical Committee, Special Interest Group, or project. It usually encompasses a specific domain of interest within the healthcare business domain like Laboratory or Pharmacy. The purpose of the DMIM is to provide a common point of reference and a description of the information content of the specific domain upon which set of trigger events and interactions can be built on.
- ***Refined Message Information Model (RMIM)*** is used to describe a related group of messages using HL7v3 conventions and methodology. The most simple analogy of a RMIM is a real-life use case, where examples would include "Insurance Eligibility Query" or "Laboratory Observation Event". It is a special version of a message information model that is used to describe information constraints that will be applicable to one or more Hierarchical Message Definitions.
- ***Hierarchical Message Definition (HMD)*** is a tabular representation of the sequence of elements (i.e., classes, attributes and associations) represented in an RMIM. The HMD defines a single base message structure - the "common" message type. It is the template from which other specific and corresponding message types are drawn. HMDs are described in the HL7v3 standard using both simple tabular and Microsoft Excel™ format files.
- ***Common Message Element Types (CMET)*** are predefined components that are re-used for several RMIMs and/or messages. They are intended to express a common, reusable pattern, and as such represent an extremely important component in the HL7v3 standard quality. Nevertheless, they are not intended to be used as a mechanism to simplify a DMIM or RMIM diagram. They are categorized based on the entry point class, which can be Act, Entity or a Role.

### 2.2 HL7v3 Composite Messaging Rules

On the highest level, every HL7v3 message is composed of three components (see Figure 4):

- HL7 Transmission Wrapper (TW) is present in every instance of an HL7v3 composite message. It includes information needed by a sending application or a message handling service to package and route the HL7v3 composite message. This wrapper also provides attributes that identify a generic messaging mode, including protocol version, sequence numbers and acknowledgement levels.
- Trigger Event Control Act Wrapper (CAW) is required for all messages except accept-level acknowledgements, for which it is not permitted. It contains administrative information like trigger event definition, author or performer or digital signature, that are related to the "controlled act". It is also the part of HL7 messages that can convey status or commands for logical operations being coordinated between healthcare applications.
- HL7 Domain Content (also called HL7 Payload) is specified by an HL7 Technical Committee, and contains domain-specific content with the purpose to satisfy a use case-driven requirement for an HL7 messaging interaction. It is required for each Trigger Event Control Act.

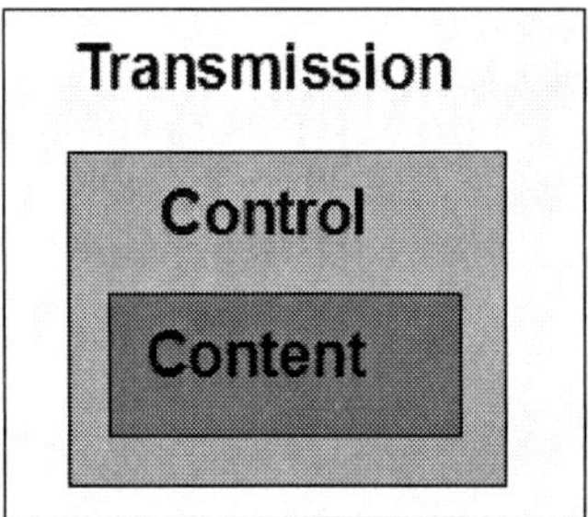


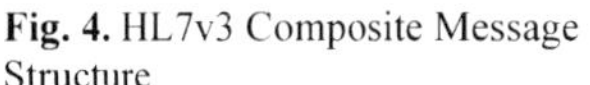

**Fig. 4.** HL7v3 Composite Message Structure

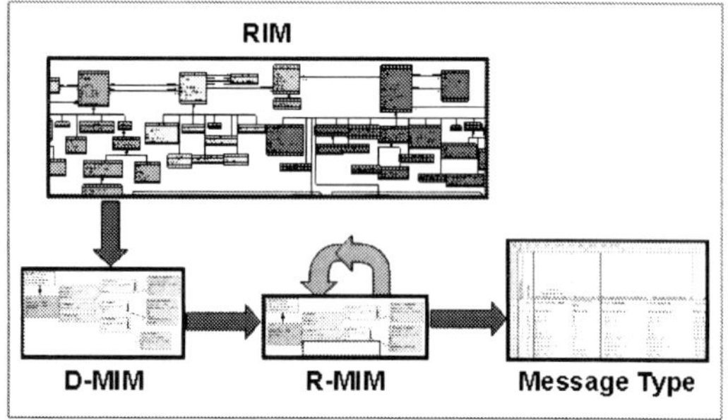


**Fig. 5.** Refinement Process for Defining HL7v3 Messages Based on the RIM

The standard also introduces XML ITS (eXtensible Markup Language Implementation Technology Specification) that provides the information on how to implement the standard using W3C XML technology [9]. XML represents an advanced, yet simple and very flexible data format that is used as the foundation for electronic data exchange between various systems. This technology is fully supported by all tools that are developed by HL7, and then used by the Technical Committees in the standard definition and implementation.

## 3. Localization Mechanisms in HL7v3 Implementation

Implementation of the HL7v3 standard in a specified setting relies on the localization process, which can include both constraining the existing models, and the introduction of new models that comply with HL7v3 standardized methodology. The constraining process reduces the optionality and uncertainty in the base models in order to make the specification more exact. Constraint methods can be applied on any level of the HL7 refinement process (see Figure 5), and can be categorized in five broad groups: (1)

*appearance constraints* determine whether a particular element must or mustn't be included from the base model; (2) *cardinality constraints* define the number of repetitions of a given element; (3) *type constraints* limit the structure of the element in question, (4) *value set constraints* limit the set of values applicable for that element, and (5) *any other constraints* stated as text to establish any local business rules. Theoretically, there are cases where the models need to be extended to accommodate the needs of local applications or realms of use. In such situations it is mandatory to follow the refinement process defined by the HL7v3 standard and modeling rules [7]. In addition to this, possible detected conflicts that potentially violate HL7 refinement and constraint rules need to be preferably avoided, since they will most probably be the cause of interoperability problems.

As specified in the standard, we have used HL7v3 refinement methods to define the information models and message types for the Croatian primary healthcare domain. In the context of HL7 domains, the scenarios and events encountered in primary care can be categorized as follows:

1. Patient Administration (PA) Domain – includes insurance eligibility checking and patient demographics queries,
2. Personnel Management (PM) Domain – includes General Practitioner (GP) and Nurse authentication and authorization procedures,
3. Claims and Reimbursements (CR) Domain – includes invoicing and GP work reports,
4. Public Health Reporting (PHR) Domain – includes reports referring to special cases that are of public health interest,
5. Infrastructure Management (IM) Domain, including Transmission, ControlAct and Query Infrastructure – includes the definition of application-level transport information content common to all message transactions.

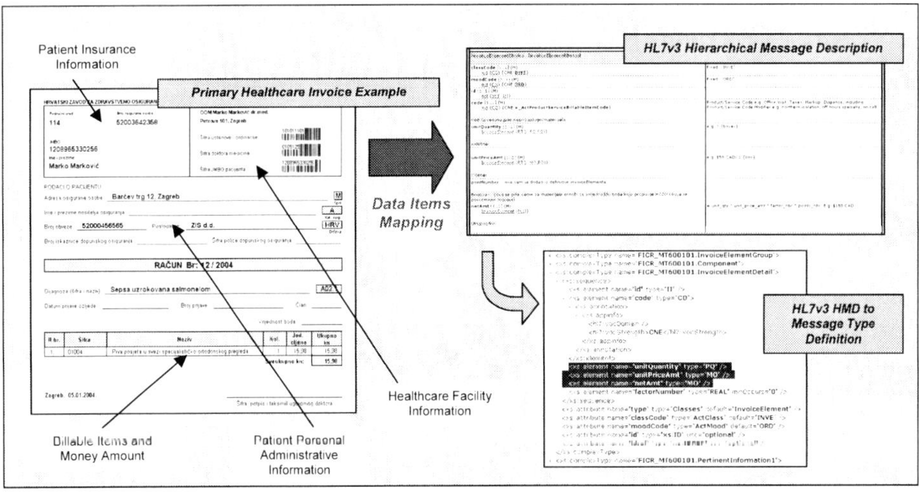


**Fig. 6.** Invoice Information Modelling

The process of HL7v3 implementation included two parallel activities: a detailed study of all Version 3 documents provided by the HL7 Inc., and close collaboration with local domain experts in the process of business and use case modeling. It is highly recommended to consult the HL7v3 specifications in the earliest phases of the system and application design, since the standard has very strong influence on business rules and information models developed by the Technical Committees. Throughout the system development phase, we have relied on the Unified Process recommendations [10] and object-oriented analysis and design, where we have used UML and design patterns as the basis for all design and implementation models [11]. These design methods and process management techniques are adopted by the HL7v3 standard as well.

To map the entire primary healthcare domain to HL7v3 artefacts, we have used different localization methods as described above (see Figure 6 for an illustration of invoice modeling). So far, we haven't been faced with the challenge to add new elements (classes, attributes, vocabularies) to existing models, in which case we would need to form an official request for standard change. This is by all means possible, and fully supported and welcomed by the HL7 Inc., but it would slow up the process of standard implementation. HL7 localization efforts can be globally grouped into three different categories according to the output artefacts.

### 3.1 RMIM Localization and Development

At the beginning of the system design phase, we have frozen HL7v3 ballot4 specifications [12], which was the latest balloting package available at that point in time (March 2003), and taken it as the requirement in application implementation. During the design activities we were faced with some inconsistencies between the local business rules and the HL7v3 information models. Furthermore, there were cases where we detected errors in the HL7 models provided. To accommodate the needs of local requirements and to solve many important implementation issues, we have conducted consultations with people from the HL7 community, using official mailing lists, workshops and meetings. Some issues were solved by using the latest balloting material available at distinct time points. For example, the ControlAct Query Request RMIM from ballot4 package could not accommodate a query using different search parameters provided in a case-by-case situation. This was solved in the ballot6 package, and we were able to use it as such. Furthermore, ballot4 is missing some important information models for different Payload domains that are needed to address the complete business process. Again, in some cases we were able to use the latest balloting material; e.g. the Patient Care Provision Request RMIM is introduced in ballot6 and can be used to accommodate a scenario when a GP requests the authorization for a patient home care provisioning. In some cases, however, DMIM and RMIM models are in the early design phases, have draft status and do not contain enough information to be used in working environments. For example, GP and Nurse authentication services are planned to be supported by a separate RMIM, but at the moment only a draft of a DMIM domain for PM is available. For that purpose, we have developed our own RMIM and defined two simple application roles just to meet our needs (see Figure 7). It is worth mentioning that the developed RMIM is based on the latest draft DMIM available (September, 2003). Following RMIM modeling, we were able to produce XML schemas using the standard tools developed and provided by HL7 Inc.

### 3.2 HMD and Message Type Localization Process

In most cases, we were able to use existing normative HL7v3 models to accommodate the needs of local applications. The common process refers to HMD models constraining to produce locally-used message types. For this purpose, we have constrained 64 different HMD definitions that include Transmission Wrappers, ControlAct Wrappers, Payloads and CMETs. Wherever possible, we further explained message types and elements, and often used a non-permitting constraint for optional elements. There were also cases where we have employed cardinality constraint mechanisms, like the number of medical personnel included in a particular event. These methods are applied in both Microsoft Excel™ tables and the HL7 repository; the former used for easier visual interpretation, and the latter for XML schema generation. This approach makes our model lightweight and minimalistic, but still fully functional and able to meet all the requirements.

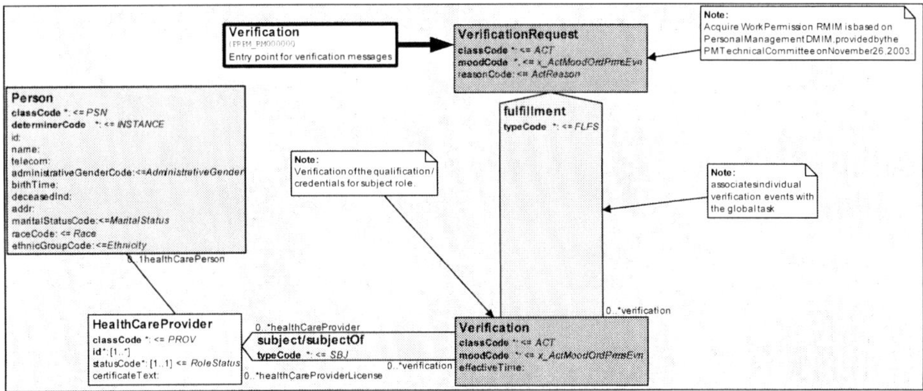


**Fig. 7.** Acquire Work Permission RMIM

### *3.3 Vocabulary Localization Process*

An especially interesting and challenging area of work refers to the HL7v3 Vocabulary domains and the coding schemes that are used in the local healthcare business processes. Since it is a proven fact that a large majority of interoperability issues refer to the terminologies used in particular domains, it is extremely important to follow the guidelines provided by the standard. There are many vocabularies used in healthcare processes for both medical and administrative purposes. For them to be implemented in a well-defined manner, the first step that must be taken is the close and detailed study of HL7v3 RIM, DMIM, RMIM and vocabulary domains concept. Thus, HL7-defined vocabulary domain tables have been developed for coded class attributes that can be found in any RIM class [7]. Here, the ***code*** attribute in Act, Entity and Role classes is quite important. It provides further classification for a particular specialization of the base class, and although it is defined as optional in most cases, we strongly recommend using it wherever possible, since this feature provides important an quality improvement when referring to semantic interoperability. The next step in the process involves the recognition of the currently-used coding schemes, and clearly distinguishing whether a particular coding scheme belongs to an *Instance Identifier* or a *Coded Element* data type (found in the base Act, Entity and Role classes as ***id*** and ***code*** elements). Our experience working with this issue is that while the distinction is perfectly clear in most cases, there are situations that this might not be fully straightforward. For example, in the case of invoice generation and formatting (Figure 6), we are required to code the drugs that are being invoiced by using the official drug list published by the Drug Agency of Republic of Croatia. This code does not belong to the ***Act.code*** element in the appropriate RMIM, which might be the first assumption. Following more detailed inspection, we have found out that it rather belongs to the ***Act.id*** attribute.

At the moment, we are in the process of coding schemes categorization and usage definitions. Prior to terminology implementation, it is strongly recommended to consult the coding system registry mechanism [13]. HL7 Version 3 defines the use of ISO Object Identifiers, known as OIDs, to identify coding systems. It also suggests their use for Instance Identifier data types to uniquely identify namespaces for identifiers. So far we have established 24 different coding schemes, of which the majority belong to the Instance Identifier group. Some of the coding schemes used already have registered OIDs, like ICD (International Classification of Diseases) codes, and some will need to be defined and registered with HL7. We haven't yet started the official code systems registration adopted by HL7; this is planned as one of future project activities.

## 4. Applying W3C XML Digital Signature in HL7v3 Messages

Requirements for the primary healthcare information system and related projects in the Republic of Croatia include enforcing the implementation of some extremely important data security mechanisms. Since all information that is exchanged between healthcare systems is extremely sensitive, data integrity must be preserved. Furthermore, the non-repudiation mechanism provides the users with the feature of transaction reconstruction that can be extremely important in cases such as audit trials.


```
<?xml version="1.0" encoding="UTF-8" ?>
- <QUCR_IN210101.Message xmlns="urn:hl7-org:v3">
    <id extension="19.3.2409.2003_20040216T131549.64Z" root="2.16.840.1.110001" />
    <creationTime value="20040216T131549.64Z" />
    <versionId>3.0</versionId>
    <interactionId extension="MCCI_IN100002" root="2.16.840.1.113883" />
    <processingCode code="P" />
    <processingModeCode code="T" />
    <acceptAckCode code="AL" />
    <applicationAckCode code="NE" />
  + <communicationFunctionSnd>
  - <controlActProcess classCode="CACT" moodCode="EVN">
      <code code="QUCR_IN210101" codeSystem="2.16.840.1.113883" />
    - <authorOrPerformer typeCode="AUT">
      - <signatureText>
        - <Signature xmlns="http://www.w3.org/2000/09/xmldsig#">
          - <SignedInfo>
              <CanonicalizationMethod Algorithm="http://www.w3.org/TR/2001/REC-xml-c14n-20010315" />
              <SignatureMethod Algorithm="http://www.w3.org/2000/09/xmldsig#rsa-sha1" />
            + <Reference URI="#resToSign">
            </SignedInfo>
            <SignatureValue>HSmG8C0hxC1tVz+8aQTm8o7Ii7re3wMQNNRAIuISjD4d176A3c8KI7S+jZVa1Ir3fXJxQBTE
              2KJScY3XGpNdAg==</SignatureValue>
          + <KeyInfo>
          </Signature>
        </signatureText>
      + <participant>
      </authorOrPerformer>
    + <subject Id="resToSign" typeCode="SUBJ">
    + <queryAck>
    </controlActProcess>
</QUCR_IN210101.Message>
```


XML Digital Signature

HL7v3 Signed Payload

**Fig. 8.** HL7v3 Digitally-signed Composite Message

The solution for these two very important requirements is based on the digital signature mechanism. In a loosely coupled environment the user has to provide all the information required to perform the security checks in an HL7 message instance, since the sending and receiving systems cannot rely on any persistent information stored in shared databases. For that reason we are enforcing the digital signing of all messages, with the support for digital certificate provisioning in CAW. In order to follow the praxis adopted by HL7, a digital signature is implemented using the W3C XML Digital Signature specification [14].

Figure 8 depicts an example of a digitally-signed HL7v3 message. By using the detached digital signature mechanism, we are signing the HL7v3 Payload only. In the process of W3C XML Digital Signature standard implementation, some inconsistencies between HL7v3 standard definition and XML data types schema have been detected; this is where we made the appropriate changes. An HL7v3 composite message signed using the W3C XML Digital Signature specification is than wrapped up in the SOAP [15] envelope and sent to the Web service that handles communication and message transfer (see Figure 9).

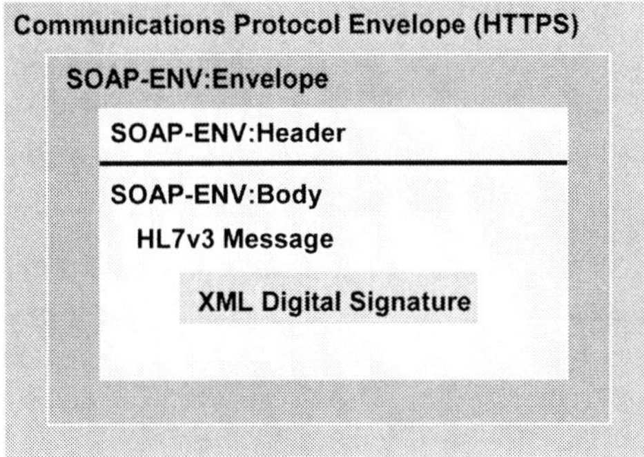


**Fig. 9.** HL7v3 XML Message and SOAP Envelope

## 5. HL7v3 Standard Conformance

The next logical question that needs to be raised is how all these localization mechanisms influence the conformance to the original HL7v3 standard. Application Roles represent the foundation of the HL7v3 application conformance testing. However, it is still very much unclear what is going to be the optimal level for Application Roles definition. If they are too complex, i.e. involved in too many trigger events, it is hard to imagine that a real-life application would need all the interactions to support its business requirements, which would lead to very few application actually needing to be HL7v3-compliant. On the other hand, low-level definitions of Application Roles would make the standard extremely complex and hard to comprehend. One idea introduced by HL7 is to use stereotypes (currently there are six Application Roles stereotypes – Placer, Fulfiller, Tracker, Confirmer, Confirmation Receiver and Notifier), and possibly inheritance and associations mechanisms for better definition and easier implementation. This concept needs to be proven in the real-life situations prior to actual standard acceptance.

For all these reasons, Application Roles are planned to be informative and not normative in the first release of the HL7v3 standard. Tooling for protocol analysis and compatibility checking is not yet developed. Feedback from early developers and implementers is expected to provide important information on the concept of Application Roles and conformance testing.

## 6. Conclusion and Future Plans

The implementation of the HL7v3 standard is very much different and much more complex from implementing HL7v2.x. Due to limited optionality and standardized methodology embedded in the HL7v3 standard, Technical Committees working in specialized realms of interest are faced with the challenging task of using normative models developed by the HL7 and localizing them in what can be a highly-specific environment. To achieve the desired level of conformance and interoperability, the profiles defined for the localized environment should clearly state how a local implementation conforms to the original standard, which is expressed in terms of constraints, extensions and other alterations to a referenced standard. Furthermore, vocabulary domains developed by the HL7 provide the basis for semantic interoperability and need to be respected by local implementations. Coding schemes used in particular domains, which in most cases are maintained by external organizations, should be implemented in a well-defined manner and possibly registered with the HL7.

So far, we have had very good experience working with the HL7v3 implementation in the Croatian primary healthcare domain. Although it is a rather complex environment, we have successfully localized the standard to cover primary healthcare business processes, where we have constrained and refined original RMIM and HMD models to accommodate the needs of the domain. We were forced to develop one additional RMIM, with close attention to the classes included in the appropriate DMIM.

Our future plans include continuous work with the Croatian HL7 Affiliate, where we are sharing our experiences in the process of defining the Croatian HL7v3 localized standard. An especially interesting area is that of vocabulary domains, code sets and schemes, where collaboration with domain experts from medical and legal areas is the foundation for achieving the desired level of semantic interoperability. In the future, we would like to extend our scope of work to hospitals, laboratories and pharmacies, where we envision the HL7v3 standard as being the cornerstone for an integrated e-health system in the Republic of Croatia.

## References


[1] HL7 Inc. Official Web Site, [Online], *http://www.hl7.org* (accessed February, 2004)

[2] International Standard Organization, Official Web Site, [Online], *http://www.iso.org* (accessed February, 2004)

[3] American National Standards Institute [Online], *http://www.ansi.org* (accessed February, 2004)

[4] European Committee for Standardization, CEN, [Online], *http://www.centc251.org/* (accessed February, 2004)

[5] HL7 Version 3 Statement of Principles, HL7 Inc. [Online], *http://www.hl7.org* (accessed February, 2004)

[6] George W Beeler and others, "Message Development Framework" Version 3.3, Copyright© HL7 Inc

[7] HL7 Version 3.0 Balloting Package, [Online], *http://www.hl7.org/v3ballot/html/index.htm* (accessed February, 2004)

[8] Andrew Hinchley, "Understanding Version 3", 2nd Edition, ISBN 3-933819-18-0

[9] W3C Extensible Markup Language (XML) 1.0 (2nd Edition), [Online], *http://www.w3.org/TR/REC-xml*, (accessed February, 2004)

[10] Phillipe Kruchten, "The Rational Unified Process: An Introduction", Addison Wesley, ISBN 0-20-170710-1

[11] C. Larman, "Applying UML and Patterns", 2nd Edition, Prentice Hall PTR, ISBN 0-13-092569-1

[12] HL7v3 Ballot4 Package, [Online], *http://www.hl7.org/v3ballot4/html/index.htm* (accessed February, 2004)

[13] HL7 OID Registry, [Online], *http://www.hl7.org/oid/index.html*, (accessed February, 2004)

[14] W3C XML Digital Signature Specifications, [Online], *http://www.w3.org/TR/xmldsig-core*, (accessed February, 2004)

[15] W3C Simple Object Access Protocol (SOAP) 1.1, [Online], *http://www.w3.org/TR/SOAP/*, (accessed February, 2004)

# Development of Teleconsultations Systems for e-Health

Vaidotas MAROZAS, Rytis JURKONIS, Algirdas KAZLA, Mantas LUKOŠEVIČIUS, Arūnas LUKOŠEVIČIUS, Adas GELŽINIS, Darius JEGELEVIČIUS
*Institute of Biomedical Engineering, Kaunas University of Technology, Studentu str. 50-343, LT 51368 Kaunas, Lithuania*
*e-mail: vaidotas.marozas@ktu*

**Abstract.** Two prototype telemedicine systems have been developed: 1) a wireless system for status assessment of cardiology patients (WSCP), 2) a system for medical image management and teleconsultations (IMTS). The former system enables the patient to record an ECG on a personal digital assistant (PDA), view it and send it via a wireless connection. The doctor on duty is then able to view the received ECG and make appropriate decisions, also to apply for consultation by sending the received ECG to the PDA of a cardiology expert. The system logs all performed operations. The hardware used in the system consists of personal computers (PCs), PDAs, analog-digital converters, ECG sensors and GPRS modems. Software consists of programs for patients, doctors on duty, cardiology experts and administration, along with a central database. The second system is intended to be used by professional doctors for management of collected images and for teleconsultations via videoconferencing in order to obtain a second opinion. The system provides an integrated environment eliminating the need to jump between many applications. By using the system, doctors are able to acquire images from analog and digital cameras, process and enhance them, as well as upload them to local or remote databases. Doctors are also able to design custom database forms. The teleconsultation part of the system supports video and audio over ISDN and TCP-IP, using both a hardware codec (Zydacron Z360) and a software codec (based on MS Netmeeting). Images are sent from one client to another using the standard protocol T.120. Images become synchronized immediately upon reception by another client.

## Introduction

Applications of state-of-the-art information and telecommunication technologies in healthcare have attracted much interest in the recent years. Health, a healthy way of living, as well as high-quality and affordable medical services are among the vital needs of the society. The average spending on health services in the European Union amounts to 8 percent of the national product, while one per cent goes to information technologies servicing the health sector. In Lithuania, a health reform is ongoing; here the entirety of telemedicine and information telecommunication technologies, called in short "e-health", could make a significant contribution to quality medical services for patients, particularly those living in remote areas [1]. "The cost of telecommunications and computing power has dropped so dramatically that the potential finally exists to unite healthcare providers with patients and purchasers in a virtual seamless system. Tele-everything through television sets and other terminals will change the way patients are treated, operated on, monitored and counseled. If patients could communicate with physicians or be monitored through the Internet, more than 20% of in-office visits could be eliminated, according to respondents in the HealthCast 2010 survey. In addition, respondents said they generally felt that more than

30% of physicians time will be spent using web-based tools by 2010", "HealthCast 2010", which was conducted by PricewaterhouseCoopers [2].

The strategy behind Lithuanian national e-health initiatives is due to be completed in the year 2004 by the Lithuanian Ministry of Healthcare [3]. The preparation of this strategy is conducted by a well-known consultancy company Tieto Enator Trigon AB (Sweden), funded by the World Bank. The strategy assesses the present status of IT technologies in healthcare, then proposes implementation principles through visions of the role of e-health in future healthcare. The strategy points out the present situation of Lithuanian healthcare and the potential role of e-health solutions [4]:

- *Patient care environment:* unequal possibilities of accessing healthcare, queues at registration, problems with remote registration, problems with free choice of health providers and physicians, no system of ensuring care accessibility and quality insurance (especially pertinent in remote regions), no patient-oriented professional information on the Internet, no practical possibilities for remote consultations, no safe storage of lifelong patient records.
- *Research and pilot developments*: underestimation of the importance of pilot projects and networks, lack of national support of international pilot activities, prevalence of purchased learning platforms with regard to domestic developments, suppression of local initiatives and underused national professional qualifications.
- *Application priorities are*: primary care, seamless and home care, telemedicine, monitoring of elderly and chronically ill patients, prevention and screening, accessibility.

The strategy stresses the role of "learning platforms", whose primary goal is to develop, implement, test and evaluate the innovative e-health applications and developments on smaller scales, and validate or reject the new ideas prior to nationwide introduction.

The Institute of Biomedical Engineering has recently taken part in several telemedicine and e-health related projects: Telemedicare (funded by EU FP5); the Swedish-funded projects Litmed I and Litmed II, and Swedish-Lithuanian projects: Baltic Medweb I and Baltic Medweb II. By working within these projects, we have conducted analysis of many systems under development [6],[7], [8],[9], and gained experience in the design and development of patient-centered vital sign monitoring teleconsultations systems, as well as image management and teleconferencing systems.

In this paper we share our experience in creating two types of teleconsultations systems: a system for remote status assessment of cardiology patients using wireless communications and an image management and teleconsultations system (IMTS) for obtaining second opinions and distance education. Our work includes analyses of possible applications and available technologies as well as design and implementation of working prototypes of the systems.

## 1. Requirements Analysis and Design Considerations

### *1.1 Modalities of Teleconsultation Systems for e-Health*

Teleconsultation systems for e-health can be categorized into several domains and applications: asynchronous and synchronous, doctor- or patient-centered. Asynchronous teleconsultations involve preparation of materials to be sent to another doctor or expert in order to obtain a second opinion in diagnostic tasks. This kind of teleconsultations is easily implemented using Web-based or regular e-mail solutions. The advantages of such systems are appreciated by expert-doctors, because they can allocate and plan their time for inspecting referrals in their available time slots. Synchronous teleconsultations put pressure on the consultants to be available when there is a need for such consultations.

Doctor-centered teleconsultation solutions are primarily dedicated for management of patient-related data and facilitating contacts with colleagues or experts in the medical field in order to get "second opinions" about specific cases. Here, the doctor is the initiator of a teleconsultation session. The basic system should be able to provide the doctor with functions for acquisition of signals and images, basic processing, enhancement and placing the images in a database together with related textual information (as patient cases). Videoconferencing capabilities should be integrated into the system and provide video, audio and as well as data communication. Data communication is needed in order for doctors to be able to send/receive images under discussion. Additionally, special care must be devoted to synchronization of remote workspaces to ensure that the same copy of a medical image is under discussion. Hardware requirements include higher-quality equipment: hardware video codecs and quality videoconferencing cameras. There are no strict requirements for system portability and mobility, weight or wirelessness. Such systems could be successfully exploited for remote education too. They are most suitable for medical specialties involving medical data in the form of images: radiology, pathology, dermatology, ophthalmology and others.

Patient-centered systems involve the patient as the initiator of teleconsultation sessions. These systems can be attached to monitoring systems too. Here the patient, being outside of the specialized medical institution, must be provided with the means for continuous assessment of his/her status by a medical professional. The system, again, must facilitate signal acquisition and communication of these signals to special monitoring centers. There are special requirements placed on the patient subsystem: the subsystem must be wireless and portable, also easy and quick to use (even in critical situations), reliable, secure, and meet the established standards. The monitoring center must provide the patient with quick responses and action plans for emergency situations. Thus, the center must possess the patient's health-related information and be able to quickly obtain additional assistance from other medical specialists or experts. Medical experts (at any time and in any place) must also be provided with patient-related information in terms of history and current data. This forces the specialist/expert subsystem to be wireless and portable as well.

### *1.2 Standard Adherence and System Flexibility*

In order to achieve a longer lifetime of the systems for e-health and related teleconsultations, strict standard adherence should be maintained where available. However, sometimes adherence to standards can decrease the flexibility of the system to adopt specific requirements, which are not predicted by the standard. In radiology, widely-used DICOM standard files include additional information, called metadata, that describes the characteristics of the image and some other data about the performed studies. Other medical specialties, such as pathology, ophthalmology and dermatology, are quite different from radiology and need to have very specific description fields, thus custom-definable database forms are sometimes desirable.

It is very important to comply with image acquisition standards, such as TWAIN, WIA (Microsoft Corp.) and DICOM. Compatibility with these standards ensures the possibility to adapt teleconsultation systems to existing and newly-obtained medical equipment.

Compliance with communication standards ensures compatibility with existing communication equipment: gatekeepers, multiconference units (MCU), gateways. Many telecommunication protocols have been defined by the International Telecommunication Union (ITU). ITU standard H.320 defines videoconferencing via ISDN networks. ISDN usage for videoconferencing and data communication decreases in step with the increasing reliability of TCP-IP networks. H.323 is most commonly used for videoconferencing and for voice-over-IP (VoIP). H.323 and SIP (SIP is a certified standard of the Internet Engineering Task Force (IETF), the global nonprofit Internet technical standards body behind HTTP and the IP Internet Protocol) are currently the two most commonly used VoIP standards. H.323 offers greater compatibility than SIP because most VoIP equipment in the field supports the H.323 protocol; thus H.323 also offers greater interoperability than SIP.

### *1.3 Database Connectivity*

Database technologies are needed in e-health teleconsultation systems for storage of different data modalities: images, signals, text information. Balancing between customization and standardization influences the contents of the databases.

Database management systems (DBMSs) come in many flavors and sizes, for all the commonly used operating systems. The amounts of data processed in IMTS are rather large: for instance, medical images acquired using modern digital cameras for pathology and ophthalmology applications can take up as much as 6MB of space (jpeg-compressed). The Olympus DP 70 camera used in pathology produces images with pixel resolutions of up to 4080x3072. Each case stored in the database usually contains several images, thus the database fills up very fast.

Several commercially-available database management systems exist: MS Access, SQL Server, Oracle, MySQL, Postgres, Sybase, etc. Microsoft Access can be used for local information storage. However, it has limitations on database file sizes - they cannot exceed 2GB. Thus, large databases must be split into multiple files, which results in switching between several databases when performing searches. The maximum file size problem can be avoided if only links to images are stored in database fields, while images themselves are stored in hard disk folders. In any case, MS Access is not suitable for the central or remote repository of information. Advanced DBMS, such as MS SQL Server or Oracle fit the increased requirements inherent in those applications.

There aren't many alternatives for DBMS in mobile and portable teleconsultation applications, where PDAs are used. Still, Microsoft provides the SQL Server 2000 Windows® CE Edition, which can be used in mobile devices running the Pocket PC operating system [10]. SQL Server CE has a small memory footprint, delivering all of its functionality in approximately 1 megabyte (MB) of RAM. Several data types are supported to ensure flexibility, and 128-bit encryption is provided on the device for database file security. SQL Server CE enables access to a central data repository whether the device is always connected or intermittently connected to the computer running SQL Server. When used with SQL Server 2000, SQL Server CE provides extended capabilities for synchronization through merge replication. Data access technologies take advantage of Internet standards, including HTTP Secure Sockets Layer (SSL) encryption, through integration with Microsoft's Internet Information Services (IIS).

### *1.4 Plug-ins*

Data management and teleconsultation systems for various medical specialties require features for advanced data processing and analysis. The best solution for integration of these features is in the form of *plug-ins*. Plug–ins can be added or removed from the main software application. Examples of plug-ins could involve interactive measurement of images, automatic recognition or calculation of specific indexes. For example, the cell labeling index (LI) is used in pathology. It is defined as the ratio of the area (or number) of brown cells and blue cells in the image. Usually, pathologists estimate this index subjectively and the estimates exhibit considerable variance among pathologists. The plug-in could help as a simple one-step action for objective estimation of LI after acquisition of the digital image.

Development of plug-ins is a time-consuming process, involving development of algorithms, testing and verification using databases. It involves researchers, software developers and doctors. Creation of the algorithm itself is usually done using a high-level language, e.g. MATLAB, Mathworks Inc. Then it is rewritten in C, compiled into a dynamically loadable library of functions and linked to the main application. However, this scenario could be shortened by using the MATLAB Compiler technology [12]. The MATLAB Compiler takes M-files as input and generates C or C++ source code as output. The MATLAB Compiler can generate C or C++ source code for combining with other modules to form stand-alone applications. Such applications do not require MATLAB at runtime; they can run even if MATLAB is not installed on the end user's system. The MATLAB Compiler can generate C shared libraries and C++ static libraries. These can also be used without MATLAB on the end user's system. In addition, the MATLAB Compiler has an extension named MATLAB COM Builder that enables algorithm developers to automatically convert MATLAB applications to Component Object Model (COM) objects. Developers can perform modeling and analysis in MATLAB and convert the models into ready-to-use COM objects. These objects can be immediately integrated with any COM-based main application.

## 2. Implementation of Prototypes

Two prototypes of teleconsultations systems for e-health have been developed at the Institute of Biomedical Engineering: a) a wireless system for status assessment of cardiology patients (WSCP), b) a medical image management and teleconsultation system (IMTS).

The first system is intended to improve medical care and service provided for cardiology patients outside specialized medical institutions. The system enables the patient to record electrocardiograms (ECG) on mobile devices, view them and send them via a wireless connection to the doctor on duty. The doctor is then able to analyze new ECGs quickly and make the appropriate decisions; also to consult with cardiology expert by sending ECGs to the experts' mobile devices if needed. The system is also able to log all operations.

The second system is intended to be used by professional doctors for management of the collected medical images in local and remote databases and for videoconferencing teleconsultations in order to get a "second opinion".

### *2.1 Design Methodology, Technologies, Development Languages and Tools*

The UML (Unified Modeling Language) technology has been extensively used for modeling of the entire systems and applications. The following diagrams have been used: use case diagrams, activity diagrams, domain field object diagrams, state diagrams, sequence diagrams, static structure diagrams and implementation diagrams (tools used included MagicDraw and MS Visio).

The modeling, prototyping and testing of image processing and recognition algorithms was implemented using the high-level MATLAB language. The developed and tested MATLAB M files were then reverse-engineered to C and compiled into accessible DLL files.

Various programming languages were used for development. C++ (Visual Studio 6.0) was used for IMTS. This was necessitated by the need to achieve a sufficient speed of the application in manipulation of large images (processing and enhancement). However, it became possible to choose the higher-level C# language for WSCP. This choice greatly accelerated development of distributed PDA- and PC-based applications.

### *2.2 User Types*

The following main classes of WSCP users have been identified: *patient* (remotely supervised heart patient), *doctor on duty* (holds responsibility for serving the patients who contact him during his duty; the doctor on duty has access to patients' medical history and other external data, as required), *expert* (cardiologist or patient's personal doctor) and *administration* (manages the medical institution operating the system).

In the case of the IMTS, there were only two main classes of users: *general practice doctor (GP)* (doctor seeking a second opinion from the expert (see below)), *doctor (expert)* (a specialist having expertise knowledge in a specific medical field (ophthalmology, pathology, dermatology, etc.))

### *2.3 Use Cases*

The associations between users and services of the system can be well expressed using UML use case diagrams. These associations also help identify system components. The use case diagram for WSCP is shown in Figure 1.

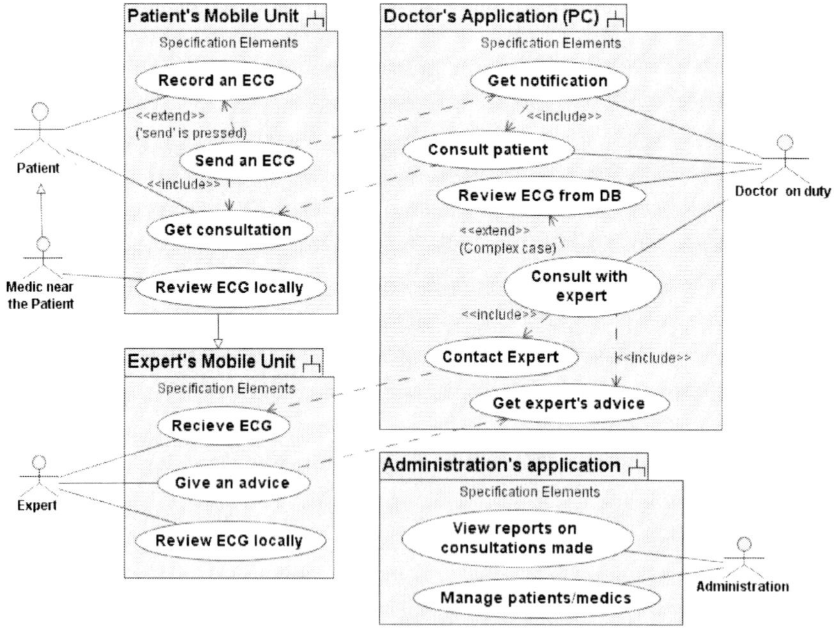


**Fig. 1.** Use cases of the ECG monitoring and teleconsultation system

## *2.4 Components of the Systems*

### *2.4.1 ECG Monitoring and Teleconsultation System*

The hardware used in the system prototype consists of PCs, PDAs (Compaq IPaq 3987), analog-digital converters (Dataq CF2), ECG sensors, and means of wireless communication – GPRS or WLAN. Software technologies used include UML, C++, C#, .NET Standard/Compact Framework 1.1 and SQL Server 2000/CE 2.0. They were chosen following careful analysis of possible alternatives. Once systems components in use cases and appropriate technologies had been identified, an architectural design of the system was created (Figure 2).

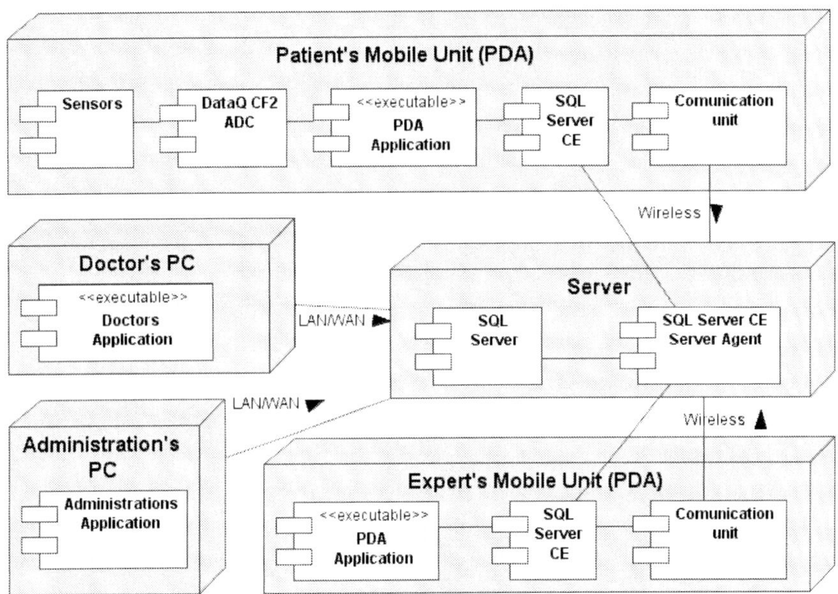


**Fig. 2.** Component diagram of the developed ECG monitoring and teleconsultation system

### *2.4.2 Image Management and the MediPAS Teleconsultation System*

The PC-based Eurotel 1telemedicine station (Euromed Networks AB (Sweden)) was chosen as system hardware. It consists of a PC with a large-screen monitor, a robot video camera (Sony EVI D31), a framegrabber (Matrox Meteor II), a video switcher (Kramer VS2081S), a video codec (Z360) and an ISDN communication card (ZC208 by Zydacron, Inc. (UK)).

The developed software uses the Matrox ActiveMIL library to control the framegrabber. A TWAIN interface is used to connect digital sources: digital cameras and scanners. The images and text-based information can be stored in a local database (MS Access 2000) or a remote database (MS SQL Server 2000). Zydacron SDK is used to integrate Zydacron videoconferencing hardware: the video codec and the ISDN communication card. The system is able to establish videoconferencing even without Zydacron hardware; it then uses Netmeeting SDK for integration of the software-based ITU H.323 videoconferencing protocol and the ITU T.120 data communication protocol.

## 3. Developed Software and Features

### 3.1 ECG Monitoring and Teleconsultation System

The developed software consists of applications for patients, doctors on duty, cardiology experts and administration, local databases for patients and experts, and a central database. Applications were built to meet non-functional requirements that are also very important. They include logins for different levels of users, user-friendly interfaces (Figure 3), security and reliable use of wireless connections. Recording, sending and storing of ECGs and logging of all activities by system users is in the scope of the system, but the consultation process itself is not, hence it is implemented by a mobile phone.

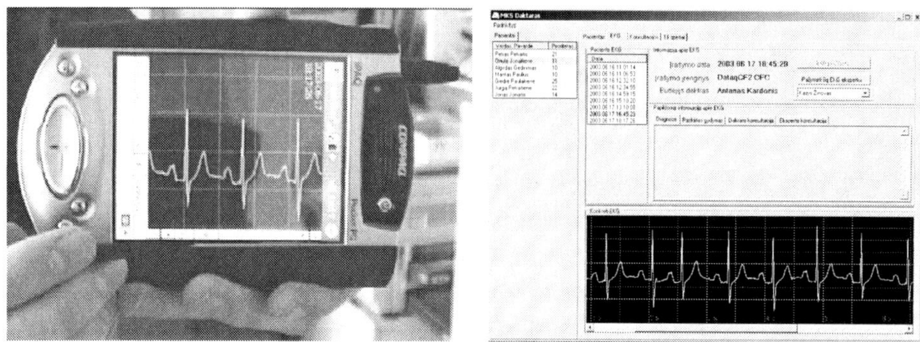

**Fig. 3.** Examples of user interface in expert and doctor applications

### 3.2 Image Management and the Teleconsultation System

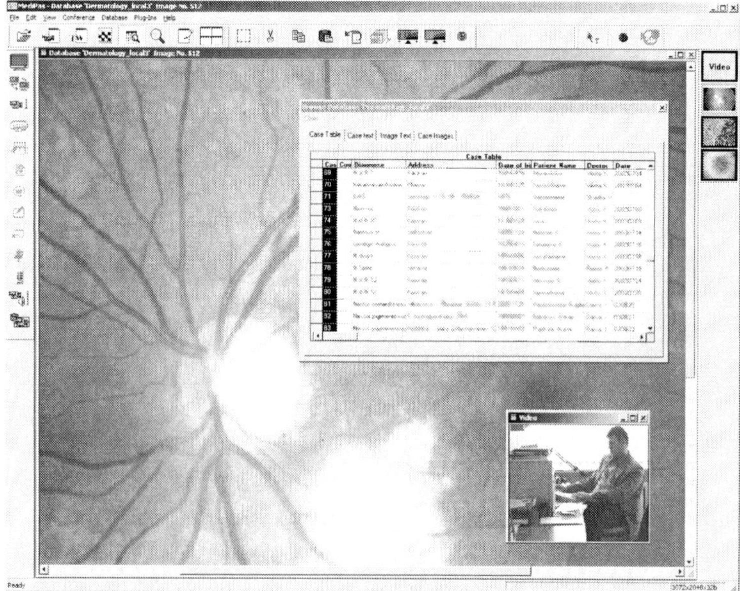

**Fig. 4.** The graphical user interface of the image management and teleconsultation system

The developed IMTS consists of the following modules: a) image acquisition, b) image editing and processing, c) database form designer, d) database browser and search engine, e) videoconferencing and data collaboration, f) plug-ins. The user interface GUI is shown in Figure 4.

The image acquisition module provides the means for acquiring images from analog and digital sources via buffers to main application workspaces. The image editing and processing module contains the most important functionality: selecting parts of the image, copying, cutting and pasting parts of image and image rotation. Basic image processing in MediPAS include: brightness, contrast, color saturation, the "undo last change" option and the "return to original image" option. In order to facilitate review of the images, the following features are implemented: list of images with thumbnails loaded in working memory, panning of the image, "left/right click" to zoom in/zoom out and comparison of images side by side. Working with databases includes the possibility of using local (MS Access) or remote (SQL Server) databases. A distinguishing feature of databases is the Database Form Administrator, which is available for both local and remote databases. By using this tool, the doctor is able to design database forms by defining ("drag and drop" actions) fields in the database according to his own requirements.

The following videoconferencing functions for teleconsultations are implemented in MediPAS: discussion on images on a common desktop, a shared pointer, synchronized drawing on the same image, storing drawings and notes in a database as new layers of information.

There are several plug-ins integrated in MediPAS: labeling index calculation in pathology images and indexing of fundus images in ophthalmology images. The obtained experience in plug-in development will be used in other medical specialties (ophthalmology, pathology, dermatology etc.).

## 4. Testing and Evaluation

One of the most important requirements for medical software and hardware systems is reliability. The systems should undergo very thorough testing and evaluation procedures. It is best if the procedures are defined during specification of system requirements. Test and evaluation procedures must define how the requirements fulfillment should be verified and what results of verification must be achieved.

A formal scenario has thus been developed for testing and evaluation of WSCP (see Figure 5). In general, each component of the system must first be tested and evaluated, following which a test of the complete system should proceed.

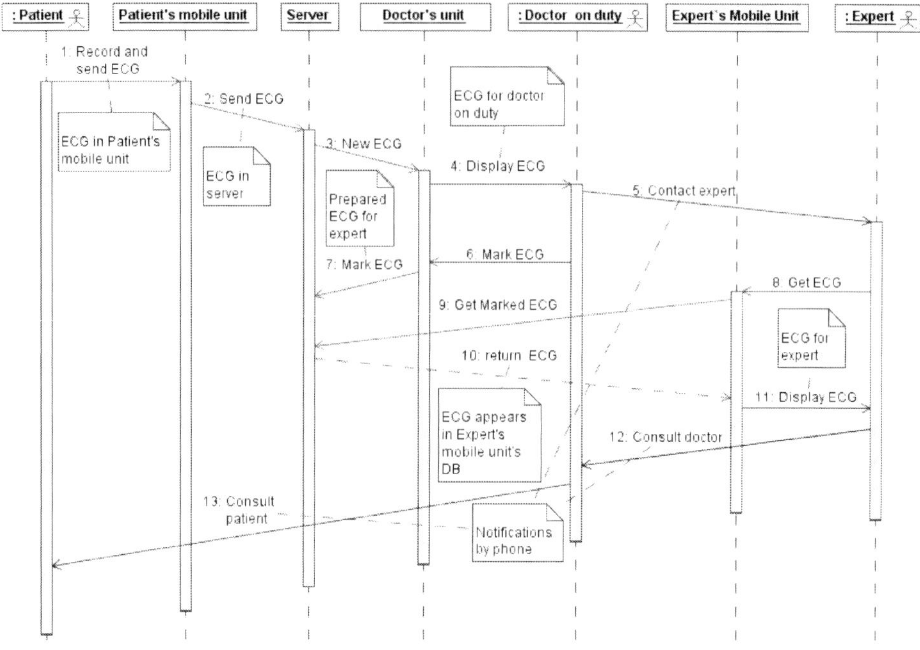


**Fig. 5.** Interactive testing methodology for the ECG monitoring and teleconsultation system

The IMTS software has been evaluated locally and internationally in second-opinion teleconsultations, remote educational seminars and lectures [12, 13, 14, 15]. Teleconsultations have generated significant interest in Sweden and Lithuania and the developed system received positive evaluations.

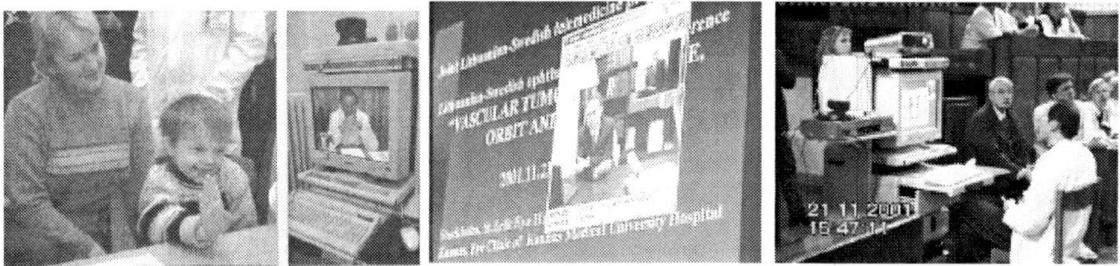

**Fig. 6.** Evaluation of the image management and teleconsultation system during seminars and lectures between Sweden and Lithuania

## 5. Discussion

Teleconsultation solutions have been designed, implemented and evaluated as learning platforms in several medical centres in Lithuania (Kaunas Medical University Hospital) as well as in partner institution in Sweden (Lund University Hospital). The medical specialities involved in the evaluation are ophthalmology, otorhinolaryngology and pathology. These specialties are perfectly suited for telemedicine because they are mostly dependent on graphical data and moving images.

Development of e-health services includes looking for solutions of technical and organizational problems. In this study we have only dealt with technical aspects

While developing WSCP we were looking for an appropriate wireless communication method. We investigated two alternatives: GPRS for long distance and WLAN for local connections. GPRS was accessed via mobile phones and special mobile packs connected to PDAs. GPRS is more expensive, though more mobile. However, our GPRS tests were not very successful in transmitting longer ECG records, although it is not very clear whether it was because of method problems or GPRS service quality. Another issue is that GPRS is usually better optimized for downloading than uploading. WLAN is ideal for operation in a smaller space, as it offers greater bandwidth and is free of charge. When using it in open spaces, distances as long as 500m can be covered, making it suitable for such applications as sports medicine. The middle layer of communication was implemented through database synchronization, using MS SQL Server CE 2.0 remote data access (RDA) technology. RDA ensures consistency of data, security, and automatic archiving of sent data, which makes it very suitable for wireless applications. However, RDA is not suitable for real-time monitoring.

While developing IMTS we investigated two approaches for videoconferencing and solutions of text and image fusion in databases. We found that hardware video codecs are expensive, yet must be used when high-quality moving images are needed for teleconsultations. Software-based video codecs are not yet adequate for these applications. The latter codecs fit audio/video conferencing requirements, only when still images are involved. Additionally, we have found that it is much more efficient to send commands between clients and to accomplish image processing locally instead of transmitting processed images.

## 6. Conclusions and Future Prospects

Development of modern telemedicine services in Lithuania is of great importance for the Lithuanian healthcare system as there is a great potential to reduce preventable diseases, improve the quality of healthcare and increase professionalism of doctors by using distant training and teleconsultations with modern telemedicine techniques.

Two learning platforms for teleconsultations in e-health have been developed and evaluated: an ECG monitoring and teleconsultations system and image management and teleconsultations system software (MediPAS).

The prototypes can be expanded and improved in the following aspects: usage of extra sensors for monitoring additional physiological parameters, improvements in security, integration of initial signal processing in mobile units, integration with existing EPR systems, optimizing the system and reusing knowledge for specific activities.

**Acknowledgements.** The wireless system for status assessment of cardiology patients is being developed as part of two R&D projects: 1) Telemedicare – an R&D project supported by EU FP5 and 2) Homotech – a project of the Lithuanian priority research and experiments program supported by the Lithuanian State Science and Studies Fund.

The medical images management and teleconsultation software MediPAS is being developed as part of the LITMED and LITMED2 projects funded by the Swedish Government through the Baltic Sea IT fund. Both projects are managed by TietoEnator Trigon AB and the MediPAS software is to be marketed in Lithuanian healthcare institutions by Euromed Networks AB.

## References


[1] TELEBALT Newsletter, Vol.2, March 2002 – October 2002, *http://www.infobalt.lt/telebalt/*

[2] "HealthCast 2010 Smaller World, Bigger Expectations", PricewaterhouseCoopers, Internet site *http://healthcare.pwc.com/healthcast2010.html*

[3] Lithuanian Ministry of healthcare, website at: *http://www.sam.lt/lt/sam/veikla/esveikata*

[4] "Strategic plan: eHealth for the development of Lithuanian Health Care 1. Introduction, starting point and vision", Håkan Håkansson, TietoEnator Trigon AB, 08 December 2003.

[5] Evy I. Karavatselou, George-Peter K. Economou, Constantine A. Chassomeris, Vassiliki Danelli-Mylonas, and Dimitris K. Lymberopoulos, "OTE-TS—A New Value-Added Telematics Service for Telemedicine Applications" IEEE Trans. on Inf. Techn. in Biomed. vol. 5, no. 3, september 2001

[6] Takahiro Y., Toshikazu S., Tatsuya F., Yutaka A., Masayuki K., Design of medical teleconsultation support system using super-high-definition imaging system, Systems and Computers in Japan, 2002, Vol. 33, Issue 8, p. 9 – 18.

[7] E. Kyriacou, S. Pavlopoulos, A. Berler, M. Neophytou, A. Bourka, A. Georgoulas, A. Anagnostaki, D. Karayiannis, C. Schizas, C. Pattichis, A. Andreou and D. Koutsouris, Multi-purpose HealthCare Telemedicine Systems with mobile communication link support, BioMedical Engineering OnLine 2003, 2:7, Published: 24 March 2003, Available from: *http://www.biomedical-engineering-online.com/content/2/1/7.*

[8] D.R. Kaufman, V.L. Patel, Ch. Hilliman, P.C. Morin, J. Pevzner, R.S. Weinstock, R. Goland, S. Shea, and J. Starrena Usability in the real world: assessing medical information technologies in patients' homes, Journal of Biomedical Informatics 36 (2003) 45–60.

[9] J. K. Pollard , M. E. Fry, S. Rohman, C. Santarelli, A. Theodorou, N. Mohoboob, Wireless and Web-based medical monitoring in the home, Medical Informatics and the Internet in Medicine, Vol.27, Number 3 / September 01, 2002, 219 – 227.

[10] Microsoft® .NET Compact Framework: Core Reference / A. Wigley, S. Wheelwright, R. Burbidge et al. – Redmond: Microsoft Press, 2003. – 896 p.

[11] Mathwoks Inc. web site: *http://www.mathworks.com/.*

[12] Swedish – Lithuanian project LITMED2 Exhibition at Telemedicine & Telecare International Trade Fair, Med-e-Tel 2004, April 21-23, 2004, "SOCIETE DES FOIRES INTERNATIONALES DE LUXEMBOURG S.A" Luxembourg-Kirchberg. *http://www.medetel.lu*

[13] An international Baltic MedWeb project: creating a data base of images of laryngeal and eye diseases / V. Uloza, A. Paunksnis, V. Marozas, R. Jurkonis, P. Severgardh // IFMBE proceedings: 12th Nordic Baltic Conference on Biomedical Engineering and Medical Physics, June 18th - 22th, 2002, Reykjavik, Iceland / Proceedings of the International Federation for Medical and Biological Engineering. Reykjavik: ISBEMF. ISSN 1680-0737. 2002, Vol. 2, p. 92-93.

[14] Teleophthalmology – cooperation between Sweden and Lithuania: The Litmed Telemedicine project, A.Paunksnis, V.Barzdžiukas, S.Kurapkienė, R.Gricius, A.Lukoševičius, L.-O.Almquist, B.Calissendorff, S.Blomdahl, E.Varnauskas, International Telemedicine Conference, 18-21 June 2001, Uppsala, Sweden

[15] An Application of International Telemedicine LITMED Project for Otorhinolaryngology, Uloza V., Almquist L.-O., Povilaitis K., Rydell R., Svensson O., Uloziene I., International Telemedicine Conference, 18-21 June 2001, Uppsala, Sweden.

# Author Index